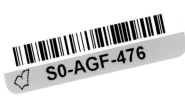

Is Breast Best?

BIOPOLITICS

MEDICINE, TECHNOSCIENCE, AND HEALTH IN THE 21ST CENTURY

General Editors: Monica J. Casper and Lisa Jean Moore

Missing Bodies: The Politics of Visibility
Monica J. Casper and Lisa Jean Moore

Against Health: How Health Became the New Morality
Edited by Jonathan M. Metzl and Anna Kirkland

Is Breast Best?
Taking on the Breastfeeding Experts and
the New High Stakes of Motherhood
Joan B. Wolf

Is Breast Best?

*Taking on the Breastfeeding Experts and
the New High Stakes of Motherhood*

Joan B. Wolf

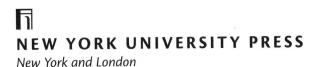

NEW YORK UNIVERSITY PRESS
New York and London

NEW YORK UNIVERSITY PRESS
New York and London
www.nyupress.org

Library of Congress Cataloging-in-Publication Data

Wolf, Joan B. (Joan Beth)
Is breast best? : taking on the breastfeeding experts and
the new high stakes of motherhood / Joan B. Wolf.
p. ; cm. — (Biopolitics : medicine, technoscience, and
health in the 21st century)
Includes bibliographical references and index.
ISBN 978-0-8147-9481-4 (cl : alk. paper)
ISBN 978-0-8147-9525-5 (ebook)
1. Breastfeeding. 2. Breastfeeding—Government policy—United States.
3. Breastfeeding—Social aspects. I. Title. II. Series: Biopolitics
(New York, N.Y.)
[DNLM: 1. Breast Feeding. 2. Health Knowledge, Attitudes, Practice.
3. Politics. 4. Public Opinion. WS 125]
RJ216.W7193   2010
649'.33—dc22   2010026254

New York University Press books are printed on acid-free paper,
and their binding materials are chosen for strength and durability.
We strive to use environmentally responsible suppliers and materials
to the greatest extent possible in publishing our books.

Manufactured in the United States of America
10 9 8 7 6 5 4 3 2 1

For Bobby and Aaron

Current truths are nothing of the sort; they are merely the best contemporary insight into a situation. And no matter how logical such insights might seem, they exist only for as long as it takes new research to prove them wrong. As a science, biology need have little concern for these mistakes; the mistakes of the past are simply stepping stones to the truths of the future. But to everybody else—all those who depend on biological advice to organize their lives and safeguard their health and future—such mistakes do matter.
—Robin Baker, *Fragile Science: The Truth behind the Headlines*, 2001

Not everything that can be counted counts, and not everything that counts can be counted.
—Albert Einstein

Contents

Acknowledgments

INTERDISCIPLINARY RESEARCH, LIKE travel in a foreign country, is unsettling. It challenges how we know the world and de-centers ways of thinking we take so for granted that we are not even conscious of them. It also can be exhilarating, especially when we recognize that much *is* shared across cultures and that we have the resources to live in, make sense of, and even contribute to our surroundings. In many instances, guidance from natives or locals can make the difference between a hazy encounter and an illuminating experience. For this book, I have been fortunate to be able to call on colleagues who "dwell" in biology, communication, English, history, philosophy, political science, psychology, public health, sociology, toxicology, and women's and gender studies. I have had provocative conversations with nephrologists, otolaryngologists, and pediatricians. I have also talked with mothers and fathers who shared with me their infant-feeding stories. Every time I complete a project, I am mindful of the debt of gratitude I have incurred; this time, I feel more than a little awed by the breadth of expertise and experience from which I and this book have benefited.

For critical feedback and moral support, my sincere thanks go to the members of my writing group: Ashley Currier, Marian Eide, Susan Egenolf, Kate Kelly, and Linda Radzik; to colleagues who also read articles and various chapter drafts: Judy Baer, Sherry Bame, Steve Ellingson, Lisa Ellis, Jan Leighley, Mary Ann O'Farrell, Jennifer Pashup, Stephanie Payne, Jim Rosenheim, Eric Rothenbuhler, Dave Toback, and Michelle Taylor-Robinson; and to those who took on the enormous task of reading the whole manuscript: Leah Devun, Marian Eide, Mike Kamrin, Kathy Miller, Katie See, Jane Sell, and Barbara Sharf. Special thanks to Gary Toback for an ongoing dialogue about medicine that, from its inception, helped me believe I could write this book; to Ron Kuppersmith and Scott Schams for their clinical observations and insight; to participants in the University of Chicago Social Theory Workshop and in conferences sponsored by the Social Science History Association and the Midwest Political Science Association; to Kathy Anderson for superior copyediting (and for lodging and terrific company during my increasingly frequent visits to Chicago); and to Cristina Duke for first-rate research assistance.

The research, writing, and publication of this book were made possible at Texas A&M University by the Women's and Gender Studies Program, the Melbern G. Glasscock Center for Humanities Research, the College of Liberal Arts, and the Office of the Vice President for Research. Once the manuscript was with New York University Press, an anonymous reviewer provided compelling suggestions for revision. Linda Blum, Anna Kirkland, and my editor, Ilene Kalish, all assiduous critics, helped me clarify crucial points and turn a rather sprawling manuscript into a more focused and readable book. I am particularly grateful for their acuity.

E. B. White once said that, "If the world were merely seductive, that would be easy. If it were merely challenging, that would be no problem. But I arise in the morning torn between a desire to improve the world and a desire to enjoy the world. This makes it hard to plan the day." The world compels us to make it better, but it is also filled with wonderful things. For me, music has been the most joyful and abiding presence. It is unlikely (and, in not a few cases, impossible) that any of those who have been an endless source of comfort and inspiration to me will ever read this book. Nonetheless, in the tradition of authors who thank their pets or local coffee shop, I would like to acknowledge a disparate group of musicians joined only by the fact that they contributed much of the soundtrack to the writing of this book: Patricia Barber, Leonard Bernstein, John Coltrane, Bill Evans, Patty Griffin, Sharon Isbin, Gustav Mahler, Brad Mehldau, Cole Porter, Dianne Reeves, Virginia Rodrigues, Dmitri Shostakovich, Nina Simone, Jessica Williams, and Cassandra Wilson.

I am especially grateful to friends and family who have supported me, in myriad ways, throughout the writing of this book: Donnalee Dox, Marian Eide, Lisa Ellis, Cherie Marcus, Jen Pashup, Katie See, the Toback family, and Allison Wolf. My heartfelt thanks to Rachel Baum for accompanying me over some very rugged terrain with fortitude, compassion, and (mercifully) humor. And finally, my deepest gratitude goes to Bobby and Aaron, my sweet boys, for teaching me two seemingly contradictory lessons: that parenting theories are for people without children and that feminist single-mothering two boys in Texas is possible. I love you both as big as a blue whale.

Preface

Why Breastfeeding?

IN CHICAGO, A counselor at a federal women, infants, and children (WIC) clinic laments the tragedy of teenaged mothers choosing to go to school instead of breastfeeding their babies.[1] The director of the neonatal intensive care unit at DC General Hospital tells mothers of infants with runny noses that the babies would not be sick if they breastfed.[2] And an anthropology professor argues that infant formula producers, "just like tobacco companies, produce a product that is harmful to people's short and long-term health."[3] Meanwhile, in Congress, Representative Carol Maloney has introduced legislation to amend the 1964 Civil Rights Act to include various protections for breastfeeding, and Senator Tom Harkin has proposed that warning labels, similar to the Surgeon General's warning on cigarette packages, be affixed to formula containers.[4] How did we arrive at a place in the United States where formula, which nourishes millions of healthy babies every year, can be likened to nicotine? Where breastfeeding her baby can be considered more important to a teenaged mother than getting an education? Where, without evidence, a doctor feels professionally and morally justified telling bottle-feeding mothers that *not* breastfeeding essentially *causes* babies' illnesses or that breastfed babies do not get sick? These are the questions that drive this book.

Hyperbole is commonplace in the world of breastfeeding advocacy, and it is staked on an overwhelming consensus that breastfeeding is the optimal form of nutrition for virtually all babies everywhere.[5] According to the most recent policy statement of the American Academy of Pediatrics (AAP), the "diverse and compelling advantages for infants, mothers, families, and society from breastfeeding and use of human milk for infant feeding include health, nutritional, immunologic, developmental, psychologic, social, economic, and environmental benefits."[6] Infant-feeding studies frequently begin with a reference to breastfeeding's well-known advantages, and in 2009, a director at the U.S. Department of Health and Human

Services' Agency for Health Care Research and Quality announced that "the debate over the relative value of breastfeeding compared with artificial means of feeding is over, as the data are unequivocal in favor of breastfeeding."[7] Even formula companies, which have a vested interest in reducing breastfeeding rates, explicitly state that human milk is the nutritional "gold standard" and advertise their products as "closest to breastfeeding." In the chaos of conflicting opinions about caffeine, epidurals, cosleeping, and practically every facet of pregnancy, childbirth, and child care, the hegemony of the "breast is best" message in public discourse is remarkable.

It is all the more so because the science behind the consensus is deeply problematic. While compelling evidence indicates that breastfeeding reduces babies' risk for various gastrointestinal (GI) infections, medical journals are otherwise replete with contradictory conclusions about breastfeeding's impact: for every piece of research linking it to better health, another finds it to be irrelevant, weakly significant, or inextricably tied to factors that are difficult to measure with the standard tools of science. While many of these studies describe a correlation between breastfeeding and more desirable outcomes—for example, some studies have found that breastfed babies have fewer respiratory infections—they rarely control adequately for what scientists call "confounding variables," factors that have not been examined but could be affecting the outcome. Perhaps most troubling, breastfeeding cannot be distinguished from the decision to breastfeed, which could represent a more comprehensive commitment to healthy living that itself is likely to have a positive impact on children's health. If mothers who breastfeed also wash their hands more frequently, keep their babies from crowded places, and expose them to fewer viruses, is it breastfeeding or careful hygiene that produces fewer infections?

Furthermore, despite numerous theories, scientists have been largely unable to demonstrate how breast milk works in a baby's body to protect or promote health.[8] In instances like this, in which the "exposure" (breast milk) and the "confounder" (the choice to breastfeed) are highly correlated and the biological processes by which the exposure has salutary effects have not been identified, determining causality is especially challenging. When studies find an association between breastfeeding and reduced risks, therefore, it is not at all clear that one causes the other, and the conclusion that breastfeeding confers health benefits is far less certain than its proponents contend. Indeed, a great deal of evidence suggests that the difference between breastfeeding and bottle feeding has little impact on the overwhelming majority of infants in the developed world.[9]

I did not set out to tell a story about science. Rather, I began this project to understand why feminists had not paid much attention to breast-feeding as a social process. Both the AAP and La Leche League International, the world's largest breastfeeding support organization, advise that babies in "the early weeks" should breastfeed eight to twelve times a day, which effectively means that new mothers will find themselves feeding nearly every other hour.[10] Even when babies begin to feed less often, breastfeeding requires an all-encompassing physical and emotional commitment from mothers. Why, I wondered, had feminists not grappled with infant feeding to the extent that they had with so many other aspects of reproduction and child care?[11] That "breast is best" I never questioned. My plan was to spend a few days reading the medical literature to learn precisely what science had determined to be breastfeeding's health benefits before I returned my focus to feminism.

As days turned into months, it became clear to me that feminism's relationship with breastfeeding was only one dimension of a much broader and more perplexing set of questions: Why, when the scientific evidence is weak and inconsistent, do almost all "experts" agree on breastfeeding's superiority? In the absence of compelling medical evidence, how have scientists, doctors, powerful interest groups, and the general public come to be persuaded that breastfeeding is one of the most important gifts a mother can give to her child? What does public discourse on infant feeding in America tell us about the relationship between mothers and children as well as about broader social practices that, at least at first glance, have nothing to do with women or motherhood? Why has breastfeeding become a potent, almost sacrosanct symbol, despite serious flaws in the scientific rationale for its health benefits?[12]

Breastfeeding literally embodies popular unease about risk, health, and motherhood; it serves as a repository for numerous cultural anxieties, many of which have little to do with infant feeding per se. In this book, I try to convey the range of these concerns and how they converge in various expert conversations about breastfeeding. To do so, I use a variety of scholarly literatures, from social theory, cultural studies, and media studies to infant-feeding science, epidemiology, and health policy, each with its own vocabulary, rules, and assumptions. I have tried to avoid overly technical language and to offer examples when my analysis seems especially abstract, but melding such diverse approaches has been an enormous challenge, one that, I suspect, will not be entirely lost on readers. It is, nonetheless, only by disentangling the sprawling roots of American public discourse on breastfeeding that we can begin to understand their equally far-reaching consequences.

This is a book about what I call a "risk culture," broadly speaking. It is also about health risks and, more specifically, the risks related to breast-feeding; about cultural expectations of mothers and how they shape per-sonal and social meanings of breastfeeding; about rules and routines in epidemiological research and the development of medical knowledge; and about how risk, motherhood, and science coalesce in the social construc-tion of healthy citizens. I pay particular attention to the various individuals and institutions, many with the most altruistic intentions, that contribute to the misrepresentation of breastfeeding as essential to babies' short- and long-term health: the scientists who conduct, publish, and review infant feeding research; the doctors, government institutions, and interest groups that proclaim breast milk's advantages for women, babies, and America; and the various media that translate scientific research for the public. My primary concern is with how women's infant-feeding choices are framed by people and institutions perceived to be authoritative. Experts formu-late recommendations in cultural, professional, and political environments that make certain accounts of breastfeeding more compelling than others, and it is these contexts that form the subject of this book.

For example, conversations about breastfeeding reflect long-standing ideas about gender and motherhood. In the spirit of Gloria Steinem's infa-mous musings about how women's monthly periods would be represented "if men could menstruate,"[13] we might fantasize about what breastfeed-ing would mean if men, instead of women, had functioning mammary glands.[14] Scientists might assure men that bottle feeding helped babies connect to multiple caretakers, a process of horizontal bonding essential to normal psychological development. Formula might be lauded as evi-dence of man's conquest of nature and mastery over his body. Supplemen-tal nursing systems, which involve taping a tube to one's nipple to help a baby "latch on," might never have been invented (and if they had, they probably would be denigrated for violating men's bodies and personal autonomy). Where Steinem imagined men embracing menstruation as the essence of their superiority, we might envision them dismissing lacta-tion as quaint and unnecessary, rather like churning one's own butter or making paper. In other words, representations of biological practices re-flect unequal distributions of power, and the significance of breastfeeding in America has its roots in long-held assumptions about femininity and masculinity.

Breastfeeding also is grounded in deep-seated beliefs about mothering. From the last decades of the twentieth century to the present, the notion of "good enough" mothering has been replaced by "exclusive motherhood," "intensive mothering," and "the new momism,"[15] or what I have termed "total motherhood." Like the new momism, total motherhood requires mothers to be experts in everything their children might encounter, to become lay pediatricians, psychologists, consumer products safety inspectors, toxicologists, and educators.[16] Mothers must not only protect their children from immediate threats but are also expected to predict and prevent any circumstance that might interfere with putatively normal development.[17] Total motherhood is a moral code in which mothers are exhorted to optimize every aspect of children's lives, beginning with the womb. Its practice is frequently cast as a trade-off between what mothers might like and what babies and children must have, a choice that frames public discourse on breastfeeding. And when mothers have "wants"— such as a sense of bodily, emotional, and psychological autonomy—but children have "needs"—such as an environment in which anything less than optimal is framed as perilous—good mothering is defined as behavior that reduces even infinitesimal or poorly understood risks to offspring, regardless of the potential cost to the mother. The distinction disappears between what children *need* and what *might enhance* their physical, intellectual, and emotional development. Mothers are held responsible for matters well outside their control, and they are told in various ways that they must eliminate even minute, ultimately ineradicable, potential threats to their children's well-being.

What makes breastfeeding especially powerful is how it resonates in ways that have nothing to do with gender, mothering, or infant feeding per se. Common assumptions about women and maternal bodies are crucial to understanding representations of breastfeeding; but expectations of mothers take shape in much more diverse social contexts, and breastfeeding has been invested with so much meaning precisely because it resonates so broadly.[18] In American public discourse, breastfeeding is a trope in causes ranging from environmental progressivism to religious fundamentalism. It is invoked by those who believe that what is "natural"— breastfeeding is perceived to be an organic process—is inherently best, but it also confirms the authority of science: research purports to demonstrate that breast milk is nutritionally optimal. It is embraced by grassroots women's health advocates as well as by institutional medicine, or the scientists, doctors, and medical associations that health activists have long mistrusted. It serves liberal, radical, and cultural feminist ends at the same time that it appeals to non- and even antifeminists. Like manna from heaven, said to taste like whatever the person eating it desires, breastfeeding appears to have virtually unlimited meaning. To be sure, bottle feeding also has rhetorical appeal, but breastfeeding reverberates across seemingly unbridgeable divides.

What links many of these discussions is what I call a "risk culture," a pervasive anxiety about the future that drives many people to build their lives around reducing all conceivable risks. What they eat, how they raise their children, and which cars they drive—nowadays so many decisions seem designed to diminish risk and optimize the future. Scientists and various other experts produce a constant stream of information about everything from health and relationships to the economy and the environment, and their advice is subject to constant revision. One day people are advised to eat more fish, and the next they are warned to avoid the environmental toxins that contaminate natural habitats. The quantity and scope of this information, however inconsistent, create a widespread but false impression that the wisdom to make perfect choices is available to everyone and that all risks, particularly health risks, can be prevented with proper calculation. Public discussions about risk are infused with an ethic of neoliberalism: scientists, doctors, and government institutions emphasize individual responsibility, and good citizens are idealized as those who take care of themselves and exercise personal control. A neoliberal risk culture is, in short, a personal responsibility culture. As I discuss at length, however, risks are omnipresent and ever present, and behavior that is risk averse in one domain is likely to create new risks in others. Choices also are socially constrained, and people without social or economic resources often are unable to behave in ways that the experts have deemed to be responsible.

Risks, moreover, can be minimized or exaggerated, and which risks we pay attention to at any given moment—which ones preoccupy experts and lay people alike—frequently depends on cultural values. In the United States, health risks, and particularly those that individuals bear the responsibility to manage, command abundant attention. This is perhaps most apparent in the nonstop barrage of information telling people how a healthy diet can protect against obesity, diabetes, heart disease, and countless other illnesses. Risks to children, and especially threats conceptualized as mothers' obligation to reduce, are prominent in public discourse as well. Indeed, while my concept of total motherhood owes much to earlier notions of the new momism and exclusive or intensive motherhood, what distinguishes it is precisely this emphasis on risk, or the insistence that mothers eliminate all risk to children at any cost. Breastfeeding, in which mothers are personally responsible for reducing health risks to babies by controlling the production and consumption of their food, is the epitome of total motherhood in a neoliberal risk culture.

What follows, therefore, is much more than an analysis of breastfeeding. It is a study of weak science, an investigation into how cherished but unsubstantiated beliefs about health become conventional wisdom. It is an exposé of motherhood and the collective fantasy that mothers can and should produce perfect children. It also is an inquiry into cultural values and the responsibility that citizens place on themselves and others, a parable of middle-class America's preference for individual instead of communal solutions to a wide array of problems, including those that have social or biological causes and those whose origin and development we simply do not understand. At its core, this is a story about how ordinary citizens, increasingly anxious in a progressively more complicated world, rely on these values to manage an unrelenting barrage of information whose complexity far exceeds any one person's capacity to grasp.

1

Monitoring Mothers

A Recent History of Following the Doctor's Orders

EVEN BEFORE THE creation of powder formulas, infant feeding was a morally charged practice. In colonial and postrevolutionary America, for example, women who did not nurse their babies were often considered to be selfish and unpatriotic. Nonetheless, many women sought alternative forms of feeding. The demand for wet nurses, socially disadvantaged women who breastfed other women's children, was constant, and human milk was among the most advertised commodities.[1] Some mothers, particularly in the middle class, found breastfeeding distasteful or immodest, while others found it exhausting. Scientists, doctors, and clergymen believed that breastfeeding was superior to bottle feeding, but they also argued that emotions, diet, exercise, and various other environmental factors could have a negative impact on the quality of a woman's milk. The belief that middle-class women were weak and unable to sustain breastfeeding, for example, "was a distinguishing characteristic of both the popular and professional medical literature."[2] Employing a wet nurse remained a possibility throughout the nineteenth century, but a growing middle-class consciousness deterred most of these mothers from turning to lower-class women to feed their babies. Doctors, too, were concerned about the moral and physical suitability of the women who served as wet nurses, many of whom were single mothers, and they also worried that these women would not submit to doctors' control. Cow's milk was the most readily available substitute, but it did not have the same ingredients as breast milk, often carried bacteria, and was extracted, transported, and stored under filthy conditions. Boiling eliminated bacteria but was also feared to make the milk less nutritious. The absence of a safe and reliable surrogate for breast milk was widely blamed for high infant death rates, which, despite advances in disease theory and diagnostic tools, actually increased between 1850 and 1900. At the turn of the twentieth century, one-third of children living in cities died before the age of five years, and overall infant mortality hovered around 10 percent.[3]

At the same time, infant feeding began to play a significant role in the development and consolidation of pediatrics as a distinct branch of medicine.[4] Indeed, as the century progressed, pediatricians were often referred to as "baby feeders," and pediatrics became synonymous with infant nutrition. As a practical matter, doctors' incomes were dependent on the number of patients they saw, and consultations regarding infant feeding provided a steady stream of revenue. Physicians presented themselves as uniquely qualified to oversee feeding and argued that infant mortality would decline only if mothers gave themselves over to their authority. They also argued that routine weight checks were essential to confirm normal growth; that the nurses, social workers, and lay reformers who dominated the child welfare movement did not have the medical training to evaluate the individual child's development; and therefore that regular visits to the pediatrician's office were necessary.[5] Meanwhile, pediatric researchers produced various milk substitutes based on calories and different percentages of fat, protein, and sugar, and their endless tinkering with proportions reflected the competition among scientists to determine whose formula was best. It also served to legitimate pediatricians vis-à-vis other physicians who did not take seriously infant and child medicine as a distinct medical specialty. Professionalization also was enhanced by pediatricians' supervision of milk stations, which distributed sterilized milk and prepared formula, and also the certification of cow's milk, both methods of making milk safer that were far more expensive than pasteurization—which doctors feared destroyed some of milk's nutritive qualities—but that guaranteed physicians' services would be essential to infant feeding.

Throughout the first half of the twentieth century, pediatricians grew increasingly fond of "artificial feeding," as bottle feeding was commonly known. As evidence developed to suggest little difference in health between breastfed and properly bottle-fed babies, pediatricians began to contend that feeding with evaporated milk or appropriately constituted formula, under a doctor's supervision, could be as nutritious as breastfeeding. They did not directly dispute the notion that breastfeeding was optimal, but they relied heavily on their clinical experience, which indicated that babies developed normally on some form of mixed feeding or on manufactured foods alone. Like their predecessors, pediatricians argued that "relief bottles" could provide a respite for exhausted breastfeeding mothers. Nursing babies should receive one bottle a day, some advised, so mothers could have a modicum of freedom; if babies grew accustomed to bottles, these doctors reasoned, they might have an easier time with weaning. In addition, anxiety could adversely affect a mother's milk supply, so bottles might even improve lactation. By the 1940s, pediatricians generally accepted the viability of generic milk substitutes, and they blamed any health problems on infants or mothers' failure to follow doctors' advice, not on the formula itself.

Regardless of its nutritional merits, supervised bottle feeding made doctors central to babies' lives. Bottled milk, moreover, gave physicians the comfort of knowing exactly what and how much babies were consuming, and this reinforced their control over infant feeding. Some openly expressed their preference for "the young mother with a nutritionally untutored mind who frankly states that she knows nothing about babies and leaves the instruction to me" over a mother who had studied nutrition in college or was aware of competing opinions. One pediatrician stated frankly that it was "easier to control cows than women," and by midcentury, some contended that an educated mother could be a threat to her child's well-being.[6] Medical schools devoted many more hours to teaching about artificial feeding than about breastfeeding, so the average physician knew more about the bottle than the breast and was ill prepared to counsel mothers struggling to breastfeed. Doctors' misgivings about manufactured baby food pertained largely to mothers who fed without professional instruction. While these pediatricians were concerned about the health of these babies, they also recognized that unsupervised feeding reduced their function and income. At the same time, commercial food companies offered doctors free samples and calculators, and they stressed in mass advertising that formula should not be used without a doctor's prescription. The American Medical Association eventually threatened to remove its seal of approval from products whose manufacturers included instructions on labels and that advertised directly to mothers. Those companies that failed to comply fared much worse than those that did. Both industry and pediatric practice ultimately benefited from the mutual affirmation that formula feeding required a doctor's supervision. By emphasizing the indispensability of medical advice, formula companies bolstered the business of pediatrics, which then guaranteed that more women would be trained to use formula.

The emergence of pediatrics as a distinct field in medicine and the consolidation of doctors' control over infant feeding reflected broader changes in the social value of science. In the latter half of the nineteenth century, as historian Charles Rosenberg argues in *No Other Gods: On Science and American Social Thought*, the "constantly shifting equilibrium between secular and religious imperatives" was tilting strongly toward the former.[7] This meant not the delegitimation of religious or ethical concerns but the increasing role of science in pronouncing what was socially desirable. In addition to uncovering the putatively natural laws of any given process, science also determined what was virtuous; a scientist should not simply ascertain what was true but should establish what was *appropriate*.[8] Doctors were perceived and understood themselves to be high-minded reformers, and they insisted that scientific expertise was needed to raise children.

The proliferation and moral elevation of science meant that mothers became subject to a reign of expertise in areas that long had been considered somewhat mundane. As homemaking became a domestic science, for example, women sought education in home economics and the science of housework. It was in this era of "scientific motherhood"[9] that scientists began to make careers of advising mothers about what women had been doing largely on their own for centuries. Experts took their place alongside—and sometimes supplanted—customary female networks composed of midwives, relatives, and friends. Exhorting mothers to "Add Science to Love and be a 'Perfect Mother,'" an advertisement for a twenty-six-part child care course in *Parents Magazine* in 1938, made clear the growing reach and appeal of scientific authority. According to the advertisement, this course was written by

> one of America's greatest Child Authorities—Dr. Grace Langdon, Specialist and Adviser to the U.S. Government on such subjects as Parent Education, Nursery Schools and Homemaking. She has 1,500 government nursery schools under her direct supervision. She has the entire wealth of the latest Scientific advances in Child Training at her fingertips—and she makes it all available to YOU!

Low-income mothers were educated at public clinics, and government information, child care manuals, and visiting nurses in rural and urban areas stressed the need for scientific advice on all matters having to do with infants and children.[10]

In the context of scientific motherhood, mothers had even more reason to believe that the advice of pediatricians was essential to infant feeding; and in the early years of the twentieth century, if physicians and other experts in the science of child care continued to advocate breastfeeding, by the end of World War I they appeared to assume that most mothers, for a variety of reasons, would bottle-feed. Doctors' visits, home economics courses, hospital routines, and advice columns were increasingly dedicated to proper artificial feeding practices, giving the impression that the bottle was just as healthful as the breast. Science was equated with medicine and scientists with doctors, and this translated into the normalization of doctor-directed bottle feeding. In practice, each woman had to navigate her own way through the counsel of experts, her mother, and friends; she was, in the puzzling formation of child care expert Dr. Benjamin Spock, to trust her instincts and follow her doctor's advice.[11] Whatever her instincts, public discourse was dominated by the recommendations of child care experts who presented bottle feeding as a suitable alternative to breastfeeding. As doctor-supervised formula feeding became the norm, pediatricians also began to see babies and young children for regular checkups. These "well checks," originally designed in the 1920s to provide education and care for immigrant mothers and children in public clinics, eventually became the envy of middle-class mothers who wanted their children to have the same care and were willing to pay for it. When pediatricians realized that well care could provide a substantial and steady income, they moved these visits to their private practices and eventually helped force the closing of public clinics. The privatization of well-child medicine marked the beginning of routine and preventive care in pediatrics, which was estimated to comprise at least half the pediatric service provided in the 1950s and became central to the mission of pediatrics in the last decades of the twentieth century.[12]

This orientation toward prevention was significant in two seemingly contradictory ways. On one hand, it provoked a crisis of boredom: many pediatricians, who already found themselves near the bottom of the physicians' pay scale, grew frustrated at the absence of challenge or stimulation in routine checkups, especially as several of the major childhood infections and diseases either had disappeared or had been brought under control. What developed was "dissatisfied pediatrician syndrome," as practitioners called it, and it aroused such profound despair that many wondered whether pediatrics would survive.[13] On the other hand, the shift in focus made it possible to conceptualize anew the mission of pediatrics. Acrimonious professional debates took place in the 1960s and 1970s over what, if anything, pediatrics contributed to the practice of medicine that could not be provided by general physicians and pediatric nurse practitioners. This dilemma, along with a new, biopsychosocial model of health developing throughout clinical medicine, resulted in a sweeping notion of well care, which eventually came to encompass children's whole well-being. A variety of childhood experiences became medicalized, or were recast as potential pathologies that required the intervention and expertise of pediatricians. "Well" children were to be physically as well as socially and emotionally healthy. By 1975, pediatricians were speaking of a "new morbidity," which included chronic disabilities, such as asthma and allergies, and also learning, behavioral, and social impairments. The framing of these challenges as illnesses, and not simply as "problems" or "difficulties," gave them a medical cachet designed in part to persuade pediatricians reluctant to stretch the boundaries of child medicine. This comprehensive concept of well care divided childhood into different components that needed constant monitoring, and in the process, it solidified pediatrics as an independent branch of medicine.[14]

Obstetrics and the Ecology of Pregnancy

Similar developments in patient monitoring also helped legitimize obstetrics as a distinct discipline and medical practice. General physicians and midwives argued that they had the skills to provide women's reproductive health care, and like pediatricians, obstetricians faced doubts about the need for the kind of specialization they represented. It was, in part, the emergence of "the fetus" as a separate patient that helped establish bounded intellectual and clinical territory for obstetricians. In the late nineteenth century, public health workers, scientists, doctors, and others engaged in social action began to speak of "infant mortality" as a specific phenomenon.[15] In the early twentieth century, "the public fetus"—"a life" with a distinct conceptual existence whose protection required the social surveillance of pregnant women—began to emerge.[16] Urban public health institutions, devoted to reducing both infant and maternal mortality, began to target the prenatal period. In 1916, for example, New York City's milk stations were renamed "baby health stations," and the new centers included care focused on the fetus.[17] By midcentury, major obstetrics textbooks were speaking of the fetus and "fetal stress." Meanwhile, the "perinatal period," which referred to the time surrounding birth, developed as a clinical concept. Reasoning that deaths before, during, and shortly after birth had similar causes, obstetricians began to focus on monitoring the fetus. The concept of perinatal mortality conjured up a living subject before and during birth and encouraged doctors to optimize fetal life in order to maximize infant health. This new subject shook the relationship between inside and outside and reoriented the pregnant woman, the living subject, and the experts charged with their care.[18]

Simultaneously, a new approach to disease, which dramatically expanded the definition of what was "medical," began to take shape. In this paradigm, health and well-being were conceptualized ecologically, which meant that everything about individual lives was potentially significant to health status or was a possible risk factor for poor medical outcomes. This shift from a biomedical to a biopsychosocial model of medicine was welcomed by most health professionals and activists as a positive step toward a more integrated notion of health; increased knowledge would enable patients to make better choices and exercise more control over their well-being. But it also meant that nothing should be shielded from medical scrutiny. Where a person lived and worked, what she ate and breathed, her personal habits and social relationships—every behavior could be measured and monitored by a medical professional. By the late 1960s, virtually all aspects of women's lives came to be viewed as potentially risky to the fetus. As William Arney argued in *Power and the Profession of Obstetrics*, obstetricians contended that "absolutely everything must be made visible to medicine, be subject to observation, and recorded," and they collected copious data from each patient as much to confirm normalcy as to identify pathology. Pregnancies and births were to be "separated, individualized, subjected to constant and total visibility, and then offered technologies of normalization to guarantee an optimal experience, not necessarily for the individual, but for the system as a whole or, more precisely, for the individual considered in relationship to other components of the system."[19]

In other words, each pregnancy was to be tracked in relation to others, and deviations were cause for concern, not because they indicated danger, but simply because they were different. As "the notion of risk was transformed from a dichotomy to a continuum," pregnant women were categorized as high or low risk, which meant that no one was without risk and every pregnancy had "pathological potential."[20] The distinction between abnormality and normality became increasingly difficult to define, and "healthy" pregnancy and childbirth became even more dependent on the obstetrician's expertise and judgment. Moreover, "whereas earlier forms of prenatal care had been about maternal health, and prenatal education about the health of infants, risk assessment was novel in its attention to the health of the fetus."[21] New specialties developed in perinatology, embryology, and maternal-fetal medicine. By the last quarter of the twentieth century, the fetus was as much the obstetrician's patient as was the pregnant woman, and obstetrical work depended to a great extent on prenatal care.[22]

The fetus also aided obstetricians confronted by a growing women's health movement. In the late 1960s and 1970s, women's health activists challenged medical authority over women's bodies. They argued that doctors were "condescending, paternalistic, judgmental, and non-informative" and that the medical profession ultimately functioned to "enforce the subordination and neglect the needs of women" and other disadvantaged groups.[23] They also accused doctors of undertaking procedures and prescribing risky drugs that were unnecessary. They urged women to reject the largely male profession's control over their bodies, and they trained women to oversee their own reproductive health. While the National Women's Health Network monitored federal agencies and health policy, groups such as the Boston Women's Health Collective, authors of the well-known *Our Bodies, Ourselves: A Book by and for Women*, provided women with information, acted as referral services, and stressed both self-care and care from other women. "We encourage women health consumers to work for woman-controlled, woman-oriented health care and to pressure medical institutions to respond more flexibly to our needs," wrote the authors in the 1976 edition.[24] Activists encouraged women to give birth at home, not the hospital; assisted by midwives instead of controlled by doctors; and "naturally" rather than with pain-relieving drugs or technology. They created women's health and alternative birthing centers that were staffed largely by nonphysicians, and these institutions encroached on the patient base and challenged the authority of obstetricians and gynecologists.[25]

The fetus gave obstetricians a moral and professional stake in prenatal care. Whereas proponents of natural childbirth tried to naturalize reproduction, obstetricians sought to pathologize it; whereas the former fought to marginalize doctors, the latter emphasized risk in pregnancy and childbirth to demonstrate that physicians were essential to healthy births. In his history of obstetrics and gynecology, Arney went so far as to suggest that obstetricians preferred to "leave their treatment of the mother-to-be out of the debate entirely, for they now had the fetus, which they could defend against all bad consequences they claimed might result if they accommodated the demands of women for a more natural birth experience for themselves."[26] Just as in the nineteenth century, when forceps and ether had simultaneously improved the experience of childbirth for many women and helped obstetricians in their efforts to displace predominately female midwives, so in the twentieth century did fetal monitoring, expanded prenatal care, and a nebulous concept of abnormality work to improve the health of pregnant women and to cement the professional authority of obstetricians. As the medical parameters of pregnancy expanded, "the hospital became the center of a system of obstetrical surveillance that extended throughout the community."[27] Everything a pregnant woman did became grist for the medical mill, and comprehensive surveillance was justified as being in the best interests of the fetus. It was the fetus that required medical intervention, and it was in their concern for the fetus that obstetricians positioned themselves as more knowledgeable and trustworthy than women and as essential to a healthy pregnancy. They turned increasingly to their monopoly on technology, such as ultrasound, fetal monitors, and newborn intensive care units, to make the case for their unique ability to manage the omnipresent risks of pregnancy.[28]

The twentieth century was an era of consolidation for both pediatrics and obstetrics, and the establishment of each field as a bona fide specialized form of medical knowledge was made possible, in large part, by expanded opportunities for patient surveillance. As a result, both obstetricians and pediatricians became increasingly engaged in their patients' lives. The ecological approach to pregnancy, in which everything about women's lives was potentially consequential for the fetus, created the possibility of pregnant women's empowerment through knowledge but also broadened the terrain of obstetrical monitoring and medical control. Both physicians and women came to believe that the health of the fetus depended on medical expertise and frequent contact between patient and doctor. After birth, surveillance shifted from the mother to the baby, and the obstetrician's continuous monitoring of the pregnant woman's body in order to optimize the fetal outcome gave way to the pediatrician's constant auditing of the baby to manage proper development. On one hand, tracking children's maturation could bypass mothers, since their bodies no longer prevented direct medical contact between doctor and patient. On the other hand, mothers retained responsibility for both ensuring that children received proper medical attention and creating and maintaining conditions that would promote growth. Just as women monitored their bodies during pregnancy with an eye toward creating low-risk fetal environments, mothers managed their own lives and their children's bodies to minimize threats to optimal development. By the last decades of the century, the professionalization of both pediatrics and obstetrics and gynecology had redefined pregnancy, birth, and childhood as medical events to be managed by doctors. This medicalization of women's and children's bodies is integral to total motherhood in a risk culture.

The Resurgence of Breastfeeding

Motivated by their Catholic faith, a commitment to correcting misinfor-
mation about breastfeeding coming from doctors, and a strong belief that
"nature intended mothers to nurse; therefore, mothers ought to nurse,"
a group of seven suburban housewives founded La Leche League (LLL)
in 1956.[29] At the heart of the LLL philosophy was (and remains today)
the principle that mothers are naturally best suited to care for babies and
to help other women with breastfeeding. The founders wrote and published the first edition of *The Womanly Art of Breastfeeding* in 1958, and
the second edition, which appeared in 1963, sold more than a million
copies before a third edition was published in 1981. The authors argue
early in the book that "breastfeeding is integral to good mothering." It is
"Nature's way," and it is healthiest for babies as well as mothers who have
become "bogged down in scales and charts and schedules" and have lost
"confidence in their own abilities." The authors advise each reader to tell
her doctor during her first prenatal visit that she plans to breastfeed. If he
disapproves, "you definitely need to be in touch with some mother who
knows the ins and outs of breastfeeding because of her own successful
personal experience." Remember, the authors stress, that "your right and
privilege as a patient is the choice of a doctor sympathetic to your needs
and desires," and this is a right protected by the American Medical Association. Above all, "don't let your confidence in yourself be shaken. We
know many women who have successfully nursed their babies and en-
joyed it thoroughly" even when their doctors have not been supportive. At
the hospital, after the baby is born, "you may need to be prepared to assert
yourself." Once home, let the baby determine the feeding schedule, and
when it comes to weaning, "let the baby do it." A baby who has received
appropriate care and attention eventually will lose the need to be breastfed. They advise mothers to "turn a deaf ear" to people who criticize them.
"This is *your* child, and you are doing what you know is best for him."[30]
    Building in part on the LLL's success, the resurgence of breastfeeding
began in earnest in the late 1960s and early 1970s. Although they distanced
themselves from LLL's broader philosophy, which deemed that *mothers*
were exclusively responsible for babies' care, many women's health advocates promoted breastfeeding as "ideally suited to a baby's need."[31] In 1974,
breastfeeding became part of an anticapitalist campaign when international
activists revealed that many babies in the developing world were dying as

a result of formula companies' deceitful promotional practices and failure to educate the women who were buying their products. These companies, including the Swiss-based Nestlé, had been hiring women with no medical training to dress up as nurses and give away formula. They also were providing hospitals with free samples whose use interfered with lactation, and new mothers often went home unable either to breastfeed or to pay for additional formula. Many of these mothers lacked basic literacy, and they did not understand the potentially lethal consequences of mixing the powder with contaminated water or diluting the concentration to make the formula last longer. In a controversial pamphlet entitled *The Baby Killers*, the British charity War on Want argued that formula manufacturers were promoting "commerciogenic malnutrition" in developing countries.[32] A few years later, in 1977, activists in the United States launched a boycott of Nestlé products that eventually spread to Australia, Canada, New Zealand, and Europe. Then, in 1981, the World Health Organization (WHO) and the United Nations Children's Fund (UNICEF) issued the International Code of Marketing of Breastmilk Substitutes, which banned formula advertising or distribution of samples. The code was approved by 118 countries.[33]

Although practicing pediatricians were free to supervise formula feeding as they deemed appropriate, the American Academy of Pediatrics (AAP) had always supported breastfeeding. In 1982, an AAP task force issued a statement reiterating the organization's support for breastfeeding but also criticizing the WHO's code for its "limited approach to an issue that is complex and involves extensive social, economic, and motivational factors . . . particularly evident for the situation in the United States." The report argued that significant differences existed between breastfeeding and bottle-feeding mothers and that the actual effects of breastfeeding were difficult to isolate. It concluded that pediatricians should "work to improve the knowledge of all potential expectant and current parents on optimal infant feeding nutrition, emphasizing the positive aspects of breast-feeding and the proper choice and utilization of breast milk substitutes."[34] In short, the AAP argued that breastfeeding was preferable but that formula was an acceptable alternative.

But controversy in the preceding decade over the marketing of formula in the developing world had generated strong antiformula sentiment and energized new breastfeeding advocates. It also had stimulated research into the health effects of different feeding practices. Five times as many studies on breastfeeding appeared in 1980 as in 1970, and nearly twice as many were published in 1990 as in 1980.[35] In 1997, the AAP declared that the superiority of breastfeeding, even for women in the industrial-ized world, was undeniable. It urged all women to breastfeed exclusively for six months, and it cautioned practitioners to "weigh thoughtfully the benefits of breastfeeding against the risks of not receiving human milk" before recommending formula or early weaning.[36] Decades of advocacy from domestic and international women's health activists certainly had helped shape this statement. But by the close of the twentieth century, the viability of pediatrics as a separate branch of medicine also was no longer in doubt. Well checks, a diffuse notion of morbidity, and preventive care had come to define the profession, and supervised infant feeding was no longer a central component of pediatric practice.[37] Some breastfeeding ad-vocates continue to argue today that pediatricians lack the knowledge and commitment to help women struggling to breastfeed and that the formula industry exercises undue economic influence over the AAP.[38] But the 1997 statement, and an update in 2005, stipulated in no uncertain terms that breast is best,[39] an assertion that few in pediatrics or medical practice in general would challenge today.

Current Scholarship and Chapter Summaries

When, for the first time, a mother provides ongoing care to her baby as a separate entity, as a body that exists outside her own, breastfeeding con-stitutes a rupture. But as a continuation of the vital connection between mother and baby, breastfeeding also prolongs the perinatal period. It is the only moment in the child's life cycle that requires surveillance of both the mother's and the baby's bodies, and as such, it is especially fraught with social meaning. Now that pediatricians and most other medical doc-tors have come to embrace breastfeeding as best for babies, scholars in the social sciences and humanities, many of whom identify themselves as feminists, have begun to ask critical questions about the social dimensions of infant feeding. In particular, these scholars have examined what breast-feeding reveals about race, class, gender, and motherhood in various social contexts, and this book owes much to their pioneering work.

One of the first texts in this field, Pam Carter's *Feminism, Breasts, and Breast-Feeding* (1995), challenges the "fact" that breastfeeding is superior. Concentrating on the United Kingdom, Carter emphasizes the importance of understanding women's varied experiences of infant feeding. She ar-gues that pro-breastfeeding policies often serve as an instrument of social control by enabling various institutions of authority to police the bodies of black, working-class, and less educated mothers, women whose mothering practices have always been suspect to the middle class. These women, she contends, struggle to reconcile their feeding choices with conflicting prescriptions for appropriate behavior in public and private spaces and with heteronormative expectations about the sexual purpose of women's breasts, social obligations that take on different meanings depending on racial and class context. Nonwhite mothers in Britain have particular difficulty appreciating the celebration of "nature" and "the natural" in pro-breastfeeding discourse, as these terms are often used pejoratively to mean "primitive" and "animalistic" in other conversations about race.

The foundational text for studying breastfeeding in the United States is Linda Blum's *At the Breast: Ideologies of Breastfeeding and Motherhood in the Contemporary United States* (1999). Blum examines breastfeeding through the lens of what she calls "exclusive motherhood," exemplified by the LLL's philosophy, according to which breastfeeding is a uniquely and naturally "womanly" art that corresponds to babies' natural need to be in constant close contact with their mother. Blum contends that this vision of "embodied" motherhood, with its emphasis on the continuous and exclusive interaction between mother and baby, is tantamount to the normalization of white, middle-class mothering, maternal practices that are inaccessible or undesirable to black and white working-class mothers for a variety of social, economic, and cultural reasons. Blum contrasts breastfeeding in embodied motherhood with a more "medical" model, in which doctors regulate and women scrutinize their behavior in order to produce perfect breast milk. Whereas exclusive motherhood is grounded in the relationship between mother and baby, medicalized feeding centers on mothers' bodies and the production of milk. Here the breast pump makes possible the constant nutritional presence of the mother, who need not be physically present. While this medical model places less emphasis on the interaction between mother and baby, it nonetheless assumes the time, socioeconomic resources, and availability of the maternal body for optimal child development that define exclusive motherhood. Breastfeeding, Blum concludes, is a class-enhancing, racialized project. Like Carter, Blum demonstrates the hegemony of white and middle-class values in various discourses surrounding motherhood. "Breastfeeding does not have inherent truth," she writes, "but meanings determined out of power relations, various disciplining practices, and conflicting needs and interests, which are inherently political."[40]

A small but growing literature has begun to build on the work of Carter and Blum, and this research bears directly on my analysis of breastfeeding discourse in the United States. Jules Law suggests that debates about infant feeding are less about breast milk and formula than about "the social, domestic, and technical arrangements conventionally associated with them." He argues that the current pro-breastfeeding literature construes different feeding forms within a framework that unquestioningly accepts a gendered division of domestic labor as both normative and universal, fails to understand mothers and babies as participants in a broader family unit, and therefore presents a skewed picture of the "benefits" of breastfeeding and the "risks" of formula feeding.[41] Glenda Wall contends that Canadian breastfeeding education material reveals assumptions about pregnancy as a moral endeavor and the importance of personal responsibility in reducing the cost of social programs.[42] Based on interviews with mothers in the United States, England, Sweden, Australia, and Canada, other scholars have raised questions about the challenges of infant-feeding decisions and practices for mothers' sense of themselves as both embodied women and "good mothers."[43] Elizabeth Murphy, for example, illustrates how different mothers narrate their feeding decisions as being consistent with a notion of good mothering, and Orit Avishai demonstrates how class-privileged women construct breastfeeding as a consumer undertaking and as a project to be managed and accomplished.[44]

Bernice Hausman analyzes cultural representations of infant feeding in the United States. Writing as "a breastfeeding advocate" who took "enthusiasm and delight in the practice," Hausman explains that she became "frustrated with feminist collusion with the idea that in order not to induce guilt in mothers who don't or can't breastfeed, we shouldn't argue for its benefits, or even acknowledge that breastfeeding has a biological benefit at all." That white and middle-class mothers are culturally and economically situated in ways that make breastfeeding more likely, she maintains, should provoke a feminist critique not of the injunction to breastfeed but of the inequitable social arrangements that make breastfeeding less possible for black and working-class women.[45] Hausman accuses feminist scholars who have criticized the advocacy of breastfeeding of a tendency "to sidestep a significant engagement with science and its findings in order to focus on political meanings." She objects to what she calls feminists' "strategy of raising questions about medical evidence in order to assert the primacy of cultural meanings of breastfeeding" and what she claims is their preference "that biological considerations be subordinated to political ones." "All the [medical] research points in the same direction," she contends, and "accepting the scientific evidence doesn't have to mean giving up on politics."[46] For Hausman, the superiority of breastfeeding is an inconvenient truth that must be recognized before feminists can think critically about its political consequences. A "significant engagement with science" means acknowledging that breastfeeding is medically beneficial, regardless of its ramifications for feminist politics.

Hausman's critique is based on several erroneous assumptions: that science has demonstrated compellingly that breastfeeding is medically advantageous, that all scientific research indeed "points in the same direction," and that any challenge to the evidence is a disingenuous effort to shift attention from breastfeeding's medical benefits to its antifeminist implications. In fact, Blum and Law identify specific methodological and interpretive problems in scientific studies.[47] They do not undertake a systematic analysis of breastfeeding research, but neither does Hausman, despite her claim to "engage with the scientific case for breastfeeding . . . on its own terms . . . as a data set crucially important to maternal and child health." Rather, Hausman cites a few articles that argue for the medical importance of breastfeeding, acknowledging but ultimately bracketing various problems in these and other studies and concluding that "scientific claims for the biological benefits of breastfeeding cannot be dismissed as only discursive."[48]

Hausman's appraisal of feminist scholarship and her defense of breastfeeding science as more than "discursive" neglect the fact that the production, publication, and dissemination of science also are shaped by culture and subject to feminist critique. Breastfeeding research is framed, conducted, and communicated within specific disciplinary paradigms that are themselves situated in social contexts, conditions that set boundaries around what kind of information can be ascertained. At every stage, from the questions that scientists ask to the strategies they use to answer them to the ensuing discussion of the results, breastfeeding research reflects, or is constrained by, what makes professional and cultural sense. "*What* we know about the world," in other words, "cannot be fully understood independent of *how* and *why* we know it—what social practices are used to establish facts and what human values, goals, and interests those facts serve."[49] This does not mean that findings of breastfeeding research are purely "discursive" or that they have no basis in material reality, but it does suggest that the contrast Hausman draws between "medical evidence" and "cultural" and "political" meaning is too stark. The best research results are partial truths that can be understood only within the parameters of their production, and a "significant engagement with science" requires situating scientific practice in its cultural, professional, and political contexts.[50] Such is the aim of this book.

In the next chapter, I explain why the scientific evidence for breastfeeding's benefits is not nearly as compelling as various advocates insist. I argue that despite overwhelming sentiment to the contrary, epidemiological research does not demonstrate persuasively that breast milk is medically superior to infant formula for most babies in the developed world. While breastfeeding does appear to reduce the risk for various GI infections, the evidence for virtually every other health measure is plagued by unexamined confounding variables, potential selection bias, and inconsistent outcomes, all terms that I explain in detail. I recognize, as do most scientists, that even the best research on any subject is characterized by some degree of uncertainty and that scientists necessarily draw conclusions based on imperfect information. Precisely because no result is ever completely conclusive, scientists have set for themselves standards for proof that must be met before findings can be interpreted, and research suggesting that breastfeeding protects against various poor health outcomes falls considerably short of these measures. The more carefully that studies control for bias and confounders, the less significant that breastfeeding becomes, and the residual benefits could well be explained by general differences in the health practices of breastfeeding and bottle-feeding parents. Health advantages attributed to breastfeeding might have more to do with behavior surrounding breastfeeding than with breastfeeding per se, behavior that, at least theoretically, could be adopted by bottle-feeding families.

Despite this possibility, which scientists commonly acknowledge in published research, the recommendation to breastfeed goes largely unchallenged, and this unanimity among health professionals has much to do with how science is conducted and findings are communicated in a risk culture committed to total motherhood. The design, execution, and interpretation of breastfeeding research take place within a "risk-factor" paradigm whose methodological parameters sharply limit the kinds of questions that can be asked and the conclusions that can be drawn. This research is shared in professional journals in which results are easily misconstrued by scientists and doctors overwhelmed by the volume and complexity of information they must master. Results are then presented to a public largely ignorant of basic scientific principles by journalists unschooled in scientific method or the meaning of risk in epidemiological research. In uncritically circulating the findings of breastfeeding research, these journalists aggravate popular fears and misconceptions about risk and reinforce the expectation that mothers have a categorical responsibility to reduce risks to their children. The practice of science, including communication among scientists and between professional science and the public, are central to the misrepresentation of breastfeeding.

In chapter 3, I outline the parameters of what I call the neoliberal risk culture in which the message that "breast is best" circulates. Here efforts to control the future, and specifically to prevent negative events from taking place, serve as an organizing principle of human behavior, and various forms of scientific expertise exercise far-ranging technical and moral authority over the choices people make. People look constantly to doctors, toxicologists, psychologists, financial planners, and other risk analysts to make everyday decisions about how to eat, breathe, raise children, improve relationships, manage money, and the like. Concerns about risk, especially about health and threats to the body, are widespread, and information about diet and disease pervade public discourse. Life is medicalized, or cast as a body project that requires the continuous monitoring and judgment of medical science, and health becomes a defining characteristic of responsible selfhood and citizenship.

In a risk culture, all manner of experts encourage individuals to assume personal responsibility for their health by subjecting themselves to assorted mechanisms of external and self-surveillance, which I explore at length. Race, class, and gender inequalities recede from visibility, and individuals are held accountable for outcomes well beyond their control. At the same time, as science is increasingly understood to be able to illuminate the path toward optimal living, the pace and uncertain effects of technological progress produce anxiety, and appreciation grows for anything perceived to be "natural." In such forms as organic foods, herbal medicine, and recycled products, nature takes on an aura of practical and moral authority. Long assumed to play a crucial role in both family and national vitality, mothers in a risk culture are assigned the onus of ensuring babies' and children's health. In conversations about motherhood, breastfeeding is coded as safe, natural, healthy, and responsible.

Chapter 4 examines how the representation and practice of infant feeding are shaped by social expectations of mothers. Here I describe what I define as an ideology of total motherhood that requires mothers to devote themselves wholly to reducing risks to their children. Before they even try to become pregnant and throughout the lives of their children, women are counseled to guard against all imaginable threats to their real or anticipated offspring. They are told by multiple authorities to monitor their bodies in order to optimize conception, pregnancy, and childbirth, and they are advised that no risk to a child is too small to eliminate and no cost is too high to bear in the effort. As girls grow into women, their bodies are increasingly conceptualized as future wombs that must be managed to create a low-risk environment for the inevitable fetus. Diet, sleep, work, thought, leisure behavior: virtually every dimension of women's lives is framed in terms of how it might affect their babies' health and well-being. Once a woman becomes pregnant, the fetus is cast in various discourses as a separate person. It becomes a distinct human entity that has needs and rights that are in direct conflict with, and take precedence over, the wants and desires of the mother, who is to remain devoted to reducing all risks to her fetus. "Natural" mothers eschew the trappings of modern life, including pain relief during childbirth and disposable diapers, that might make their lives easier but that they believe could put their children at risk for anything from delayed development to diaper rash. Pregnancy guides eventually give way to baby and toddler manuals and a voluminous library of child-raising advice that assumes mothers will subjugate their own needs, often cast as desires, to those of their children. Breastfeeding is integral to total motherhood. Advised that it reduces risks to babies' physical, emotional, social, and cognitive well-being, mothers are expected to undertake any sacrifice necessary to breastfeed. They are to track what they eat, reduce stress, suppress emotional needs, and restructure employment to accommodate breastfeeding. No matter how high the cost to the mother or how marginal the risk to the baby, breastfeeding is imperative in a risk culture committed to total motherhood.

Chapter 5 brackets the question of whether research has sufficiently demonstrated the advantages of breastfeeding in order to ask whether, even if proven, such benefits would be strong enough to justify the rhetoric of contemporary advocacy. Here I analyze as a case study the National Breastfeeding Awareness Campaign (NBAC), sponsored in 2004–2006 by the U.S. Department of Health and Human Services, and I argue that the campaign distorted both the putative risks of bottle feeding, such as increased GI infections, and the costs or trade-offs of breastfeeding. "You'd never take risks before your baby is born. Why start after?" asked televised public service announcements over images of pregnant women logrolling and riding a mechanical bull. The campaign, and particularly its fear-based approach, exploited the dynamics of a culture consumed by risk and total motherhood. Based on weak and inconsistent research, it capitalized on the public's misunderstanding of risk and risk assessment by portraying infant nutrition as a matter of safety versus danger and then creating misleading analogies. In telling mothers that not breastfeeding put their babies in danger, it misrepresented statistics. It manipulated deep-seated common assumptions about the responsibility of mothers to protect their babies and children from harm, and it offered little to redress the psychological, socioeconomic, and political concerns of women themselves. Crucially, it ignored the risks and trade-offs of breastfeeding itself, costs that are overwhelmingly shouldered by mothers. In most infant-feeding research, and in all the research cited by the NBAC, the putative benefits of breastfeeding for babies are calculated against the potential costs of formula feeding for babies, not the costs of breastfeeding for women who, as mothers, are presumed not to have needs that might diverge from those of their babies. A nexus of flawed medical research, fears about and misapprehension of health risks, and an ideology of maternal responsibility, the NBAC revealed breastfeeding as a microcosm of total motherhood in a neoliberal risk culture.

In the conclusion, I situate breastfeeding in the context of debates about other contemporary health risks. In particular, I explore the ongoing campaign against America's "obesity epidemic" as another example of the limits of epidemiology, neoliberalism, and framing health behavior as risky. As numerous scholars have demonstrated, the fact that obesity is correlated with poor health outcomes does not provide evidence that extra weight—adiposity, or the fat itself—*causes* sickness or, by extension, that losing weight reduces many of these health risks. Yet the admonition to be thin, like the injunction to breastfeed, has become a guiding principle for those who seek to be healthy, responsible citizens. The obsessions with thinness and breastfeeding stem from a glut of health information that reflects a misunderstanding and misuse of the concept of statistical significance in both science and the popular media. As moral agendas, they reveal a certain blindness to how what is labeled "healthy" reflects social privilege, and they give rise to fearmongering and hyperbole, or what one lactation scientist who advocates breastfeeding nonetheless calls a "netherworld of drivel created by advertising and political posturing."[51] Research is far from demonstrating that, in the words of one academic advocate, "adequate consumption of human milk as an infant is a power-ful guarantor of health and long life."[52] In truth, no such guarantee exists, and examining the false elixirs that all societies create reveals a great deal about their values. As Diane Eyer wrote about early theories of maternal-infant bonding that were widely accepted but eventually rejected:

> For researchers in the social sciences, it is a matter of self-defense to understand how seemingly carefully constructed research findings can be distorted and why. For clinicians it is important to understand the implications of basing practice on research findings. And for parents and potential parents, it is important to sort out what is fact and what is fiction in the advice they receive on childbirth and child rearing.[53]

2

The Science

Does Breastfeeding Make Smarter,
Happier, and Healthier Babies?

AT THE CORE of the "breast is best" message is the notion that breast-feeding—the substantive properties of breast milk, the interaction between breastfeeding mother and baby, or some combination of the two—is medically superior to bottle feeding for babies. That is, breastfed babies are physically, cognitively, and emotionally healthier than their bottle-fed counterparts, and their relative well-being can be attributed to one or various dimensions of the breastfeeding process. There is broad disagreement on the extent to which employers and public institutions should make accommodations for breastfeeding, and scientists have not established any consensus on the long-term health effects of breastfeeding for women who lactate. But few in either the medical community or the public, including critics of the rhetorical and political tactics of some more ardent activists, question the biological "fact" that, as the American Academy of Pediatrics (AAP) has argued since 1997, "human milk is uniquely superior for infant feeding."[1] Yet the evidence for breastfeeding's health benefits is far more equivocal than the AAP implies. Indeed, an analysis of the epidemiological research on breastfeeding—how studies are designed, carried out, interpreted, and communicated among scientists and between medical professionals and the public—indicates that while breastfed babies, on average, do appear to be slightly healthier, the science does not demonstrate compellingly that breast milk or breastfeeding is responsible.

Although scientists have recently begun to examine the biological consequences of breastfeeding for women, breastfeeding research has focused overwhelmingly on its potential effects on babies, the consumers of breast milk. In these studies, scientists have looked at the association between different modes of infant feeding and various physical, mental, social, and emotional health outcomes. These include asthma and allergy, bed-wetting, various childhood cancers, cardiovascular disease, celiac disease, child abuse, diabetes, diarrhea, eczema, growth pains, leukemia, necrotizing enterocolitis, inflammatory bowel disease, intelligence, mother-infant bonding, obesity, otitis media, postneonatal death, preterm infant health, respiratory infection, sleep-related breathing disorders, social mobility, stereoacuity, stress, sudden infant death syndrome (SIDS), and urinary tract infection. PubMed, a database of medical research maintained by the National Library of Medicine, indicates that 1,155 articles with "breastfeeding" or "breast-feeding" in the title or abstract were published in 2009 alone. The scientific literature is voluminous, and I do not intend that this chapter be a comprehensive review.

Rather, I concentrate on the health outcomes for babies that have generated the most attention in scientific journals with relatively high "impact factors," or rates of citation. I also incorporate the evidence cited by the National Breastfeeding Awareness Campaign (NBAC), sponsored by the U.S. Department of Health and Human Services between 2004 and 2006, and articles in journals determined to contain "the best evidence relating to clinical pediatric practice."[2] I do not include material from journals devoted specifically to breastfeeding, including *Breastfeeding Medicine, International Breastfeeding Journal*, and the *Journal of Human Lactation*. All these are peer reviewed and have editorial boards composed of research scientists, but their editorial policies make clear that each journal's mission is to promote breastfeeding.[3] I offer a plausible rival explanation for breastfeeding's benefits: that behavior associated with breastfeeding, not breastfeeding per se, explains any relationship between breastfeeding and better health. I argue that methodological and interpretive problems are pervasive at every step of the research process, from the design of the studies to the communication of their results; that as is often said, correlation does not equal causation; and that except in the case of gastrointestinal infections, the biological mechanisms by which breastfeeding promotes better health have not been demonstrated. In short, I contend that the unfounded certainty about breastfeeding's benefits in both scientific and popular culture is rooted in the discourse of breastfeeding research.

Observational Research

The success of epidemiological studies depends not on their ability to explain how diseases are acquired and controlled, ostensibly the mission of epidemiology, but on their establishment of a statistical relationship between a variable or a set of variables, such as obesity or the consumption of dark chocolate, and a particular outcome, such as heart disease or high blood pressure. Variables linked with disease, such as high cholesterol or residency in a highly polluted area, are termed "risk factors." In the past decade, epidemiological research has been "going through a soul-searching period" during which critics have argued that this approach conceals more than it reveals.[4] Epidemiologists, they contend, search for antecedents to disease at the individual level based on the dubious assumption that these factors "can be linked to outcomes without necessity for intervening factors."[5] They strive to be parsimonious, or to arrive at the simplest explanations, but in their effort they often obscure both what precedes putative risk factors, such as genetics, and the mediators linking these factors with disease, such as behavior. While correlations are provocative, they reveal little about process, such as why fat tissue is detrimental to the cardiovascular system or why the flavonoids in dark chocolate reduce blood pressure. The explanation for the associations, in other words, "resides in linkages along a causal chain whose detection is hindered by the very structure" of risk factor epidemiology.[6] Epidemiology, therefore,

> is never able to establish "causation" in either direction. All that it can show is "association," a much-misunderstood term. . . . When all goes well in an epidemiological study, one finds an association between two things. No more, no less. And that's true even of the best of studies, those that are methodologically rigorous and carefully constructed.[7]

But in a research domain that emphasizes measurability over analysis at the same time that it purports to explain how diseases proliferate, what results is a "continual confusion of observational associations with causality" in which researchers employ "more and more advanced technology to study more and more trivial issues."[8]

Infant-feeding research also is limited by its reliance on "observational" methods. Because the medical community largely assumes that breastfeeding is medically superior to formula feeding, researchers consider that it would be unethical to construct randomized controlled trials (RCT) in which babies were randomly assigned to either breast or bottle. Instead, they systematically observe people who have chosen, for their own reasons, to breastfeed or bottle-feed. The results of observational investigations are often at odds with one another, and the ability to replicate such studies is much lower than for RCTs.[9] One powerful reason for this is that observational research frequently fails to adequately weigh crucial confounding variables, unexamined factors in a study that plausibly could explain differences in outcome. Confounding makes it difficult to isolate the protective powers of breast milk itself, or to rule out the possibility that something associated with breastfeeding is responsible for the benefits attributed to milk. Hypothetically, if most mothers who breastfeed also eat low-carbohydrate diets or exercise five times a week, it would be difficult to determine whether the different health outcomes in breastfed babies stemmed from breastfeeding or from the nutrition or exercise associated with breastfeeding. As the number of years between breastfeeding and the measured health outcome grows, so too does the list of potentially influential factors, which means that the challenge of isolating cause and effect is magnified when trying to evaluate long-term benefits. While consideration of confounding is always a challenge in observational research, it is of "paramount importance" when correlations are not strong or when causal pathways "involve not just biological but also behavioral steps that need to be understood and measured to demonstrate a logical sequence between intervention and outcome."[10]

Research on siblings is one way to reduce the confounding that results when preexisting dissimilarities between people in control and experimental groups can explain distinct outcomes. A recent sibling study that examined breastfeeding and bottle feeding reported that "nearly all of the correlations found in the between-family model become statistically insignificant in the within-family model." The one exception, a positive correlation between breastfeeding and cognitive ability, is itself ambiguous, as the authors acknowledge, "because of unobserved factors that lead a mother to feed two infants differently."[11] For example, does a breastfed child have a higher IQ than her bottle-fed brother because her mother had the time and energy to breastfeed, and perhaps to consistently engage with, only her daughter? Two additional sibling studies reached contradictory conclusions about breastfeeding's impact on obesity but agreed that within-family investigations have not controlled for "why a mother chooses to breast-feed one sibling and not another" or why she might breast-feed one child longer than another.[12] Said differently, breastfeeding cannot be clearly distinguished from the decision to breastfeed; the choice to initiate and continue breastfeeding might signal a variety of health-promoting behaviors on the part of the child's caretakers, and the decision to breastfeed could represent an approach to child care that is far more important than breastfeeding itself. When behavior that is associated with breastfeeding has the potential to explain much of the statistical advantage attributed to breast milk, the scientific claim that breastfeeding confers health benefits, or that not breastfeeding increases risk, is precarious.

The Evidence

Does breastfeeding reduce later obesity, defined by many scientists and health professionals as one of the most pressing public health problems facing the United States today? To date, the evidence is not compelling. Multiple studies have addressed the effects of different modes of infant feeding on various indicators, including weight gain in the first week of life and infancy (and the impact of this initial weight gain on later weight), trajectories of body fat and body mass index (BMI) throughout childhood and the life course, and overweight and obesity in young children, adolescents, siblings, African American and Latino youth, and low-income children. These studies reveal the problems that characterize most breastfeeding research. They inconsistently measure the amount, duration, and exclusivity of breastfeeding; depending on the study, a baby can have been "breastfed" if it received only breast milk, some milk, or mostly milk for a few days, weeks, a month, or several months. They rely on mothers to recall information about infant-feeding practices that took place long before the studies are conducted. One investigation even asked mothers of adult daughters to recall their breastfeeding protocols from as long as forty years earlier.[13] Some studies find no benefit from breastfeeding,[14] and the strong majority of those that do find an association between breastfeeding and reduced overweight and obesity offer some form of qualification: that any inverse relationship between breastfeeding and overweight is small, that it disappears in regression analysis, and/or that the relationship could be explained by unexamined confounding variables.[15] Literature reviews,[16] meta-analyses,[17] and commentaries[18] echo the conclusion that breastfeeding's protective effect for obesity is small and/or inconclusive. "Mean BMI is lower among breastfed subjects," concludes a meta-analysis in the *American Journal of Clinical Nutrition*. "However, the difference is small and is likely to be strongly influenced by publication bias and confounding factors. Promotion of breastfeeding . . . is not likely to reduce mean BMI."[19]

Two articles published in the *Journal of the American Medical Association* (*JAMA*) in spring 2001 reveal the challenges of determining whether breastfeeding reduces the risk for obesity. One study finds "inconsistent associations among breastfeeding, its duration, and the risk of being over-weight in young children," while the other concludes that "infants who were fed breast milk more than infant formula, or who were breastfed for longer periods, had a lower risk of being overweight during older child-hood and adolescence."[20] The first expressed concern that any associa-tion between breastfeeding and risk for obesity "may be confounded by unmeasured sociodemographic or intervening familial factors," and in an effort to control for two such factors, diet and exercise, the second asked its adolescent subjects to complete a mail-in survey that included ques-tions about eating habits, physical activity, and television viewing during the previous year.[21] That the authors attempted to consider the impact of energy consumed and expended on body weight indicates their awareness that these might well obviate any protective effect of breastfeeding. Their data, however, are questionable. Researchers have argued that "no single problem has been more formidable to nutritional epidemiology than the measurement of dietary intakes" and that the difficulties are "notorious" because people are inclined to "'fudge' their answers" or "lie outright."[22] This might explain why a frequently cited study found that full-fat milk products, sweet desserts, butter, and breakfast cereals were consumed less frequently by overweight children. The authors suggest that this surprising association "reflects avoidance of these products by children who are over-weight,"[23] although it is at least equally plausible that respondents did not answer the questionnaires truthfully. Additional studies have found that self-reports of diet and activity are poor indicators of actual BMI and that parents' and teens' reports of weight perception are weak indices of ado-lescent obesity.[24] Diet and exercise are sensitive subjects for most Ameri-cans, and the ability of preteens and teenagers wrestling with their body image to provide unbiased information is perhaps even more doubtful. Given the cultural and generational pressures to be thin, the overweight subjects might have been more likely to overstate exercise and underre-port caloric intake, which would skew relationships with some other vari-able, such as breastfeeding. Conclusions based on these accounts should therefore be drawn cautiously.

In the discussion section of the second *JAMA* article, furthermore, the authors acknowledge that "residual and unmeasured confounding are always of concern in an observational study where the subjects choose the level of exposure and not all covariates are measured with optimal precision."[25] The data they provide, in fact, support another explanation: that parental behavior explains the apparent weight differences between breastfed and bottle-fed children. According to this interpretation, mothers who choose to breastfeed for its purported health advantages might also have both the desire and the means to promote a healthy lifestyle, which would include a balanced diet and physical exercise. If heavier adolescents, who in this study were more likely to have been bottle-fed, were not encouraged to eat well and be active, the lower incidence of obesity among breastfed children would have less to do with breast milk than with mothers and/or fathers who promote healthy living. Epidemiological studies have failed to rule out the possibility that caretaker behavior associated with breastfeeding explains any correlation between breastfeeding and reduced overweight and obesity. Because the self-reports are unreliable, and because the authors did not eliminate the potentially salient behaviors associated with breastfeeding, the lower incidence of obesity among breastfed children and adolescents cannot be convincingly attributed to breastfeeding.[26]

Does breastfeeding make babies smarter? Some studies, meta-analyses, and reviews have found breastfeeding to be associated with increased cognitive development and higher IQ.[27] As in obesity research, these investigations are methodologically problematic, as they define "breastfeeding" differently, employ different outcome measures, and generally find that the advantages associated with breastfeeding are small and could be explained by confounding variables, such as maternal IQ and/or behavior.[28] Critics routinely point to a "lengthy and probably impossible to complete" list of potentially confounding variables, including "the possibility that mothers who breastfeed may also promote academic success in other ways."[29] In a *JAMA* article finding "a significant positive association between duration of breastfeeding and intelligence," the authors acknowledge that "behavior predicts behavior, and even within each different social class and educational level, it may be that mothers who spend more time breastfeeding during the first year of life also spend more time later interacting with the child."[30] If this were the case, any increase in intelligence among breastfed babies would be attributable not to breast milk but to behavior linked with breastfeeding, and bottle-fed children with caretakers who were able to invest more time with them would be equally likely to have higher scores on intelligence tests. A study that controlled for maternal IQ and parenting skills found that "the observed advantage of breastfeeding on IQ is related to genetic and socioenvironmental factors rather than to the nutritional benefits of breastfeeding on neurodevelopment."[31] Other studies that controlled for maternal verbal abilities,

IQ and education produced similar results.[32] Two separate review articles argued that most of the existing investigations failed to satisfy basic methodological standards, including implementing appropriate controls. One, published in the AAP's journal *Pediatrics*, concluded that "no convincing evidence exists regarding the comparative effects of breastfeeding and artificial feeding on intelligence."[33]

Does breastfeeding protect against various ear infections, or otitis media? Here again, the results have been mixed.[34] The more tightly these studies controlled for confounding variables, such as the number of other children to whom the study subject was exposed, the less significant breastfeeding became and the more plausible the salience of healthy behaviors practiced by the caretakers of breastfed babies was as an explanation for the residual benefit. In a review of outcomes associated with breastfeeding, the Agency for Healthcare Research and Quality in the U.S. Department of Health and Human Services confirmed a relationship between breastfeeding and reduced infection but also explicitly stated that causality could not be inferred from observational studies that did not control for "behavioral factors intrinsic in the desire to breastfeed."[35] The Clinical Practice Guideline for Diagnosis and Management of Acute Otitis Media (AOM), issued by the AAP and the American Academy of Family Physicians, mentioned breastfeeding only once, saying that "the implementation of breastfeeding for at least the first 6 months also seems to be helpful against the development of early episodes of AOM."[36] To support this recommendation, it cited only two publications. One was a review stating that "if breast-feeding reduces [otitis media] incidence and prevalence, several alternative explanations exist for its benefit." The other was a study concluding that "the protective effect of breast milk is, at best, limited."[37]

Attendance at a day care facility is the environmental variable most consistently associated with a higher incidence of otitis media. The authors of the preceding study state that "a strong positive relationship [exists] between the occurrence of otitis media and the number of other children to whom an infant is habitually exposed, whether in day care or at home," and "what appears to matter most is not where but how many."[38] Ear infections are secondary and not contagious; they most often result when the eustachian tube becomes swollen from a cold or respiratory illness, thereby trapping fluid in the middle ear and creating painful pressure on the eardrum. More contact with other children means increased susceptibility to colds and respiratory infections, the precursors to ear infection, so parents who limit their babies' exposure to other people—in grocery stores, shopping malls, and the like—might also be reducing their vulnerability to ear infection. The same is true for parents who closely monitor the behavior of people who spend time with their babies, those who require, for example, frequent hand washing and other hygienic practices unrelated to feeding method.

Does breastfeeding protect against diabetes? At least two review articles argue that studies of insulin-dependent diabetes have neglected confounding factors, produced "little firm evidence of the significance of nutritional factors in the etiology of type 1 diabetes," and appear to be vulnerable to bias.[39] Confounding is a particularly entrenched problem in research on non-insulin-dependent (type 2) diabetes. One frequently cited investigation that found exclusive breastfeeding for the first two months of life to be linked to a significantly lower rate of type 2 diabetes failed to point out that the decision to bottle-feed also was correlated with less exercise and more central obesity, both independent risk factors for the disease.[40] Other studies measured outcomes in teenagers and adults with little to no attention to behavior or events that take place after breastfeeding.[41]

Does breastfeeding protect against asthma and respiratory infections? The science on infant feeding and asthma has produced widely varying results. Although some research indicates that breastfeeding reduces risk for asthma,[42] several studies found that breastfeeding increased the risk.[43] The evidence is especially at odds regarding the type of asthma (atopic or nonatopic), the duration of either the protective or harmful effect, and the identification of which babies and children stand to benefit or suffer.[44] Studies of respiratory infections variably measure the effects of siblings and child care and often contradict each other on the precise outcomes (e.g., lower- or upper-respiratory tract infections), beneficiaries (e.g., girls or boys), and duration of breastfeeding's advantages.[45] Although many studies have found breastfeeding to be associated with fewer infections,[46] they are subject to the same methodological limitations and biases as are investigations of infant feeding and ear infections. Some research, including a relatively carefully controlled study that inspired widespread praise from breastfeeding researchers, has found no significant reduction in respiratory tract infections in babies more likely to have breastfed longer and more exclusively.[47] A review that specifically examined environmental and demographic risk factors for respiratory syncytial virus (RSV), the most common cause of lower respiratory tract infections in infants and children, found that breastfeeding did not in itself appear to decrease the risk of infection. In fact, the author suggested that if studies linking breastfeeding with a lower incidence of respiratory disease applied rigorous methodological standards, including systematic multivariate analyses, breastfeeding itself would likely not be a protective factor, a conclusion that echoed earlier research.[48]

Parental behavior is the most significant confounder for which infant-feeding studies have failed to account. As one study notes, differences in behavior and interactions with babies in mothers with different feeding practices "are extremely difficult to measure and virtually impossible to control for in observational studies,"[49] and this is especially true when the period between exposure (type, initiation, exclusivity, and duration of bottle feeding or breastfeeding) and outcome (such as obesity or IQ) is lengthy. Moreover, while multiple studies indicate that women with higher educational attainment and income are more likely to breastfeed,[50] controlling for education and income does not eliminate health behavior as a confounder. One study found that women who breastfed were, as a group, more likely to be of higher socioeconomic status and to expose their babies to less group day care. It also found that women of higher socioeconomic status were, as a group, more likely to have their babies in group day care earlier and for more hours per week.[51] This study makes clear that breastfeeding mothers behave differently in at least one way that has a direct effect on babies' health: their use of group child care, which suggests that other actions are worth examining.

For example, the decision by less-educated, lower-income women to breastfeed might well signal both a commitment and the resources to behave in ways more commonly associated with higher education and income, healthy habits directly correlated with breastfeeding but with effects independent of breastfeeding per se. In one study that controlled for maternal education, the authors concluded that "in addition to having more illnesses, formula-fed infants cost the health care system money," around $400 per baby, and that increased costs were associated not with differences in educational attainment but with formula.[52] Yet in another study, low-income women who chose to breastfeed were more than twice as likely as their formula-feeding counterparts to cite its benefits to their babies' physical and psychological development as having contributed to their feeding decision; they were more than five times more likely to say it mattered "a lot."[53] A reasonable hypothesis is that women who breastfeed because of its ostensible health advantages, regardless of their income or education level, are more likely than women who choose formula to promote healthy living in other ways. The cost savings associated with breastfeeding then would not be explained by breastfeeding but by health routines more commonly practiced among breastfeeding mothers that cannot be reliably measured by controlling for socioeconomic variables. Until epidemiological research evaluates this possibility, health behavior remains a plausible explanation for most of the benefits attributed to breastfeeding.

PROBIT

The Promotion of Breastfeeding Intervention Trial (PROBIT) was, among other things, designed to address the problem of selection bias. Thirty-one urban and rural maternity hospitals and polytechnic clinics in the Republic of Belarus[54] were randomly assigned to participate in either an experimental program, in which health care workers assisted women with initiating and maintaining breastfeeding and lactation and provided postnatal breastfeeding support, or a control program that continued existing breastfeeding practices and policies. From October 1996 through December 1997, more than 17,000 mother-infant pairs were then randomly assigned to the two programs. The study compared the prevalence of any breastfeeding at three, six, nine, and twelve months and of exclusive or predominant breastfeeding at three and six months. It also compared the annual incidence of gastrointestinal (GI) and respiratory infection, otitis media, and atopic eczema. To reduce selection bias, or to neutralize differences that might have existed between mothers who chose to breast-feed or formula-feed, the study restricted participation to those mothers who had expressed an intention to breastfeed when they were admitted to the postpartum ward. The authors reasoned that if the intervention group, which received enhanced lactation support, had longer and/or more exclusive breastfeeding rates and better health outcomes, a protective effect could be attributed to breastfeeding with more certainty. In a 2001 *JAMA* editorial that preceded the published results, Ruth Lawrence, the author of the widely used *Breastfeeding: A Guide for the Medical Profession* and one of the best-known breastfeeding advocates in the medical community, called PROBIT "masterful."[55]

The study found that the mothers in the intervention group breastfed longer and more exclusively than did the mothers in the control group. At three months, 60 percent of mothers in the control group and 73 percent in the experimental group continued to breastfeed. Seven times as many mothers in the intervention group were breastfeeding exclusively at three and six months. The study also found that 13.2 percent of babies in the control group but only 9.1 percent in the intervention group contracted one or more GI infections in the first year, a clinically significant relative risk reduction of 40 percent. It also determined that the intervention reduced the risk of eczema in the first year of life, although data classification problems caused the authors to warn that this result "should be interpreted with caution."[56] Conversely, reductions in risk for various respiratory tract infections were not statistically significant, as babies in both groups had roughly the same incidence of upper respiratory tract infection, otitis media, croup, wheezing, and pneumonia. PROBIT II, representing 81.5 percent of the children originally randomized and tracked, compared the children in the two groups at 6.5 years of age. It found that longer and more exclusive breastfeeding had no protective effect on allergy and asthma;[57] that it did not reduce adiposity or blood pressure or affect height and weight;[58] that it had no effect on dental caries (tooth decay); and that it neither reduced nor improved emotional difficulties, hyperactivity, or conduct or peer problems.[59] The intervention group, however, did have higher mean scores on all measures of intelligence, and the study concluded that "prolonged and exclusive breastfeeding improves children's cognitive development."[60]

PROBIT publications consistently and accurately describe the study as "the largest randomized trial ever conducted in the area of human lactation." But PROBIT randomly assigned mother-infant pairs to breastfeeding support, not to breastfeeding itself, and therefore did not eliminate the problem of confounding. By restricting participation to mothers who were committed to initiating breastfeeding, the study was able to eliminate the choice to breastfeed as a confounder. It did not, however, similarly exclude the decision to breastfeed for a longer period of time or without supplementation. PROBIT did not address whether or how preexisting differences between mothers who breastfeed longer and more exclusively, on one hand, and those who initiate breastfeeding but eventually do not continue or do so only partially, on the other hand, reflect differences in overall health behavior that themselves contribute to better outcomes.

Having been told by obstetricians, pediatricians, the media, and advice books that breast is best, for example, large numbers of women in the United States commit to breastfeeding. But many ultimately find the physical, emotional, and time demands of nursing overwhelming, and they then abandon or reduce breastfeeding earlier than they originally intended.[61] Evidence from the Centers for Disease Control and Prevention (CDC) indicates that 25 percent of babies who were breastfed were supplemented with formula within two days of birth and that almost 40 percent of breastfed babies were also receiving formula at three months.[62] Among the roughly 10 percent of mothers who remain committed to exclusive breastfeeding for six months, the period recommended by the CDC and AAP, are no doubt those whose feeding experiences, on balance, have been positive. But likely among these women committed to breastfeeding are those, too, who for various reasons are more able to tolerate the challenges of breastfeeding for the putative health benefits it provides. These mothers, along with their partners, might be exceptionally devoted to hygiene, high levels of interaction, and other behaviors that could have positive health effects. They might have resources, such as money or extensive support networks, that enable them to ensure that their babies are provided care by people with similar priorities. As most breastfeeding advocates argue, if duration and exclusivity are more important than intention and initiation in health outcomes, they might also reveal more about the lengths to which different mothers are able to go to optimize their children's health. Behavioral differences, in other words, might be associated not simply with the choice to breastfeed but with the decision to breastfeed longer and more exclusively as well.

That the duration and exclusivity of breastfeeding were enhanced in the PROBIT intervention group indicates a plausible association between intensive breastfeeding support and extended and full breastfeeding. But the finding that babies in the intervention group had a lower incidence of GI infections and improved cognitive development cannot be reliably attributed to breastfeeding because mothers who breastfeed longest and exclusively might also be more likely to adopt other significant health-promoting routines. Nonetheless, in the case of GI infection, the overall evidence for breastfeeding's protective effect is strong, consistent, and plausible. Moreover, and crucially, the biological mechanism that offers such protection can be observed. Breast milk is packed with antimicrobial proteins, specifically secretory IgA and lactoferrin, which act as protective agents in the gut.[63] A breastfed baby ingests these antibodies, which line the stomach and combat the various bacteria in the GI tract. This process suggests that reduced rates of GI illness among breastfed babies in both developed and developing countries result at least partially from the ingestion of antimicrobial properties in mothers' milk.[64] It does not disprove the hypothesis that parental behavior contributes to fewer infections, but it does indicate that breastfeeding has independent benefits. Therefore, a sound medical case can be made that breastfeeding reduces the risk for GI infection, and PROBIT confirms this effect.[65]

Research on breastfeeding's impact on intelligence, however, has produced widely varying results, and hypotheses about breastfeeding's biological impact on cognitive development have not been rigorously demonstrated.[66] Furthermore, if mothers who breastfeed longer and more exclusively also promote intellectual development in other ways—they and other caretakers read, speak, and engage more with their children and encourage cognitively stimulating activities—the effect of breastfeeding itself will be difficult to isolate.

Communicating Breastfeeding Research: Medical Journals

Infant-feeding studies are problematically designed and executed, but scientists also communicate with one another in ways likely to minimize the significance of methodological shortcomings and exaggerate breastfeeding's protective powers. Scientists and physicians, for example, often lack the time and/or training to read and evaluate original research. One study examining the electronic version of the *British Medical Journal* found that narrative reviews and editorials were accessed far more frequently than were original research articles or systematic reviews in the first week after their publication. This result, the authors write, "may disappoint those who believe that it is important for readers to critically appraise the primary research data."[67] Another study found that review articles published in "throwaway journals"—those without original research, not published by medical societies, high in advertising, and provided free of charge—were judged by physicians to be more relevant and more likely to be read than those in peer-reviewed journals.[68] Internal medicine residents in one investigation expressed low confidence in their ability to evaluate research, a concern that was validated when they scored an average of eight out of twenty, or 40 percent, on a biostatistical survey. Nearly one-third of the participants indicated that they had never received biostatistical training during their medical education. A greater number of senior residents performed worse than junior residents, suggesting that time away from medical school lowered statistical competence. Doctors' failure to evaluate study data critically, the authors warn, could lead to misguided advice to patients and "erroneous applications of clinical research."[69]

The standard format of articles in medical journals also interferes with the careful evaluation of research. Published studies are divided into four sections: the background, which usually explains a gap in the scientific literature, followed by an explanation of the methods employed, the results, and a discussion of the conclusion. An abstract briefly outlining the main points of each section generally appears on the first page, either alongside or before the beginning of the article. Research on the reading habits of physicians and scientists suggests that abstracts are read far more regularly than original articles. According to one study, internists read abstracts twice as often as full articles. Respondents, whom the authors contended had underestimated their reliance on abstracts, also expressed the need for accessible clinical summaries and the expectation that journal editors would ensure methodological rigor and quality.[70] Other doctors, including pediatricians, have been found to have similar reading habits.[71]

It is not unusual, moreover, for an abstract to contain information inconsistent with the article itself. An investigation of six major general medical journals, for example, found that from 18 to 68 percent of the abstracts contained data that were irreconcilable with or were not mentioned in the article itself.[72] The author of a study on carcinogens in breast milk later indicated that he had made a mistake in the abstract, an error that probably overestimated an already dubious attribution of deaths from formula feeding by about 65 percent.[73] The abstract of a study finding breastfeeding to be associated with reduced overweight concluded: "Prolonged breastfeeding is associated with a reduced risk of overweight among non-Hispanic white children. Breastfeeding longer than 6 months provides health benefits to children well beyond the period of breastfeeding."[74] The first statement accurately represents the research presented in the article; the second is unwarranted and reflects the conflation of observational associations with causality against which thoughtful epidemiological researchers have cautioned.

Even readers well trained in statistical methods who read only abstracts will be unable to assess the methods used, which in breastfeeding research are often disputable, and will also miss the discussion, which usually addresses the confounding variables and the study's attempts to eliminate them. In the case of breastfeeding, the discussion is where the behavioral factors so difficult to rule out are often mentioned, and a failure to read this section can lead to a misunderstanding of the results. For example, in the JAMA study finding a connection between breastfeeding and cognitive development, the authors state clearly in the discussion that the association of certain types of parental behavior with breastfeeding and their impact on intelligence "is an open question." Nonetheless, the abstract's conclusion states the following: "Independent of a wide range of possible confounding factors, a significant positive association between duration of breastfeeding and intelligence was observed."[75] The conclusion is technically accurate, but it is meaningful only in the context of the discussion, which many readers are unlikely to examine. That confounding is a problem in infant feeding research is an open secret; most studies concede the uncertainty created by unmeasured variables. But this acknowledgment rarely makes its way into conclusions or abstracts, which is where most readers get their information.

The wording of both the titles and the texts of articles can be misleading as well. An editorial accompanying the two conflicting investigations regarding childhood overweight was entitled "Breastfeeding May Help Prevent Childhood Overweight," even though one of the studies concluded that the "duration of full breastfeeding does not appear to be predictive of or necessarily have preventative properties for overweight in early childhood, and encouraging breastfeeding for overweight prevention would not be as effective as moderating familial factors in preventing early childhood overweight."[76] Here the title of the editorial is technically correct but deceptive. Unless readers have read the two studies as well, they are likely to regard the protective effects of breastfeeding as greater than reported. In another example, the authors of a commentary on a study suggesting that breastfeeding might actually increase overweight[77] argued that "the extent to which breast-feeding protects against obesity is not settled," as if the question of whether breastfeeding were in fact protective had already been resolved. Their statement that "the best evidence to date does show a reduction in risk" was not supported by a footnote, so it is unclear which research was "the best."[78] One study found "no statistically significant effect of predominately breastfeeding compared with predominately formula feeding on neurodevelopmental outcomes" but nonetheless concluded that "supporting parents to breastfeed preterm infants may maximize the potential advantages of early nutrition in neurodevelopmental outcomes of [very low birth weight] infants."[79] On the relationship between breastfeeding and higher intelligence, an editorial accompanying one study pointed out that "despite the difficulties in establishing a causal relation between breastfeeding and improved cognition," researchers should use even information they are skeptical about "as an important additional advocacy tool."[80] As Jules Law, a rare critic of breastfeeding science, writes, all too often negative or inconclusive studies recommend breastfeeding "on the grounds that its virtues are already established in any case."[81]

When researchers consistently eliminate the explanatory power of potentially significant variables, including behavior, through inadequate controls, faulty conclusions become operating assumptions. Once a variable has been correlated with a positive health outcome, a discourse develops that encourages further investigation of its protective powers. Since the early 1980s, when the AAP first officially weighed in on the relative benefits of breastfeeding, infant-feeding research has been divided into roughly three periods. Between 1982, when the AAP suggested that "subtle, built-in" differences between breast and formula-feeding mothers made "interpretation of cause and effect . . . extremely difficult,"[82] and December 1997, when it claimed without qualification that "human milk is uniquely superior for infant feeding,"[83] the National Library of Medicine database indicates that a yearly average of 192 studies were published with "breastfeeding" or "breast-feeding" in the title. Between January 1998 and January 2005, just before the AAP's next policy statement, the yearly average rose to 297, or a 50 percent increase in seven years. From February 2005, when the AAP reiterated its support for breastfeeding, through December 2008, the average was 420 articles, an additional 40 percent increase in just under four years.[84]

To navigate this increasingly vast and labyrinthine terrain of research, scientists and physicians rely on conventional wisdom, and the more they do so, the more conventional the wisdom becomes. Trained in and habituated to risk-factor research and accustomed to news of breastfeeding's powers, they reproduce and have little reason to doubt positive findings. Routine controls, however inadequate, are accepted as valid, and repeated correlations are presumed to represent further evidence of a causal relationship between breastfeeding and good health. The evolution of conventional wisdom about breastfeeding exemplifies what economists call "informational cascades," a process of information-diffusion in which an individual accepts the judgment of another person or a critical mass of others largely because the costs of making his or her own evaluation in regard to time, money, or intellectual energy, are too steep.[85] In today's risk culture, in which information develops quickly and exponentially, scientists and physicians face the practically insurmountable task of keeping abreast of current research. One study estimated that primary care physicians would need to consider 7,287 articles each month "to comprehensively and systematically update the primary care knowledge base."[86] Informational cascades and reliance on colleagues to evaluate information outside one's narrow range of specialty are virtually inevitable. Indeed, in infant-feeding research, articles commonly open with references to the "well-known" advantages of breastfeeding, benefits that the authors assume to be compelling but have not verified and lack either the time or skills to do so. Unable to master the expansive literature on breastfeeding, individual researchers are likely to assume that breastfeeding is superior because so many others have already made that judgment.

The abstract conclusion of one investigation, for example, stated that "breastfeeding does not appear to prevent asthma, delay its onset, or reduce its severity. However, breastfeeding is still recommended for its many other benefits."[87] Another study that examined the impact of breastfeeding on the development of ear infections found that "the protective effect of breast milk is, at best, limited. Nonetheless, the findings may be viewed as further supporting the undisputed desirability of breast milk feeding."[88] Studies finding no association between breastfeeding and obesity argue strenuously that breastfeeding still has many benefits. "It cannot be too strongly emphasized that breastfeeding has numerous attributes that render it the preferred feeding choice for almost all infants," emphasized a study finding no association between breastfeeding and obesity.[89] A 2007 investigation concluded that while breastfeeding does not reduce obesity, it "promotes the health of the mother and child."[90] In a National Institutes of Health press release stating that breastfeeding had only a minor effect on reducing childhood overweight, the director of the National Institute of Child Health and Human Development claimed that breastfeeding was nonetheless "extremely valuable for infants—boosting their immune systems and their mental abilities, and reducing their risk for infection."[91] And an editorial explaining why further research was needed on the association between breastfeeding and obesity observed that "for many other reasons, breast-feeding is the clear best choice for almost all mothers and infants. Thus it makes sense to add potential obesity prevention to the list of breast-feeding's benefits."[92]

Articles often begin with a statement about breastfeeding's well-established benefits, and scientists frequently refer to its putative advantages, even though the outcomes on which consensus exists remain unclear. That breastfeeding helps prevent ear infections is assumed by those who judge that it has no impact on asthma, while its protective qualities against asthma are accepted by those who find no connection between breastfeeding and ear infections.[93] That breastfeeding is superior is so widely assumed that studies now try to determine the risk factors for bottle feed-ing. That is, choosing not to breastfeed has now assumed the status of a disease for which certain mothers are "at risk."[94] "The irony," writes risk scholar Cass Sunstein about cascades and fear, "is that if most people are following others, then little information is provided by the fact that some or many seem to share a certain fear. Most are responding to the signals provided by others, unaware that those others are doing exactly the same thing."[95] In the meantime, the concern the AAP expressed in its 1982 statement, that differences between breastfeeding and formula-feeding mothers might explain divergent outcomes, has been neither systemati-cally pursued nor resolved.

Communicating Breastfeeding Research: Popular Media

The media tend to present the results of breastfeeding research uncriti-cally. As early as 1997, Lawrence Gartner, a pediatrician and the chair of the AAP working group on breastfeeding, was quoted in *Newsweek* as stat-ing, "It's hard to come out and say, 'Your baby is going to be stupider or sicker if you don't breastfeed.' But that's what the literature says."[96] Alan Lucas, one of the authors of a study associating breast milk with a lower incidence of heart disease, estimated to the Reuters News Agency that "hundreds of thousands of deaths in the western world could be pre-vented by breastfeeding" and that "more could be prevented if the uptake in breastfeeding was higher." It was not clear how he had arrived at this number, but the story was featured prominently on the Yahoo!News page and was reported in major newspapers shortly after the study results were announced.[97] In reporting the study, Dr. Emily Senay of CBS's *The Early Show* called breastfeeding "the gift that keeps on giving even later into life" and added, "I could be here all day and pretty much talk about the ben-efits of breastfeeding."[98] She listed allergies, eczema, ear and other infec-tions, and childhood cancers as conditions for which breastfed babies are at reduced risk and also said that breastfed babies had higher IQs.

Journalists share scientists' tendency to highlight breastfeeding's su-periority, even when writing or talking about studies demonstrating no advantages to breastfeeding. A story reporting research showing no as-sociation between breastfeeding and obesity, published in the *New York Times* and the *Washington Post* and on ABC.com and CNN.com, opened by drawing attention to breastfeeding's "many benefits." "I'm the first to say breast-feeding is good," even if it has no impact on obesity, emphasized Karin Michels of Harvard Medical School, the study's lead investigator, while the story's author stressed that the obesity finding "doesn't take away the other benefits of breast-feeding, such as building immunity to disease."[99] Both the authors and the critics of a study linking breastfeeding to higher IQ lamented the media's "fervent and dangerous response" and the "distressing and potentially harmful" conclusions drawn in the lay and medical press, which were reporting that breastfeeding made children smarter.[100] In 2008, Yahoo!News ran a front-page story entitled "Breast-Feeding While on Seizure Medicine Doesn't Harm Babies." Although the study in question examined only the impact of anti-epilepsy drug treatment on children's cognitive abilities, the headline suggested that the overall safety of breast-feeding while on this medication was no longer in question.[101]

Even under the best of circumstances, the phrasing that scientists use can be easily misconstrued. That breastfeeding has a "significant" relationship with a particular outcome, such as a reduced incidence of diabetes, is a statistical finding; it does not indicate that the relationship is causal or medically important. When breastfeeding "is associated with" fewer infections, it does not mean that breast milk prevents illness; nor does the assertion that breastfed babies tend to have higher IQs mean that breastfeeding increases intelligence. The statement that breastfeeding "is protective against" a disease, assuming a persuasive study, would mean that breastfed babies have a reduced risk for getting sick, not that they are literally protected from contracting the illness. When science journalists present research conclusions without explaining either the empirical or the discursive context in which they were derived, the results are essentially incomprehensible to consumers. To be communicated effectively, research must be rendered "in terms which have meaning to those who are the subjects of study, as well as to those by whom or for whom the study was done."[102] Journalists, in other words, are not simply reporters but interpreters.

> Much like it makes more sense to translate the French *il fait froid* to the English "it is cold," rather than to a literal translation, such as "it makes cold," so the translation of science for the public must be informed by an understanding of the "idiomatic" use of scientific language.[103]

Yet when scientists fail to use their own language correctly or to follow their own rules, consumers have little hope of receiving accurate information.[104]

How the media present research on breastfeeding reflects broader problems in science journalism. Few media outlets can sustain substantial science staffs. Even at major newspapers, such as the *New York Times*, a small number of science reporters are expected to cover "everything from anthropology to astrophysics to atherosclerosis."[105] At the same time, scientific research is becoming increasingly specialized, making it even more difficult for reporters to achieve competency in the areas about which they write. Although government policymakers and the public learn more about risks from the media than anywhere else, most health and science reporters have no formal training in the sciences or in interpreting health statistics. Those who do are often freelancers who are dependent on university and corporate assignments. The *Boston Globe*, considered to have one of the stronger weekly health/science sections, at one point employed a staff of eight, most of whom had humanities or other liberal arts degrees and none of whom had a science degree.[106] In one study of television health reporters, only 5 percent had a degree in a science-related field, and only one-third were assigned exclusively to the health beat.[107] With little expertise, medical reporters have to make sense of scientific language under deadline pressure and at the expense of attention to complexity and uncertainty. Editors worried about space or time frequently shorten reports and omit crucial information.[108] According to science writer and journalism professor Jon Franklin, "editors ignorant of science tend to handle paragraphs they don't understand by taking them out."[109]

Research also demonstrates that medical journalists are more likely to allow certain subjects, such as doctors or scientists, to state hypotheses unopposed; that they rarely question methodology, a starting point for evaluating research; and that they tend to rely on syndicated news packages and media information produced by health centers, drug companies, and other vested-interest groups.[110] One study found that press releases from prominent medical journals circulated to reporters "frequently presented data in exaggerated formats, and failed to highlight study limitations or conflicts of interest."[111] At the same time, more than half the broadcast journalists surveyed in a different investigation said they were most likely to cover a story if they had received press releases or some other form of public relations communication.[112] High-profile media give substantial coverage to papers delivered at scientific meetings, half of which are never published or appear in low-impact journals. Presentations that receive front-page newspaper coverage are no more likely to be published than others.[113] In a long critique of medical news, published in the *New England Journal of Medicine*, Timothy Johnson, medical editor at ABC News, advocated that medical journalists somehow be required to demonstrate competence in biostatistics and epidemiology. "If we think it is important to certify hairdressers and massage therapists, might not it be important to certify those who transmit medical news day in and day out?"[114]

At the same time, much of the public lacks the tools to understand general science and medical information. Standardized exams are imperfect measures of ability, but the evidence they do provide suggests that schools at all levels are not teaching students basic skills. In 2005, only 27 percent of fourth- and eighth-grade public school students performed at or above proficiency level on a national science exam; 35 percent of fourth graders and 29 percent of eighth graders were proficient or better in mathematics.[115] In a study of science aptitude in more than three hundred first- and second-year university students, the average participant correctly answered fewer than half the questions, expressed a certainty bias in responses regarding truth status, conflated cause and correlation, and confused explanations of phenomena with the phenomena themselves. University students performed no better than high school students, yet they offered very positive assessments of their ability to read and understand scientific writing.[116] Only small percentages of people understand the concept of a scientific study, the significance of experimentation and control groups, or the determination of probability.[117] The 2003 National Assessment of Adult Literacy established four categories of health literacy (below basic, basic, intermediate, and proficient) and found that although more than half of Americans fall in the intermediate category, more than one-third have only basic or below basic health literacy. Moreover, much of the health information that people encounter requires proficiency skills that only 12 percent of Americans possess.[118] People frequently misunderstand the purpose of medical tests. For example, millions of women who no longer have a cervix still undergo Papanicolau (PAP) smear screening.[119] Research demonstrates that people have trouble understanding risk and need quantitative assessments to be explained in context. One critic went so far as to warn of an impending "epidemic of limited health literacy," and nearly all stress the need to improve all forms of health communication.[120]

Future Research

Whether breastfeeding reduces the risk for various negative health outcomes remains an open question. Except in the case of GI infections, the
biological mechanisms that might offer protection have not been demonstrated and cannot be reliably assumed.[121] Selection bias and residual
confounding provide plausible explanations for the benefits attributed to
breastfeeding, and epidemiological research on infant feeding has failed to
adequately measure the impact of parental behavior on children's health.
The socioeconomic variables most commonly employed, such as income
and education, do not address whether the decision to breastfeed or the
commitment to breastfeed longer represent an orientation toward parenting that itself is good for babies' health.

To compellingly evaluate the influence of parental behavior within the
risk-factor paradigm, researchers would need to construct quantifiable
variables that could serve as valid proxies for the kind of behavior that
might affect outcomes. Measuring hand washing and other indicators of
hygiene, as well as time spent reading to or verbally engaging babies and
older children, might begin to address the impact of behavior on infections and cognitive development. Conversely, to reliably assess whether
breastfeeding is superior, regardless of social context, a study might have
to abandon the methods of risk-factor epidemiology altogether, which
likely would be a labor- and time-intensive undertaking. As one pediatrician wrote more than a decade ago regarding the lack of appropriate
controls in SIDS research, such studies are improbable because "funding
agencies are unwilling to make the necessary large financial investments;
nor do capable investigators in need of academic enhancement have the
patience to tackle projects where results might not be forthcoming for
many years."[122]

Still, epidemiologists have long recognized the limitations of risk-factor
research, and they have been engaged in extensive and, at times, acrimonious debates about the need for a paradigm shift. Toward precisely what
the field should turn is unclear, and it is probable that specific questions
will require nuances in different directions. Now focused on describ-
ing the association of specific modes of feeding with different outcomes,
breastfeeding researchers might begin to investigate breastfeeding as part
of a cluster of variables often associated with better health. This clustering
might be more significant than any one variable in itself, and it might be

caused by intricately connected "upstream" forces, at the population level, and "downstream" influences, at the individual level, variables that are not always easily quantified or plotted in regression analysis. For example, the experience of racism or poverty cannot be captured by coding study participants as "white" or "black" or measuring income. Wide levels of social inequality, low social status, and weak social networks often lead not only to living in neighborhoods with low social capital, exposure to environmental pollutants, and unhealthy behaviors but also to chronic stress. Protracted anxiety is harmful to the body's stress response system and can be detrimental to the health of mothers and fathers, and therefore babies, from conception. It also is likely to affect the environment in which babies and children are raised.[123] Accounting for its impact with the methods of risk-factor epidemiology might not be possible.

Perhaps epidemiological research could be supplemented by qualitative analysis, such as ethnography, an anthropological method of observing people in their everyday lives. Ethnographers might study families in which children are breastfed and formula fed with an eye toward identifying behaviors that are distinct to each mode of feeding. If, indeed, different habits do exist, research should then address the extent to which this behavior is enabled and constrained by class and other social structures. If breastfed babies are healthier than those who are formula fed, it might be largely because their caretakers have the resources—money, extended support networks, strong partnerships, job flexibility—to create healthy environments. It might also be that these parents experience lower levels of the chronic psychosocial stress that can lead to organ and tissue damage and other illness and that make devoting energy to routine health practices difficult. Healthy behaviors, in other words, are often not a matter of choice, and they can be code for privilege. Therefore, to be meaningful, health research must analyze the social and economic contexts of people's choices. Although building a body of compelling qualitative research would require an enormous amount of time, labor, and interdisciplinary cooperation, such data could shed light on critical questions that have not been addressed effectively with existing methods and that must be answered in order to understand the relative effects of breast and bottle feeding.

In the meantime, continued research with the same methodological flaws has costs. While these studies might provide new ways of thinking about how breastfeeding could act in the body to improve babies' short- and long-term health, history suggests that they also will be misinterpreted by doctors and scientists already overloaded with information as further evidence of breastfeeding's superiority. A *JAMA* editorial regarding research on infant diets and type 1 diabetes argues that "too many signposts point to an uncertain future" and that "further investigative trials should not be undertaken until more insight into underlying disease mechanisms has been acquired."[124] A similar cautionary note might be struck in the case of breastfeeding. Myriad studies suggest possible health advantages, and investigation into the underlying processes by which breastfeeding might be beneficial should be emphasized over further observational research. Proof of breastfeeding's benefits depends not on additional findings of association between breastfeeding and improved outcomes but on demonstrations of *how* breastfeeding contributes to better health.

3

Minding Your Own (Risky) Business

Health and Personal Responsibility

IN DECEMBER 2005, the *New York Times* ran an op-ed piece in which writer Karen Karbo poked fun at HarperCollins, publisher of a new edition of the popular children's book *Goodnight Moon*, for digitally removing a cigarette from a photo of Clement Hurd, the illustrator. Alongside a redrawing of one of Hurd's illustrations depicting the inside of Bunny's house, Karbo pointed to other "potentially harmful" messages that HarperCollins had not addressed. "How long has this bowl full of mush been sitting here?" she queried. "A single drop of sour milk contains more than 50 million potentially fatal bacteria. At the very least, Bunny is in danger of contracting irritable bowl syndrome. Not to mention mush is low in fiber. Suggested change: Digitally remove." She continued. "A fire blazing in the fireplace while Bunny sleeps? Suggested change: get rid of it. At the very least, digitally add a fire extinguisher to the wall. And hello? Where are the smoke detectors?" As for the knitting rabbit who is babysitting, the "quiet old lady whispering hush," Karbo suggested that her apron be emblazoned with a message indicating that she is a citizen, hired from a reputable agency, who has passed a criminal background check. "Penetrating injuries to the chest by knitting needles are not uncommon," she admonished. "Also, someone could lose an eye. Suggested change: Digitally remove. The quiet old lady is not getting paid to knit, anyway."[1]

The target of Karbo's parody is an American preoccupation with risk, especially threats to children, a virtual obsession that shapes how scientists, public health officials, and advocacy groups present breastfeeding to the public. Australian sociologist Deborah Lupton identified at least six major categories of risk apprehension in Western societies, including the United States:

"Environmental risks," or those posed by pollution, radiation, chemicals, floods, fires, dangerous road conditions and so on; "lifestyle risks," those believed to be related to the consumption of such commodities as food and drugs, engagement in sexual activities, driving practices, stress, leisure and so on; "medical risks," those related to experiencing medical care or treatment (for example, drug therapy, surgery, childbirth, reproductive technologies, diagnostic tests); "interpersonal risks," related to intimate relationships, social interactions, love, sexuality, gender roles, friendship, marriage and parenting; "economic risks," implicated in unemployment or under-employment, borrowing money, investment, bankruptcy, destruction of property, failure of a business and so on; and "criminal risks," those emerging from being a participant in or potential victim of illegal activities.[2]

David Ropeik and George Gray, former directors of the Harvard Center for Risk Analysis and coauthors of *Risk: A Practical Guide for Deciding What's Really Safe and What's Really Dangerous in the World around You*, list forty-eight commonly feared sources of risk, including artificial sweeteners, caffeine, cell phones, electrical and magnetic fields, mad cow disease, microwaves, asbestos, carbon monoxide, DDT, lead, mercury, pesticides, radon, antibiotic resistance, mammography, vaccines, and X-rays.[3]

Indeed, the desire to avoid risk is apparent everywhere. Supermarkets offer complimentary wipes to disinfect shopping cart handles, and hand sanitizers are practically ubiquitous. Restaurants flag the heart-healthy, low-fat, low-carbohydrate meals on their menus, and consumers' demand for organically produced foods has shown double-digit growth for more than a decade.[4] Children can wear unremovable bracelets that transmit location data in case they are kidnapped. Some schools have banned tag and touch football, claiming that students could be injured while playing, thus raising the ire of those concerned that sedentary children are at greater risk for obesity. As the baby-boomer generation ages, anxieties about health risks and personal safety abound, and news about obesity, diabetes, and Alzheimer's disease seems to be in the headlines every day. Meanwhile, the federal government is criticized for both its under- and overregulation of risk. Experts on one side clamor for more oversight of day care centers, drugs, automobile safety, and food production. Known risks must be eliminated, they argue, regardless of the cost. Better safe than sorry. Experts on the other side point, among other things, to the proliferation of academic journals devoted to studying risk and to the increasing popularity of risk officers in business and government organizations as evidence that excessive regulation is stifling progress and consuming resources that should be devoted to innovation. These critics disparage many risk concerns as "worry candy" that prevents the public from paying attention to potentially more serious problems.[5] Western societies, they lament, are attempting "the risk management of everything" at the expense of growth and good sense.[6] Ironically, as society expends more and more effort to make life safer and healthier, many in the public become more, rather than less, concerned about risk.[7]

A diverse group of social scientists has assembled a prodigious body of research on risk. To speak of a "risk literature," however, is at once to recognize the cogency of risk as an analytic concept and to exaggerate any consensus on its meaning. As a group, risk scholars fail to agree even on whether risks exist in any real sense: whether they are concrete, calculable outcomes or cognitive constructs whose animation can be imagined only under particular social and political circumstances. On one hand are "realist" views that emphasize how objective risks are assessed by professionals and gauged by the population at large. For example, what is the statistical risk of serious injury while riding in a sport utility vehicle, and how do consumers weigh that risk in deciding what kind of car to purchase? On the other hand are "constructionist" perspectives that stress the social processes involved in creating, identifying, and experiencing risk. For example, how and by whom have undergoing epidural anesthesia in childbirth or drinking tap water come to be perceived as risky endeavors, and what do they accomplish by treating them as such?[8] Whereas some people are concerned with sharpening measurement tools, others understand the calculation of risk as inseparable from its production. While the former tend to be preoccupied with whether individual decision making is logical, the latter often challenge the very notion of rationality and seek instead to understand how choices make sense in specific social contexts. Fundamental divides exist even within each camp. Little effort has been made to connect these contrasting approaches, to knit together disparate strands of risk scholarship.

This chapter is just such an effort, albeit a modest one with a very specific agenda. The following discussion is explicitly selective, and readers desiring either a comprehensive analysis of risk scholarship or a resolution of its contradictions will be disappointed. My aim is not to reconstruct any particular theory or discourse in its integrity but instead to plot pieces of divergent analyses in an account of risk that can lend coherence to the many meanings of breastfeeding in the United States today. To be sure, different approaches are grounded in apparently irreconcilable assumptions. If many more people who smoke develop lung cancer and die, the

health risks of smoking cannot be meaningfully described as "constructions." Still, how various experts and the public think about smoking is a
result of cultural contingencies, including the development of epidemiological science around "risk factors," inattention to culturally unimagina-
ble or politically sensitive risk factors for lung cancer, and the meanings
of "cancer" in both scientific parlance and the popular imaginary. Risks
are multidimensional. They can be simultaneously real, to the extent that
they represent concrete danger, and constructed, in the sense that both
knowledge and communication about risks are dependent on conventions
in scientific research and cultural values that are reflected in language and
framing. This is especially clear in matters of health, in which the anxieties
of a culture preoccupied by risk are manifold and the dynamics of breastfeeding advocacy have their strongest roots.

A second caveat: nowhere in this book has the onus of synthesizing a
broad spectrum of esoteric scholarship, in relatively few pages and for a diverse audience, been more challenging than in the following discussion of
risk. Yet the task is essential because this literature illuminates the broad
parameters within which breastfeeding has been constructed as a health
imperative. The feeding of babies takes place in what I call a "risk culture"
marked by the constant production of scientific information about risks,
especially health risks, and a pervasive neoliberal sentiment that every individual has a personal responsibility to make sense of this information,
prevent health problems, and act as a good citizen. This risk culture shapes
how scientists evaluate the relative risks of formula and breastfeeding. It
also structures how maternal responsibility is defined in public discourse,
how breastfeeding advocates make claims about risk, and how the government uses fear to persuade women to breastfeed.

A Risk Culture

Recent theorists have argued not simply that people in the developed
world seem more consumed with risk than in the past but that risk is the
cornerstone of a new modernity. German sociologist Ulrich Beck, for example, contends that advanced industrial democracies are becoming "risk
societies" in which individual subjectivity and social relationships are increasingly defined by people's proximity to various risks. Conflicts over the
distribution of wealth that characterize class society, or industrial modernity, are slowly being replaced by struggles over the distribution of risk in

what Beck calls a "reflexive modernity." Today, the unavoidable potential for catastrophic risks—nuclear annihilation, environmental destruction, terrorism—which are largely invisible and to which everyone, regardless of class status, is vulnerable, creates a risk consciousness that is rapidly taking the place of class as the primary organizing principle of social life.[9] British social theorist Anthony Giddens writes of "high modernity" in which "trust and security, risk and danger . . . exist in various historically unique conjunctions" and "the concept of risk becomes fundamental to the way both lay actors and technical specialists organize the social world." As the amount and complexity of scientific information dramatically increase in high modernity, family, religion, and class lose their power to shape meaningful life narratives and people must make choices with little guidance from the institutions that once helped them frame their lives.[10]

If Beck is careful to note that "we do not *yet* live in a risk society," he also argues that we are *becoming* a risk society, that class hierarchies, though still in place, are declining in significance and will soon be vestiges of an older modernity.[11] Beck acknowledges but necessarily minimizes the continued influence of class and other social institutions in his effort to cast risk as the foundation of major social change, or a new modernity.[12] The result is that too often, risks appear in his work to have consequences independent of the social hierarchies within which they circulate. For example, Beck's claims that "*poverty is hierarchic, smog is democratic*"[13] and that the axis of social life is shifting from class status to various forms of security dramatically exaggerates the decline of both socioeconomic differences and scarcity. Indeed, the mere contemplation of risk can be a reflection of privilege. Whether a man can afford to be screened to determine his risk for prostate cancer could radically impact how he chooses to live. Should that man be black or poor, he might not be advised that such a screening test exists. Poorer neighborhoods are often more polluted, which puts their residents at greater health risk. Yet, for lower-income citizens, housing decisions are based largely on cost, not air quality. If new social risk positions are developing—even the wealthy and powerful are not safe from pollution or potential ecological disaster—they are not practically separable from a person's location in the race, class, and gender hierarchies of industrial modernity that Beck argues is on the decline. The "we are all in the same boat" rhetoric discounts differences in how exposure and ability to respond to risks are socially stratified, or rooted in power.[14] Risks, in other words, might create a broad-based community of fear, "but it is *not* . . . a democracy."[15]

Even as society continues to be deeply stratified by class, gender, race, and other social markers—as key components of industrial modernity not only persist but remain forceful structuring principles—the expansion of risk calculations into ever increasing domains of life constitutes a qualitatively new situation that requires individuals to think and act in novel ways.[16] My aim is to employ Beck's thinking on risk *society* to outline the parameters of a risk *culture* within which breastfeeding takes on political meaning.[17] By positing a risk culture, I am suggesting that a risk consciousness–generalized anxiety about the future, concern about rationalizing and optimizing, fear of worst-case scenarios—is increasingly at work even when danger or harm seems remote. What clothes to wear, cleanser to use, food to eat—optimizing and avoiding harm have become more conscious and deliberate in virtually every facet of life. Status, moreover, bears heavily on the extent to which a person actively participates in a risk culture. That is, an individual's ability to make choices within a risk frame, to be an agent in a risk culture, and to adopt putatively risk-averse behavior is contingent on his or her social and economic resources. Those who literally cannot afford to adopt what is socially defined as risk-averse behavior might nonetheless be judged by the standards of those who can. A risk culture is at once autonomous, possessing a certain logic of its own, and situated, or meaningful only in its connection to gender, class, and other social processes.[18] In this book, therefore, risk is essential to understanding public discourse on breastfeeding less as it is poised to supplant other structuring principles of social organization, and thus to serve as the foundation for a risk society, than as it has become a principle in its own right, *a* determinant of human behavior, a new consciousness at the center of a risk culture.

What, then, are the central characteristics of a risk culture? For those who have the social and economic resources to consider and adopt putatively risk-averse behavior, living in a risk culture involves a never ending process of making choices to avoid potentially negative future events. While most people recognize that the future is intrinsically unknowable, incapable of being completely harnessed, they also approach it anxiously as a territory that must be "colonized" or subjected to a "reign of calculative reason."[19] That is, they devote themselves to optimizing every dimension of the future through deliberation and careful planning. In a risk culture, science is ubiquitous, as is the tendency for people to use science to plan and rationalize their lives.[20] Education, retirement, child raising, career trajectory, diet, partner choices, sexual relationships—in a risk culture, almost every aspect of human action and interaction is subject to scientific analysis and framed as more or less risky. Because risks are inherently hypothetical—they have not occurred and might not ever take place—they are ethereal and difficult to grasp. Yet because they have concrete effects in the present—they shape current behavior—they are quite tangible. Risks are "the not-yet-event as stimulus to action," a "kind of virtual, yet real, reality."[21] They demonstrate what Niklas Luhmann called the "paradox of time," in which the future exists only as we have imagined it and only in the present.[22]

In a risk culture, various sciences produce information that serves as the means by which risk is managed. The public depends on science—in such forms as medicine, engineering, and psychology—not only to generate this information but also to determine what is most important, including what constitutes a risk. In this process of framing and naming particular phenomena, these sciences essentially "create" risks, or make them real. Progress, too, engenders risk. Harnessing alternative forms of energy creates nuclear threats; more cheaply manufactured automobiles increase ownership and traffic accidents; and advances in pharmacology produce new health risks. Computers might increase efficiency but undermine the social bonds that are essential to a civilized society; medication might reduce the pain of arthritis but increase the risk of heart attack. Each new scientific development is fraught with benevolent and malevolent possibility. Unable to control or calculate the effects of the progress it sets in motion, science is a primary producer of risks.

In fact, Beck writes, risks do not have meaning until science has identified them. They "*require the sensory organs of science–theories, experiments, measuring instruments–in order to become visible and interpretable as threats at all.*"[23] Public awareness of risk, in other words, is dependent on what different sciences choose to analyze as such. What people know, in the most literal sense, is inseparable from the idiosyncrasies of particular disciplines and different fields of research, including the ways in which research is designed, executed, and interpreted, conceptual categories are created and employed, and measurement devices are constructed and applied. Risks are determined by myriad routines in sciences ranging from chemistry to criminology: disciplinary norms, including rules for gathering, analyzing, and reporting on data; funding biases, especially those risks that public and private agencies are willing to support; and diverse cultural conventions, such as gender roles, dominant forms of transportation, and preference for individual or communal solutions to social problems, all of which shape both the practice and public understanding of science. In a risk culture, in which sciences are authoritative, these conditional circumstances become more influential in framing reality.

Embedded in professional, disciplinary, and cultural contexts, the practice of science also is subject to reflexivity, what Anthony Giddens defines as "the susceptibility of most aspects of social activity, and material relations with nature, to chronic revision in the light of new information or knowledge."[24] Reflexivity is twofold: it describes how scientists continuously revisit and revise research results as well as how scientists reckon with the unintended consequences of their own accomplishments. Reflexive science, including risk analysis, extends the principle of doubt, or skepticism, to its own conclusions and unintended consequences, "scientizing" not simply nature and people but also "itself, its own products, effects and mistakes."[25] In a process of perpetual revision, reflexive science undermines the certainty of any knowledge: no sooner are the conclusions of one study evaluated than new results destabilize their meaning; no sooner are the wonders of an innovation celebrated than its risks are laid bare and their management necessitated. On one hand, this is not a historically new phenomenon. Facts have always been subject to revision, and societies have always been compelled to manage the inadvertent repercussions of progress. On the other hand, as Beck stresses, the current pervasiveness of science and its sequelae have made reflexivity and the control of fallout from progress an everyday task for both scientists and the public. The expansion of science and the sheer increase in the volume of possible threats create a risk consciousness that requires qualitatively new ways of making choices.

Because nothing is immune from scientific analysis and information is abundant, the possibility of perfect decisions seems possible; but because information is constantly changing, choices have to be perpetually revisited. Asbestos causes cancer and must be eliminated; asbestos removal creates greater risks and should be halted. Dietary fat is bad; some fats are good. In fact, fats are not as dangerous as the carbohydrates that have replaced them, and individuals must now manage the health problems associated with the shift to low-fat, high-carbohydrate diets. What becomes clear is not that science is necessarily evil or wrong but that its meaning is transitory, or indeterminate. At best, it can offer "better *accounts* of the world," or "situated *knowledges*."[26] In the unremitting stream of scientific findings, people find themselves "waiting for the latest technological development to catch up with the negative consequences of the previous innovation"[27] or for scientists simply to change their minds. Ironically, reflexive science creates radical doubt and anxiety by demonstrating that science itself is always under revision.[28] Hence science in a risk culture occupies a rather precarious position of authority: its methods are generally revered as the most compelling tools of analysis, the most reliable means to manage risk and control the future, but its conclusions have an inherently temporal value whose expiration is palpable long before it takes place. Science, as Beck writes, is both "*in*dispensable to and *in*capable of truth."[29] The proverbial emperor with no clothes, it inspires both fealty and mockery.

What is more, the various sciences, each with its own methods and routines, cannot arbitrate among the many risks they identify. They cannot determine which risks people should find more alarming or what degree of risk people should tolerate. That society and individuals must choose which risks to pay attention to, or which hazards are more dangerous, therefore, is "not merely empirical fact" but "a conceptual inevitability."[30] Consciously or not, people select among the competing possibilities of action provided by different knowledge systems, most of which are esoteric and accessible to only a narrow range of scientists. Even within particular disciplines, what is accepted as fact is necessarily based on a certain arbitrariness and suspension of skepticism. As one critic noted:

> The sheer complexity and volume of material a scientist must deal with make it impossible to examine critically the evidence bearing on all major theories. At best scientists can investigate thoroughly only narrow subfields. But knowledge is interrelated, so a scientist is forced to accept useful ideas and theories because *others have done so*.[31]

What this means for the public is that risks are "open to infinite social constructions—to being dramatized, marginalized, or changed—based on alternative knowledges," and science becomes a "self-service shop" where customers can browse for the evidence that best suits them.[32]

Both scientists and the public must evaluate which risks to address, and these choices necessarily involve attention to some risks at the expense of others. What science turns into an object of research reflects what its tools can accomplish and also the kinds of progress and judgments that make moral sense to scientists as well as citizens. The questions that scientists ask and that institutions are willing to support disclose the value that both the scientific community and the broader public place on particular behaviors and outcomes.[33] Among the many risks that science identifies, those that society embraces or rejects as matters of concern reveal its moral commitments. Risk assessment and the action based on it therefore reflect what Beck calls a *"quantitative, theoretical and causal implicit morality."* They are "the moral statements of a scientized society."[34] The regulation of sport-utility vehicles, mammogram recommendations, and the use of pesticides all are weighted with moral freight, with value decisions about safety and automobiles, women's bodies and health resources, and industry and the environment. They are statements about which risks various experts have determined are more or less tolerable. The risk of losing a crop to a parasite must be weighed against the health risks of pesticides. The risk of breast cancer must be weighed against the risks of mammography, which include the possibility of other illnesses that are not detected because resources are allocated to mammographic technology. This moral dimension of risk analysis is invisible, however, when risks are presented in isolation or when risk assessment is understood as anything other than an evaluation of trade-offs. Risk is inescapable; choices deemed "risk averse" simply foreground some risks at the expense of others. Consciously or not, every action is a pronouncement about which outcomes are least desired and which are, at least hypothetically, bearable. That the consequences of only certain behavior are perceived as risky, or that the risks of other actions are discursively invisible, demonstrates a society's inevitable moral biases.

In these value calculations, Beck argues, *"the production (or mobilization) of belief* becomes a central source for the social enforcement of validity claims."[35] Diverse sciences become politicized by markets, professions, interest groups, mass media, and others. "Social stations of risk amplification,"[36] risk professions,[37] and various media politicize risk by interpreting science for the public. Environmental groups, public health officials, and political scientists, professing expertise in soil quality, bodies, or national security, help people manage the oversupply of information by making claims about which risks are most threatening and how best to manage them. The media—and frequently journalists with limited scientific training—pay selective attention to risks and therefore make some appear more "real" than others. Risk entrepreneurs create heuristics, imagery designed to provoke intense hope or fear, and when their self-interest is at stake, they can be expected to exploit people's emotions and stress worst-case scenarios.

The most compelling risks are those that are readily "available"—that is, easily imagined, familiar, and salient. As risk scholar Cass Sunstein writes, "visualization makes the issue of probability seem less relevant or even irrelevant," and when strong emotions, such as fear, are involved, "people tend to focus on the adverse outcome, not on its likeliness. They are not closely attuned to the probability that harm will occur," and when they emphasize worst-case scenarios, "social processes are probably ensuring that they do so."[38] This tendency toward what risk analysts term "probability neglect" is not restricted to interest groups vying for membership or politicians seeking election. "Public-spirited political actors," such as children's advocates or environmental activists, "no less than self-interested ones, use probability neglect so as to promote attention to problems that may or may not deserve public concern."[39]

At the same time, reflexivity problematizes decision making for both scientists and the public. For many people, the fact that science is fluid, that it is always changing, creates the illusion that all science is equally flawed and likely to be wrong. Reflexivity essentially immunizes all points of view, no matter what their basis, against enlightened scientific claims, since science cannot be fully trusted. Politics and civic life become incoherent, battles in which each side presents a doctrine "paired and mixed with scientific detailed findings, radical criticism of science and faith in science."[40] Critical judgment is all the more difficult and emotions are more easily manipulated because so many current threats—toxins, radiation, germs—are nearly invisible. When risks cannot be visually apprehended, when they are feared to be lurking but incapable of being seen even when present, both scientists and the general population develop what psychologist Jerome Kagan labeled as "a more permissive attitude toward empirical truth"[41] in which any assertion that is conceivable, or not absolutely refutable, merits concern. Everything, and nothing, is believable.

For some people, a new "naturalism" provides something of a counterweight to offset the interminable and unnerving vagaries of science. While science is constantly changing, abstract, and elusive, nature is perceived to be fixed, concrete, and knowable. Whereas technology is fragmented and constructed, nature is holistic and pristine. Innovation is risky and fraught with ethical dilemmas, but nature is safe, ontologically superior, and morally unambiguous. When risks develop from human intervention in the natural world, from the desire to master nature, nature becomes an absolute good, "a kind of trump card against which there can be no defense." People then assume that they "can make uncomplicated choices between natural things, which are good, and unnatural things, which are bad. . . . [They] appeal to nature as a stable external source of nonhuman values against which human actions can be judged without much ambiguity."[42]

This naturalism, however, ignores the reality that the residue of human activity is ubiquitous: air, landscapes, ecosystems—nowhere does nature exist uncontaminated by human intervention. "In nature," writes Beck, "we are concerned today with a highly synthetic product everywhere, an artificial 'nature.' Not a hair or crumb of it is still 'natural,' if 'natural' means nature being left to itself."[43] The fantasy of pure "nature" and the failure to understand the scope of the human footprint skew perceptions of risk. Critics have demonstrated that lay people overestimate "man-made" carcinogens and underestimate "natural" ones, that they are more afraid of radiation from cell phones or nuclear waste than from the sun, and that they falsely assume that "natural" substances, such as herbal supplements, are risk free.[44] They fail to understand that nature cannot be morally or analytically positioned in opposition to science or be free from politics.[45]

Constructing Identity in a Risk Culture

In a risk culture, Giddens contends, people must navigate a sea of information to construct a coherent self, to create a narrative integrity through apparently trivial but essentially fraught practices.

> Each of the small decisions a person makes every day—what to wear, what to eat, how to conduct himself at work, whom to meet with later in the evening—contributes to such routines. All such choices (as well as larger and more consequential ones) are decisions not only about how to act but who to be.

These decisions, Giddens argues, are based on "abstract systems": forms of knowledge or discourse, such as medicine, engineering, and psychology. The proliferation and increasing complexity of these abstract systems in a risk culture challenge customary ways of knowing, "disembed" individuals from traditional meaning-making rationales, and provide new contexts for individual choice.[46] Traditional scripts based on religion, family ties, and class become less compelling in the face of science. The life course no longer follows standardized paths, and individuals must choose, consciously or not, which abstract systems will be their guides. As the range and complexity of information required for everyday living continue to expand, and as choices seem increasingly laden with consequences, people learn to live with anxiety and insecurity "in the form of low-grade intensities that, like low-grade fevers, permit us to go about our everyday lives but in a state of statistical stress."[47]

In a culture preoccupied with risk, identity is a reflexive project in which each person becomes a real-time and strategic autobiographer. As individuals think about who they are and how to behave consistent with that identity, they confront constant choices that will bolster or detract from the integrity of the identity they claim. Should I eat meat? Was the cow whose milk I am drinking mistreated? Mad? If I care about the environment, what kind of car should I drive? What should a parent drive? What if I am a parent who cares about the environment and lives in Michigan? Am I contributing to global warming or violence against women by wearing clothing produced in a Mexican factory? What damage to the ozone layer will result from the disposal of my shampoo container? Should I use soap and water or hand sanitizer? Which is better for the environment? For my health? Because information and experience are in constant flux, narratives of self-identity are inherently fluid and precarious. Identity in a risk society, writes Beck, requires interminable choice and "a *vigorous model of action in everyday life*" in which every decision seems fraught with significance for personal integrity.

It is not only that buying coffee in the shop on the corner may perhaps become complicit in the exploitation of the plantation workers in South America. And not only that given the omnipresence of pesticides a basic course in (alternative) chemistry is becoming a prerequisite for survival. Nor only that pedagogy and medicine, social law and traffic planning presume active "thinking individuals," as they put it so nicely, who are supposed to find their way in this jungle of transitory finalities with the help of their own clear vision. All these and all the other experts dump their contradictions and conflicts at the feet of the individual and leave him or her with the well intentioned invitation to judge all of this critically on the basis of his or her own notions. With detraditionalization and the creation of global media networks, the biography is increasingly removed from its direct spheres of contact and opened up across the boundaries of countries and experts for a *long-distance morality* which puts the individual in the position of potentially having to take a continual stand. At the same moment that he or she sinks into insignificance, he or she is elevated to the apparent throne of world-shaper.[48]

Many decisions, by necessity, are routinized. "Fateful moments," however, are particularly meaningful. These occasions—decisions to marry or divorce, to seek institutional care for an elderly parent, to invest one's savings in a new business—are fraught with risk, with both predictable and unforeseeable consequences. At these times, an individual stands at a crossroads in her existence, faced with decisions that bear heavily on her self-identity. Furthermore, she does so less tethered to traditional systems of meaning, such as religion or social class, that historically have provided direction at precisely these moments. Fateful decisions can produce not just guilt but shame. Guilt is a relatively mundane emotion that arises when one's decisions are at cross-purposes with the chosen self: I should not have done that. Shame, in contrast, develops when either the integrity of that self-concept or one's ability to sustain it comes seriously into question: I have failed at or I am not capable of being the person I am supposed to be. Guilt, Giddens writes, derives from specific acts and feelings of wrongdoing, and shame has to do with "the integrity of the self" and "fears that the narrative of self-identity cannot withstand engulfing pressures on its coherence or social acceptability."[49] Guilt is transient, but shame is enduring. Although guilt can lead to shame, the two are not the same.

Individuals in a risk culture approach their lives with what Beck calls a "double gaze"[50] that stems from the sense that invisible danger looms everywhere and that choices have unexpected consequences that will become apparent only in retrospect. People often find themselves haunted by nagging "what if" questions and therefore are compelled to engage in what Giddens terms "trust." Aware that they are not competent to understand or evaluate all the information they have, individuals arbitrarily give themselves over to particular diets, economic forecasters, or spiritual guides, which provide decision-making maps. In a modernity in which science and the decisions based on it are constantly scrutinized and revised, this kind of trust provides a "protective cocoon,"[51] an ontological security without which individuals would be paralyzed or immersed in interminable reflection. People align with the science, the "truth," that confirms what they want to believe, based on personal values; what they are socially inclined to embrace, based on such ascriptions as race, class, or gender; and what they are disciplined to believe, based on their various professional and communal commitments. Trust, therefore, is personal and subjective. As Giddens suggests, "various attitudes of scepticism or antagonism towards abstract systems may coexist with a taken-for-granted confidence in others,"[52] and these perspectives necessarily stem more from economic and social affinities and personal sensibilities than from a critical evaluation of competing scientific analyses.

If identity in a risk culture is fashioned through personal choice, the process is nonetheless shaped by important ideological forces. American culture, for example, is infused with a neoliberalism that structures how personal narratives are composed.[53] Neoliberalism draws on traditional liberal philosophy's concern with personal freedom, but with two fundamental changes. Whereas liberalism in the classic sense advocates limited government and the maximization of individual rights, neoliberalism calls for paternalist political authority and personal responsibility. Whereas classical liberals seek maximum freedom from government, neoliberal individuals are perpetually responsive to the state's engineering of their environment. In the former, government is idealized to the extent that it stays out of people's lives, thereby maximizing individual choice; in the latter, the state creates the conditions that enable people to choose to behave in ways it has determined are best for the collective good, thereby manipulating individual choice. Liberal individuals do what they want, and neoliberal individuals choose to do what they are supposed to do.

In American risk culture, neoliberalism operates along the lines of what Foucault termed "governmentality":[54] institutions of authority generate and then communicate knowledge about the population in an effort to make society operate more efficiently; people are then free to do as they please, but responsible citizens will behave as experts recommend. If the U.S. Department of Health and Human Services (HHS) recommends a low-fat diet, good neoliberal citizens will consume less fat. If the National Institutes of Health (NIH) says that children who watch little television perform better in school than those who watch more, neoliberal parents will reduce screen time. In a neoliberal risk culture, individuals practice a regulated autonomy and have responsibilities to the collective.[55] In both classical liberalism and neoliberalism, the individual is the primary social agent, but in the latter, today, personal rights are intimately tied to obligation: individuals have a *responsibility* to take care of themselves so that they are not a burden to society. Neoliberalism "calls upon each individual to enter the process of his or her own self-governance through processes of endless self-examination, self-care and self-improvement."[56] Risk management is privatized, or left to "active citizens" who internalize norms of appropriate behavior, assume the onus of self-administration, and expect the same from others.[57] Neoliberal citizens, in short, take care of themselves.

Health and Responsibility in a Risk Culture

Medicalization occurs when choices are analyzed in terms of their health implications and are subject to medical expertise, and nowhere are the burdens of individual responsibility more evident than in the accelerating medicalization of matters that at first glance have little to do with the body. In current public debate, increasing spheres of life are conceptualized in terms of medical risk, and the road to good health seems to pass through virtually everything. Sociologist Nikolas Rose described medicalization as

> biopolitical concerns with the minimization of risks to health—control of environmental pollution, reduction of accidents, maintenance of bodily health, nurturing of children—[become] intrinsic not just to the organization of health and social services, but to expert decisions about town planning, building design, educational practice, the management of organizations, the marketing of food, the design of automobiles and much more.[58]

Medicalization reflects what one critic calls a "paradox of proportion." Now that many major health challenges, such as infectious diseases, have been largely controlled, "the bar has been lowered and the elimination of increasingly smaller health risks takes on proportionally larger significance."[59] Psychotropic drugs, assisted conception, hormone replacement therapy, Viagra: today, remedies exist for biological states that once seemed immutable. According to Rose:

> Life now appears to be open to shaping and reshaping at the molecular level: by precisely calculated interventions that prevent something happening, alter the way something happens, make something new happen in the cellular processes themselves. As the distinction between treatment and enhancement, between the natural and the prosthetic blurs, the management and maximization of life itself have become the life's work, not only of each individual, but of their doctors, together with the scientists, entrepreneurs and corporations who make the reworking of life the object of their knowledge, inventions and products.[60]

Disease and even death seem more avoidable because their causes can increasingly be identified and, at least theoretically, circumvented. This heightened sense of control means that poor health no longer is attributed to luck or chance but is the personal responsibility of each individual to avoid.[61] When "healthy" signifies "responsible," sick people are increasingly praised or condemned in psychological or moral terms.[62] Information, control, and responsibility exist in dynamic relation;[63] lifestyle decisions are perceived to reflect conscious risk analysis; and good health represents self-discipline, somatic responsibility, and, ultimately, good citizenship.

Risk management is personalized, moreover, at the same time that public health discourse blurs the distinction between "healthy" and "sick" and makes "prevention" the guiding principle in healthy living. In a risk culture, because everything is potentially risky, everyone is always at risk, which means that "health no longer exists in a strict binary relationship to illness, rather health and illness belong to an ordinal scale in which the healthy can become healthier, and health can co-exist with illness."[64] The identification of risk factors and genetic predispositions tells people that they are on the verge of becoming sick, that they are almost ill. Predictive genetic tests demonstrate that "although we are ostensibly healthy now, we probably will become ill in the future and are therefore in fact already ill."[65] An advertisement from Memorial Sloan-Kettering Cancer Center lists in large print "the early warning signs of colon cancer": "You feel great. You have a healthy appetite. You're only 50. You feel fine. Nothing seems to be the matter." The ad continues: "Unfortunately, those are the same symptoms thousands of Americans had last year before they were diagnosed with colon cancer."[66] To be normal, in other words, "is to be in a state of risk, a state that at some inevitable future time will be fulfilled as a state of disease or death," a state of "statistical panic."[67] No one is truly healthy, and healthy behavior is rewarded not with an absence of sickness but with an ineradicable "semi-pathological pre-illness at-risk state."[68] Indeed, according to some critics, "what's making us sick is an epidemic of diagnoses."[69] In such a context, prevention becomes the dominant health project. The philosophy of prevention dictates that bad health is always on the horizon, a future that can be prevented only by making responsible choices in the present. To fulfill the obligations of "health citizenship,"[70] individuals are called on by various experts and the media to undertake constant self-surveillance: to demonstrate continuously their competency to take care of their bodies, and in the process, to be good citizens.[71]

Risks, however, are often framed in ways that mask the value assumptions implicit in health rhetoric. Should an individual be expected to overcome a hereditary predisposition? Can a person choose to have will power?[72] In a neoliberal discourse, in which personal responsibility is a first principle, such questions go largely unasked. Furthermore, the quantification of risk and risk management often neglect social differences. When the prescriptions according to which individuals should live their lives are abstracted from risks calculated at the population level, the hierarchies within a population disappear, and both the degree of and capacity to respond to risk for any particular individual are skewed. Public discourse about genetic conditions is often governed by a similar ignorance of inequality. All people— "rich and poor, black and white, young and old—they are all subjected to the dictate of the genes, a perspective that renders the question of social power relationships irrelevant" and effectively "blots out the social context."[73]

In a risk culture, moreover, every choice is doubly marked: an individual experiences not simply the safety or nutritional effects of one selection over another—the Toyota or the Ford, the carrots or the potato chips— but the responsibility for what those choices communicate about who she or he is. As Beck observes, "even where the word 'decisions' is too grandiose, because neither consciousness nor alternatives are present, the individual will have to 'pay for' the consequences of decisions not taken."[74] Whereas in the past, risks were perceived as more random and inescapable—floods and disease were neither predictable nor controllable—today, risks are often considered to be foreseeable and avoidable. Fate, that is, appears to be subject to individual control. If a course of action may lead to better health, increased safety, and an overall decline in exposure to danger, all that remains for the responsible person is to follow it.

Yet not everyone can be "responsible." Regular exercise is a practical impossibility for people working two jobs to survive, and preventive care is not available to those who do not know it exists or do not have the means to pursue it. Nonetheless, in a neoliberal risk culture, social problems are often individualized and internalized, and crises linked to poverty or prejudice are perceived and lived as personal failures. Given the sheer number of abstract knowledge systems and the complexity within and between them, risk management is a formidable life task for everyone. For those without the necessary resources to participate consciously in a risk culture, it can be nearly impossible, and they are likely to be judged harshly by others. In other words, if gender, race, and class—what Giddens and

Beck refer to as the traditional narratives of modernity—appear to be less rhetorically compelling, they are not necessarily less salient in determining the range of options practically available to each individual. That social structure shapes which information is accessible and which choices are possible (and which risks scientists investigate) is obscured by the premise that good citizens assess information, exercise control, and act responsibly. This expectation is predicated on two erroneous assumptions: that information diffusion is democratic, and that everyone has the capacity to behave in putatively risk-averse ways.

The almost unanimous admonition against overweight and obesity demonstrates that the dynamics of health in a risk culture are most pronounced when advice is offered and consumed as if it were devoid of uncertainty. At these moments, individuals' expectations of themselves and others intensify, and the pressure to behave responsibly becomes more acute. Today, the imperative to be thin has become almost a moral absolute. Like smoking, whose health risks have been rigorously demonstrated, obesity is widely perceived to be a serious threat to a person's health. HHS claims that obesity is a risk factor for various illnesses, including type 2 diabetes, hypertension, coronary heart disease, stroke, and some cancers, and that annual medical spending on obesity-related problems is well over $100 billion.[75] The NIH and the Centers for Disease Control and Prevention (CDC) admonish American citizens to make sure their body mass index is within "normal" range, whose definition has shifted downward as concerns about obesity have intensified. The CDC estimates that Medicare and Medicaid receipts constitute roughly half of all states' medical expenditures on obesity,[76] thus underscoring the responsibility that each person has to his or her fellow citizens to maintain a healthy body weight and to avoid burdening already strapped public assistance programs.[77] *How* people should lose weight, however, is highly contentious. Perhaps no example better demonstrates the reflexivity necessitated by health advice than dietary recommendations. Nowadays it is almost impossible to read or listen to the news without encountering new information about food and its various impacts on the human body. Fats, carbohydrates, antioxidants: research exists to confirm and refute virtually every piece of nutritional advice, and doctors, nutritionists, diet creators, the pharmaceutical industry, and research scientists battle endlessly for media and public attention. Uncertainty, doubt, and arbitrary trust are inescapable as individuals determine to control their weight and at the same time confront constantly changing information about how best to do so.[78]

In a neoliberal culture, "the pastoral positioning of the subject of health care—the subject as the recipient of health care for his/her own good or the good of a collectivity—represents a form of authoritarianism intrinsic to modern biopolitics."[79] This authoritarianism is built not on the threat of physical force but on discursive coercion, and the consequence of resistance can be social ostracization. Indeed, a sick person is expected by fellow citizens to make every reasonable effort to get well soon as compensation for the privilege of being excused from work or of receiving increased care.[80] Because the solvency of insurance plans depends on healthy subscribers and social policies are paid for by all citizens, people who "choose" to be unhealthy constitute a social problem. "The individual whose conduct is deemed contrary to the pursuit of a 'risk-free' existence is likely to be seen, and to see themselves, as lacking self-control, and as therefore not fulfilling their duties as a fully autonomous, responsible citizen."[81] For each individual, the failure to meet the requirements of good health may not lead to guilt (I made poor food choices today) but to shame (I am an irresponsible person and an unworthy citizen). Shame threatens the virtue and soundness of self as such. It stems from the internalization of a public ethic of individual responsibility and from anxiety that bad choices reflect an insurmountable and personal moral deficit. It can be the result of an individualization of problems with external and often structural roots. As "biological identity becomes bound up with more general norms of enterprising, self-actualizing, responsible personhood,"[82] developing a disease becomes tantamount to a failure to have prevented it. Good health becomes "a secular moral framework for society" in which "the personal is the medical"[83] and the biological, therefore, is the political.

Breastfeeding in a Neoliberal Risk Culture

In the United States, public discourse on breastfeeding reveals the neoliberal cultural emphasis on personal responsibility. When each person in a risk culture is responsible for his or her own well-being, every mother is uniquely accountable for the health of her babies and children. This is not an entirely new development, as women in Western societies have long been represented as citizens in regard to their obligation to raise children and to provide care for husbands and other family members.[84] Since the colonial period, when "republican mothers" were charged with raising patriotic children committed to liberty and self-sacrifice for the new republic,[85] through the nineteenth century, when the welfare of children became a governmental, or public, concern, the site of the family has provided a link between the care of individual bodies and the health of the social body.[86] Today, as the concept of health and the medicalization of life have become increasingly comprehensive, opportunities to protect children and expectations of mothers have multiplied as well. What is new in a risk culture is not the centrality of care to maternal citizenship but the scope and complexity of that responsibility and its framing in terms of risk: the expanse of children's lives over which mothers are obligated to exercise care, or the sheer volume of risks they must address; and the reach and precision of the sciences on which demands of mothers are founded.

The injunction to breastfeed is rooted in three institutions—science, motherhood, and public health—and in the dynamics of these institutions in a neoliberal risk culture. Risk-factor epidemiology, which is the basis of research comparing breastfeeding and formula feeding, is governed by rules that make sense only in a certain scientific paradigm. These methods, along with the social values of scientists and the broader public, restrict the kinds of questions asked, or the potential risks worthy of investigation, and therefore the conclusions drawn, or the risks that will be further explored. Breastfeeding research has focused on a narrow set of questions that can be answered within a risk-factor paradigm, and it has been unable to rule out rival hypotheses that require alternative methods to evaluate. The constraints and biases implicit in the conduct of this research are concealed by the putative objectivity of agreed-upon rules, and the ideological biases encoded in the results are not visible to either scientists or the public. Driven by different political and professional agendas, various risk communicators then invest this research with meaning and authority that extend far beyond the narrow confines of the knowledge system within which it was produced. The dominant paradigms of science, the methods and agendas of infant-feeding research, and the language used to communicate science provide the structural foundation for the various representations of breastfeeding in a neoliberal risk culture.

Ideas about risk and mothers also shape public discourse on breastfeeding. Long before they consider pregnancy and continuing through childbirth, girls and women are subjected to an endless flow of information about how to reduce risks to their future offspring. These data, targeted largely at women's bodies, are ephemeral, and they produce infinite opportunities for choosing and second-guessing decisions once they have been made. Conception and pregnancy advice suggests that every woman can choose to have healthy children, that producing healthy babies is largely within the individual woman's control, and that healthy children are produced by disciplined mothers. Responsible women, moreover, are responsible mothers. The neoliberal woman who is socially obligated to maintain her health becomes a neoliberal mother who must keep her baby healthy for the sake of the community. Healthy children are mothers' obligation to cultivate, and women who fail to make wise choices, regardless of their socioeconomic constraints, are at fault for producing anything other than healthy offspring. The paradox of proportion that directs attention to increasingly smaller risks is apparent in the societal expectation that good mothers will reduce all risks to their children, no matter how remote the threat or how great the investment required to address it.

The guiding principle of contemporary motherhood is that women who are mothers must act first *as mothers* and that their self-identity is dependent on optimizing their children's lives. Infant feeding is a fateful moment, one fraught with consequences for self-identity and opportunities for shame. Each woman is told that breastfeeding is superior to formula feeding because it reduces physical, emotional, and cognitive health risks to her baby. Having spent her pregnancy managing risks to her developing fetus, the new mother is told that she should continue monitoring her body—what she eats, thinks, and feels—while breastfeeding, and that surveillance now also extends to her baby, who must be constantly observed for any sign of potential disequilibrium. Breastfeeding is also part of a broader discourse criticizing "artificial" intervention in reproduction and child raising and encouraging mothers to practice "natural" family living. Pregnant women and mothers are frequently advised that the "skill to be natural" should take precedence over "the will to be artificial" and that good mothers can postpone their babies' encounter with technology and prolong their "natural" existence by making good choices, including breastfeeding.[87]

The values of American risk culture, particularly the focus on individuals, the celebration of health as an individual accomplishment, and the attribution of children's health to individual mothers, figure prominently in public health campaigns. Neoliberal governments are concerned with the health not of individuals but of the general population, and they establish parameters of healthy living that each responsible citizen is to observe for the sake of the community. These boundaries represent a selective mobilization of science, or the identification by public officials of behaviors that they believe to be most conducive to the nation's health. In a risk culture, in which people are always almost sick, good citizens devote themselves to prevention; responsibility for the health of babies is privatized, or assigned to mothers; and social and economic impediments to healthy babies are deemed to be the task of mothers to surmount. State institutions advise that breast is best for babies and that therefore good citizen-mothers will breastfeed. Cultural reasons for not breastfeeding are treated as obstacles, and economic circumstances become barriers that each mother must be persuaded to overcome. Scientific uncertainty disappears, choice becomes overdetermined, and breastfeeding emerges as central to civic motherhood.

4

From the Womb to the Breast

Total Motherhood and Risk-Free Children

IN *FREE-RANGE KIDS*: *Giving Our Children the Freedom We Had without Going Nuts with Worry*, humorist Lenore Skenazy offers parents an "A-to-Z Review of Everything You Might Be Worried About," including "Animals, Being Eaten By"; "Death by Stroller"; "Eating Snow"; and "Walking to School (or at Least the Bus Stop)." Today's parents, she writes, have lost all perspective on safety and danger, overanalyze the significance of everyday decisions, and ultimately can do more harm than good by neither teaching nor modeling good judgment for their children.[1] British sociologist Frank Furedi concurs, lamenting that parenting today "is not so much about *managing* the risks of everyday life but *avoiding* them altogether."[2]

While it might be true that risks to children seem omnipresent and that they strike a particular emotional chord, this notion of risk-centered parenting neglects the division of labor that assigns moral and practical responsibility for the protection of children to *mothers*. As Susan J. Douglas and Meredith W. Michaels, authors of *The Mommy Myth: The Idealization of Motherhood and How It Has Undermined Women*, contended, a "new momism" holds mothers accountable for producing ever more perfect children.[3] Moreover, as others have argued regarding "exclusive motherhood" and "intensive mothering," ideas about what children need are enmeshed in largely unexamined beliefs about mothers.[4] That is, the push to insulate children from danger and to optimize childhood reflects not just a greater investment in children but also increasing expectations about what mothers can and should provide.[5]

Defined within the broad parameters of a risk culture, breastfeeding is shaped more proximately by an ideology of "total motherhood." Total motherhood incorporates tenets of the new momism and exclusive and intensive mothering but stresses the near ubiquity of science and risk analysis to prescriptions for good mothering in a risk culture. Total motherhood stipulates that mothers' primary occupation is to predict and prevent all less-than-optimal social, emotional, cognitive, and physical outcomes; that mothers are responsible for anticipating and eradicating every imaginable risk to their children, regardless of the degree or severity of the risk or what the trade-offs might be; and that any potential diminution in harm to children trumps all other considerations in risk analysis as long as mothers can achieve the reduction. This last proviso suggests that risks to children (or potential children) are both most apparent and most alarming when they can be "laid at mother's doorstep"[6] or when they can be construed as the obligation of mothers to eliminate. It also suggests that when specific threats require sacrifice or intervention from others—fathers, communities, government—they are more likely to be discursively invisible, rationalized, or framed as something other than risky. The notion that risks to children are particularly salient when they are mothers' burden to reduce informs advice from a range of authorities about preconception, pregnancy, childbirth, and infant and child care. It also structures epidemiological research on and public health advice about infant feeding.

Total motherhood is rooted in the traditions of domesticity and "scientific motherhood."[7] What historians have called a "cult of domesticity" began to emerge around the middle of the nineteenth century as a commercial economy developed and distinctly public and private lives began to take shape. In this process, men were increasingly identified with a public sphere that rewarded competitiveness and self-interest, and women were expected to maintain home life as a respite from the moral coarseness of the market. In the evolving new middle class, which differed from the upper class in that its status had to be continually reestablished from one generation to the next, children's education came to seem too important to be left to servants. While fathers earned the family income, mothers were responsible for raising the children and teaching them life skills. Around the same time, the notion of what constituted good mothering began to shift from innate and God-given maternal instinct to acquired skills that required training from experts. As the century progressed, mothers were faced with a new genre of published scientific advice. Child care manuals, women's magazines, and home-health columns in other publications offered instruction about everything from infant diet and bathing to thumb sucking and bed-wetting. The fundamental principle of scientific motherhood was that mothers needed the help of medically and scientifically trained experts to raise their children properly.[8] Of course, neither domesticity nor scientific motherhood was within reach of the majority of women: poor, working class, rural, African American, and immigrant mothers who were constrained by illiteracy, lack of access to physicians, slavery and racial discrimination, language barriers, and/or the demands of economically essential maternal employment. Total motherhood, which is grounded in these earlier projects, is also a largely middle-class project that assumes all mothers have the resources, such as time, access, and money even to consider, much less act on, expert advice. Located in a risk culture that simultaneously valorizes scientific expertise and minimizes the power of social structures to limit choices, total motherhood assigns individual mothers unique responsibility for their children's welfare.

On one hand, total motherhood is simply the late twentieth- and twenty-first-century incarnation of domesticity and scientific motherhood. On the other hand, science has now become so central to the planning, organization, and optimization of preconception, conception, pregnancy, and child care that total motherhood marks a significant cultural shift. Never before has information been so comprehensive and widely available and reached so far into individual lives, holding out the promise of manipulating increasingly narrower details of existence. At no other point in history have the need to turn data into knowledge and the obstacles to doing so been more profound. Total motherhood, which circulates in a culture in which risks are omnipresent and the field of putative control is virtually without boundaries, bridges domesticity and scientific motherhood with the social dynamics of risk. It sets women, future mothers, and then mothers the impossible task of gathering, evaluating, and acting on information about an infinite number of risks that might interfere with not just normal but optimal fetal and child development. Rooted in deep-seated but reclassified convictions about maternal responsibility, it is a moral code in which individual mothers are ultimately held responsible for any harm that befalls their children.

Total motherhood reveals the vexations of a risk culture: the fixation on planning and the ongoing drive to control the future through the proper selection and application of scientific knowledge; the individualization and privatization of responsibility for lifestyles, particularly in matters of health; overlapping reverence and disdain both for science and technology and for all things natural; the inescapable moral dimension of risk analysis; and the reflexive construction of self-identity. Total motherhood also reveals how people in a risk culture often fail to appreciate the omnipresence of risk and the inevitability of risk trade-offs. In various discourses about mothering, babies' "needs" expand to include anything that could be beneficial, and need-satisfaction becomes indistinguishable from optimization. As a result, the resolution of conflicting maternal-child needs and desires tends to minimize or ignore the costs that mothers incur to reduce risks to their children. Total motherhood, furthermore, reflects the neoliberalism of American risk culture in its presumption that mothers as individuals are responsible for their children until (and even when) they can be held responsible for themselves. If good health represents a woman's commitment to being a good citizen, healthy pregnancy and children reflect a mother's responsible choices. Before conception, during pregnancy and childbirth, and throughout child rearing, mothers are charged with gathering and interpreting information, monitoring bodies and behavior, anticipating needs, and preventing danger. Although advice about children is sometimes directed at parents, the kind of information available, the opportunities for maternal surveillance, and the needs and dangers on which public discourse fixates demonstrate that the risks Americans are conscious of, the ones they most fear and are inclined to address, are those that can be reduced by mothers.

Optimizing Pregnancy

For most of human history, "women had babies without any notion of choice. Pregnancy happened and a baby arrived."[9] Women who were unable to conceive could appeal to fertility goddesses and midwives, consume herbs and minerals, or visit mineral springs, but they had little scientific understanding of how they might become pregnant. Miscarriages were understood to be either God's will or, by the nineteenth century, the result of malfunctions in individual women's reproductive machinery that were not subject to human intervention. Childbirth itself was part of the natural order of the universe, a process that could be attended but not controlled. For the most part, women feared less for their babies than for their own lives. Indeed, until the last part of the twentieth century, maternal comfort and safety were the primary concerns of women and physicians alike. Dietary changes, exercise, surgery, alcohol avoidance, even exorcism—these and other strategies were at various times assumed to increase fertility and reduce birth defects. Little evidence, however, indicates that women thought they could systematically engineer conception or manipulate pregnancy to improve the health of newborns.[10]

Today, children are planned in ways that reflect the dynamics of a risk culture. They are biopolitical constructions, products of a neoliberal ethic stipulating that "responsible women ought to control their reproductive functions, indeed, that this is what constitutes responsibility where reproduction is concerned."[11] Women are both subtly and explicitly advised that the risks of pregnancy, childbirth, and child raising are calculable and, therefore, preventable; that they must be vigilant about their bodies even before conception in anticipation of pregnancy and motherhood; and that it is every woman's individual responsibility to continuously monitor her babies and children in order to maximize their mental, emotional, and physical health. Reproduction and child care are reflexive: women are confronted with an abundance of far-reaching and often highly contested knowledge about how to create optimal wombs and then to monitor their fetuses, babies, and children in order to reduce the risks of anything deemed undesirable. This unrelenting stream of information can be both empowering and maddening. Through a process of normalization, mothers internalize a sense that they can and should control their bodies and that responsible mothers produce healthy outcomes. As more and more dimensions of daily life are medicalized, that is, turned into potential pathologies that require medical attention, mothers are asked to make decisions with little consciousness of either the moral dimension of risk analysis or the implicit values that frame their choices. In a risk culture in which particular opprobrium is assigned to those who put others at risk, these decisions have consequences that extend well beyond health and child development. While reproductive freedom and choice have increased, women are being constrained in new ways by expanding medical definitions of their reproductive responsibility.[12]

The flow of information about pregnancy begins long before conception. Advice from a variety of scientific authorities, including the national government, is directed at "women of childbearing age," a category so broad that all women past puberty, regardless of their age or plans for children, are trained to think of themselves as future mothers. Both the National Institute of Child Health and Human Development and the American Academy of Family Physicians instruct women to seek preconception care well before they try to get pregnant.[13] The Centers for Disease Control and Prevention (CDC) advises health care providers to "assure that all women of childbearing age receive preconception care services . . . that will enable them to enter pregnancy in optimal health" and to "encourage every man, woman, and couple to have a reproductive life plan."[14] Since 1987, the CDC has operated the Pregnancy Risk Assessment Monitoring System (PRAMS) "a surveillance project . . . [that]

collects state-specific, population-based data on maternal attitudes and experiences before, during, and shortly after pregnancy."[15] In 2006, the CDC issued formal recommendations regarding how to improve preconception health and health care, the first of which called for "Individual Responsibility across the Lifespan" and defined the target population as "women, from menarche to menopause, who are capable of having children, even if they do not intend to conceive." All the recommendations "emphasize individual behavior and responsibility for improving preconception health"[16] and demonstrate the neoliberal orientation of contemporary risk culture.

Women are repeatedly advised to act with an eye on their maternal future. The American College of Obstetricians and Gynecologists (ACOG) recommends that "all women of childbearing age should take 0.4 milligrams of folic acid daily" to reduce the risks of neural tube defects.[17] This recommendation is based on compelling science, and the medical result of increased folic acid intake has been a dramatic reduction in the incidence of spina bifida and related disorders.[18] The psychological effect of such advice is to have women thinking as mothers well before they conceive. Most pregnancy guidebooks now include a pre-pregnancy section, and a relatively new genre is devoted specifically to the period before conception. Among the latter are such books as *Before You Conceive: The Complete Pregnancy Guide*, *The Pre-Pregnancy Planner*, and *Getting Pregnant: What You Need to Know Right Now*.[19] These titles suggest that responsible women will seek out and follow advice about appropriate conduct and indeed that women who want to become pregnant in the future must adopt prescribed behaviors in the present. Women must plan for pregnancy even before they decide whether to pursue it; they must monitor their lifestyles and behave as if they will try to become pregnant, regardless of how pregnancy fits into their plans. The very terms of the discussion— "pre-pregnancy," "pre-conception," "women of childbearing age"—define women in their relation to motherhood, as though pregnancy were normal and everything else were biologically deviant. In health matters, the distinction between women and mothers can be elusive.

Women who seek preconception advice are both subtly and explicitly advised on how they can control their fertility. Whether they chart their cycles with pen and paper or track ovulation with expensive monitors, they are propelled into a reflexive contemplation and routine assessment of how their actions might affect their ability to conceive. Women are cautioned that stress can inhibit fertility and advised to seek ways to relax.

Nearly all guides mention the importance of "a healthy diet," advice that women trying to become pregnant have been hearing since at least the middle of the nineteenth century but whose effects on conception and pregnancy, other than in the case of malnutrition, are far from clear. "Everything you put into your body is connected to your ability to conceive!" admonishes Modernstork.com.[20] Women are repeatedly warned that the risks of infertility and genetic abnormalities increase with gestational age, and those who choose to postpone having children have been the subject of bitter public debate about women's responsibility to produce healthy offspring and the ethical uses of reproductive technology. Despite media attention that focuses overwhelmingly on women's fertility, however, only about one-third of infertility cases can be attributed to problems in women's reproductive functioning. Another one-third stem from men's health problems, and the remaining one-third are caused by a combination of factors or remain unexplained.[21] The irony is that male infertility treatment almost invariably involves medical interventions on women's bodies, and it is largely on women that public discourse and medicine focus.[22] In infertile couples, women who want to be mothers, but not men who want to be fathers, confront complex and invasive regimens: they must track menses and ovulation, undergo blood tests and sonograms, give themselves medication and injections, and submit to a range of procedures from artificial insemination to in vitro fertilization.

Pregnancy guidebooks offer self-surveillance programs in which women can regulate their behavior to raise their chances of producing a healthy baby. The immensely popular *What to Expect When You're Expecting*[23] offers pregnant women month-by-month advice on how to track their changing bodies and developing fetuses and how to reduce potential risks. In response to complaints that the book was unnecessarily scaring women by focusing on remote risks and complications, the authors made significant changes in the third edition. Accordingly, a section that was entitled "Playing Baby Roulette" became "Putting Risk in Perspective," and the "Best-Odds Diet" was renamed the "Pregnancy Diet." Yet even though some of the language was deliberately changed, the emphasis on preventing risk and the message of danger remain. In the second edition, women are warned that

> every bite counts. You've got only nine months of meals and snacks with which to give your baby the best possible start in life. Make every one of them count. Before you close your mouth on a forkful of food,

consider, "Is this the best bite I can give my baby?" If it will benefit your baby, chew away. If it'll only benefit your sweet tooth or appease your appetite, put your fork down.[24]

In the third edition, women are similarly cautioned:

Every bite counts. You've got nine months of meals and snacks with which to give your baby the best possible start in life. Try to make them count. As you raise fork to mouth, consider, "Is this a bite that will benefit my baby?" If it is, chew away. If it isn't, see if you can't find a bite more worthy.

Additional recommendations include adding green plants to homes to help purify the air, not standing in front of microwaves to reduce fetal exposure to radiation, and eschewing hair dyes and permanents (even though "the risk is only theoretical").[25] Other books—*How to Prevent Miscarriage and Other Crises of Pregnancy: A Leading High-Risk Doctor's Prescription for Carrying Your Baby to Term, Avoiding Miscarriage: Everything You Need to Know to Feel More Confident in Pregnancy,* and *Preventing Miscarriage: The Good News*—suggest that diligent women can prevent pregnancy loss, even though the causes of individual miscarriages are largely speculative.[26] Implicit in the titles is the notion that women who do suffer miscarriages could have avoided them if they had informed themselves properly.

At prenatal visits to the obstetrician, routine testing helps identify potentially serious problems, such as diabetes and preeclampsia, but also further enmeshes pregnant women in the information-control-responsibility dynamic of a risk culture. Obstetricians track blood pressure and weight, urine for sugar or protein, and feet and hands for swelling. Doctors also are likely to palpate and measure the abdomen to verify the size and shape of the uterus, to listen for a fetal heartbeat, and to test for gestational diabetes and anemia. In addition, the ACOG now recommends that all pregnant women be advised of options for testing that might indicate fetal abnormality. As their bodies are continuously monitored, pregnant women must become conversant with what anthropologist Rayna Rapp, one of the first academics to examine couples' experiences of prenatal screening, calls the "resolutely medico-scientific" language of genetic counseling. These consultations are problematic, not least because counselors are often insensitive to the class, ethnic, and racial contexts in which women must weigh the risks of prenatal tests against those of potential fetal anomalies and then interpret and act on the results based on abstract probabilities.[27]

Women who undergo testing might well confront scenarios that are fraught with moral implications: Should a positive blood test for Down syndrome be followed by a more definitive amniocentesis, a procedure that carries a slight risk of miscarriage, a risk that might well stem from a Down fetus and not the amniocentesis itself? Should the discovery of an operable abnormality lead to fetal surgery, which poses risks to the fetus and the expectant mother? Or should such a pregnancy be terminated? What kinds of personal and social supports would be available to care for a child with special needs? In a neoliberal risk culture focused on prevention, testing makes disability less a collective problem—"What will *we* do to embrace and accommodate those among us with disabilities?"—than one for individual women to manage: "What will *she* do to avoid having a baby with a disability" or to provide appropriate care for this baby once it is born.[28] Each pregnant woman is "positioned in a web of surveillance, monitoring, measurement and expert advice that requires constant work on her part: seeking out knowledge about risks to her fetus, acting according to that knowledge."[29] At the same time, dangers to women themselves are far less well known. For example, pregnant women are more likely than other women to experience domestic violence, and pregnant victims of violence are at increased risk for a variety of poor maternal outcomes, including femicide.[30] At times, a responsible pregnancy appears to require reducing risks to the fetus and making choices that lower the costs for everyone but the pregnant woman.

Medically, legally, and culturally, the fetus has developed into a distinct subject vulnerable to a hazardous womb, a viable human exposed to varying degrees of risk depending on the behavior of its mother. Ultrasound photography—"shooting the mother"—provides visual evidence of the fetus as a complete person,[31] and advances in this technology, now a standard component of prenatal care, have led to remarkably detailed imagery. Mothers-to-be can take home three-dimensional pictures of their fetuses during the second trimester. The market for fetal products and prenatal services, brimming with tools to help jump-start babies' emotional and intellectual development, offers additional opportunities for fetal surveillance. The implicit message is that parents who do not avail themselves of these resources put their fetus at a comparative disadvantage. Advertising for the Wombsong Prenatal Sound System, "based on the latest in prenatal and brain research and developed by a team of medical professionals," advises that "a baby's brain cells multiply rapidly, making connections that may shape a lifetime of experience and learning," and recommends using the system every day "to stimulate your baby and enhance brain development." Embryonics toys, sold at Toys "R" Us and Amazon.com, provide a "Learning System from Womb to Classroom."[32] The Institute for Perinatal Education, featured on CBS's *The Early Show*, teaches "prenatal parenting . . . the concept of actively parenting, with forethought and directed attention, your unborn child." Frederick Wirth, a neonatologist, professor of pediatrics and the institute's president, offers a set of prenatal parenting techniques based on "the fact" that a mother's emotions "are carried across the placenta by messenger molecules impacting the baby's brain development [which] can affect a child's emotional character for life."[33] Such "messenger molecules" have never been demonstrated.

While some prenatal exposures are known to be harmful to the fetus, many others, including some that are well publicized, are largely hypothetical. Certain medications, folic-acid and vitamin-D deficiencies, and the failure to control serious maternal health problems increase the risk of birth defects or ailments later in life, and pregnant women have benefited enormously from prenatal research. Nonetheless, when a good mother is expected to reduce any *conceivable* risk to her fetus, all manner of conjecture about pregnancy behavior can become prescriptive. The developing "fetal programming" hypothesis, which proposes that health problems throughout life stem from exposures in the womb, is one example that has received extensive media attention. Reporting on a widely publicized study of prenatal diet in rats, for example, *U.S. News & World Report* offered this lead:

> Most pregnant women wouldn't dream of belting back cocktails or lighting up. But what about that Big Mac and daily Krispy Kreme doughnut? In a Freudian twist, a growing number of researchers now contend that if Junior eventually battles middle-age spread, hypertension, and diabetes, Mom's diet during pregnancy will bear some of the blame.

The article was accompanied by a photo of a baby bottle nipple.[34] "Moms Eat Junk Food, Kids Get Fat" was the headline for a CBS.com story on the same study.[35]

A *Los Angeles Times* report on fetal programming demonstrates the ways in which women's control over their wombs is both obligatory and impossible. Experts are not suggesting that "pregnant women take every possible precaution for fear of dooming their children," the article cautioned, but "many fetal programming experts say reproductive-age men and women need to know that they probably have more control over their children's future health than they realize." It quoted a scientist at the National Institute of Environmental Health Sciences: "You can't help but be a little scared of everything that could go wrong. There are a lot of things outside of your control. But I was surprised to learn how much is in my control." Yet precisely what could be controlled was not clear. "Stress is probably really important. Infections during pregnancy may be important. Any kind of environmental influence could perturb programming."[36] The article's message to pregnant women was this: everything is potentially risky. You have control over fetal development, but we do not know how. Actions that you think are innocuous are probably harmful, but we cannot tell you which ones. This behavior might be more problematic at certain times in pregnancy, but we do not know when. It can produce either disastrous or moderately negative effects, but we cannot predict either one. Critics of prenatal science and the sense of responsibility and control it often inspires have noted that "womb-centric predictions of a child's future—whether rooted in supposed genetic disparities, gestational maternal-fetal conflict, eating habits during pregnancy, or whatever else—always undersell the role of one's later environment."[37] Nonetheless, armed with this kind of conditional information, pregnant women are warned that even mundane decisions can have irreversible consequences.

From forced caesarian sections and fetal homicide laws to the prosecution of women for drug use during pregnancy and the highly racialized and much publicized "crack baby" epidemic—which researchers now have demonstrated dramatically exaggerated the number of babies possibly affected and the teratogenicity of cocaine itself[38]—social panics have concretized an image of the fetus as imperiled by its mother.[39] Pregnant women who drink alcohol are held in particular contempt, although the overwhelming majority of women who consume alcohol during their pregnancies give birth to babies unaffected by fetal alcohol syndrome (FAS). Only about 5 percent of women who drink *heavily* give birth to babies exhibiting signs of FAS, and "there is no consistent, reliable evidence . . . to indicate that alcohol categorically affects fetal development regardless of level of exposure or timing of exposure, or absent other factors," including poverty and malnutrition.[40] But pregnant women who eschew alcohol reap the rewards that come with exercising self-control and behaving in socially responsible ways. An outgrowth, in part, of the antiabortion movement, the discourse of "fetal rights" suggests that babies have the right to be born with a sound mind and body, and the logic of neoliberalism in a risk culture suggests that social institutions will hold individual pregnant women responsible for protecting this right when possible.[41] In total motherhood, poor fetal outcomes are individual, not social, problems.

Meanwhile, men and fathers are largely absent from discussions of fetal rights. Pregnant women are warned about FAS, along with toxoplasmosis, salmonella, and listeriosis, but not about domestic violence, whose effects on maternal and fetal outcomes have been amply documented.[42] Critical links between fathers and fetuses are either ignored or disregarded. For example, while acrimonious debates surround women who choose to postpone childbearing, a growing body of research pointing to a higher incidence of autism and schizophrenia among children fathered by older men provokes little public discussion.[43] Cynthia Daniels, author of *Exposing Men: The Science and Politics of Male Reproduction*, demonstrated several gender disparities in the research and public discourse on fetal rights. Studies associating male reproductive exposures with miscarriage, fetal abnormalities, birth defects, and other health problems have been dismissed for methodological problems that are routinely tolerated in research on female exposures. In scientific journals, evidence for maternal risks to a fetus is presented as certain, compared with studies of male risks, whose conclusions tend to be tentative and qualified. In the media, science indicating male reproductive exposure risks is presented as idiosyncratic and less credible than female exposure risks. Women are portrayed as negligent and uninformed, whereas men are almost never presented as uniquely responsible. Involuntarily exposed to potentially harmful substances, unwitting conduits of harm, men appear as victims in much the same way as fetuses. "Debates over fetal rights are not so much about the prevention of fetal harm," Daniels argues, "as they are about the *social production of truth* about the nature of men's and women's relation to reproduction."[44] Less about "unborn children" than about mothers' obligation to guarantee fetal health, public discourse on the fetus is the epitome of total motherhood.

"Natural" Mothers

The recourse to "the natural," too, is a microcosm of total motherhood. In a risk culture, when virtually everything from conception through childbirth can ostensibly be either controlled or optimized, nature becomes a beacon, a respite from the complexity of a highly specialized world. The romanticization of what is organic, and therefore somehow more pure or authentic, provides an alternative to the pervasive and highly technical language of science, a discourse that threatens to take "the nature out of Mother Nature" and to upset "the 'natural order' of life."[45] Those who oppose interference in what they view as a natural reproductive process encourage pregnant women to "re-frame their thinking in order to regain their natural authority," to avoid routinized invasive procedures that "externalize the mother's body and wisdom, keeping her distanced from the trust she might otherwise learn to develop in herself," and to dispel "the negative messages we have all internalized—for example . . . that our bodies are not trustworthy [and] that our intuitive awareness is inferior to science and technology."[46] Natural mothering tells women that only they have the capacity to properly care for their babies, and in so doing it affirms the most basic principle of total motherhood: that mothers—not families or other institutions—are uniquely responsible for their babies' and children's well-being.

Critical of a society overly invested in consumerism, science, and individualism, advocates of natural mothering and family living nonetheless embrace these very institutions. Natural baby catalogs and mail order businesses, for example, offer nursing wear, noncompetitive toys, and other merchandise designed to enhance natural living and to satisfy consumer urges. These products, in addition to advice that natural mothers will make their own baby food, wash cloth diapers, and constantly "wear" their babies in slings, ignore the time, income, and flexibility necessary for natural mothering, resources that are unavailable to single or working mothers or families dependent on two incomes. In natural mothering advice, furthermore, the virtues of nature are filtered by science and expertise, and much of what opponents of medical intervention champion is less a rejection than a selective embrace of scientific authority. Natural childbirth and parenting are mediated by classes and experts, and books are written by authors whose credentials are prominently displayed next to their names. *The Natural Parent: Parenting from the Heart* was written by "parenting specialist" Jan Hunt.[47] Naturalmom.com offers articles and advice from "Pregnancy and Fertility Expert Herbalist" Susun Weed, whose books are recommended by "expert herbalists and well-known women's health physicians such as Susan Love MD, Christiane Northrup MD, Rosemary Gladstar, and David Hoffman."[48] Peggy O'Mara, editor and publisher of *Mothering*, the popular magazine of "natural family living," claims that her book, *Having a Baby, Naturally*, is based on "a register of over 9,000 controlled studies from almost 400 medical journals, in 18 different languages, from 85 different countries."[49]

Dubbed "America's pediatrician" and credited with coining the term "attachment parenting"—a concept that promotes each mother's constant physical and emotional attachment to her baby—William Sears offers counsel predicated on the belief that the best mothering is practiced independent of medical expertise, advice that actually draws its legitimacy from precisely that authority.[50] The eponymous Sears Parenting Library, composed of books written by Sears and his wife Martha, a nurse, is itself an example of the expert culture that infuses the discourse of total motherhood and about which Sears advocates a conscious skepticism.[51] These books on pregnancy and baby and child care frequently appeal to scientific research that highlights the potential risks of medical intervention. For example, Sears and Sears make sure to note that their objection to ultrasound screening is supported by a professor of obstetrics and gynecology at Harvard Medical School who chaired a National Institutes of Health task force on diagnostic ultrasound, that is, a scholar from a most prestigious medical school whose authority qualified him to chair a government committee.[52] The back cover of *The Baby Book* similarly seeks to establish Sears as an authority in pediatric science. He and his wife are "the pediatrics experts to whom American parents are increasingly turning for advice and information on all aspects of pregnancy, birth, child care, and family nutrition. Dr. Sears was trained at Harvard Medical School's Children's Hospital and Toronto's Hospital for Sick Children, the largest children's hospital in the world. He has practiced pediatrics for nearly thirty years. Martha Sears is a registered nurse, certified childbirth educator, and breastfeeding consultant." Sears' website adds that he is a fellow of the American Academy of Pediatrics (AAP) and the Royal College of Pediatricians.[53] In challenging women's reliance on emissaries of science, Sears and his wife position themselves as just such authorities.

The discourse of natural pregnancy and childbirth reveals the inevitability of science in a risk culture. "Natural" mothers dismiss trust in abstract authority and assume singular responsibility for their children, both hallmarks of total motherhood. They are liable for wading through a morass of information, ensuring optimal fetal development, managing pain in labor, and raising healthy and well-adjusted children. They are repeatedly advised to rely on their intuition when interacting with authorities and not to interfere with their bodies' natural reproductive functions. For these mothers, "good mothering practice is predicated on *trusting* that nature will resolve all parenting dilemmas,"[54] and the rules of nature constitute the kind of "abstract system" that Anthony Giddens argues has replaced the institutions of knowledge, such as class or religion, that dominated earlier modernity.[55] The surplus of both information and interpretive frames in a risk culture requires that people choose what to believe, and a philosophy of "the natural" is one among the many abstract systems of knowledge in which mothers can place their trust. At the same time that they wrest control from "science," mothers give themselves over to the logic of "nature," and in submitting to this authority, they resemble the scientifically oriented mothering they explicitly reject.[56]

Proponents of natural pregnancy also fail to understand that risk is omnipresent, that it inheres in every action, and that nothing is risk free. Sears and Sears suggest that even hypothetical risks should be avoided. They approvingly recount a story about their daughter-in-law's refusing to allow her obstetrician to use the Doptone monitor, which records the fetus's heartbeat, without explaining the full range of its costs and benefits. "Can you guarantee it won't harm my baby?" she asked the doctor. "Nobody knows for sure" if the monitor is safe, write the Sears, who embrace the recommendation of another obstetrician that "in the face of even theoretical risks, where there is no benefit, then the theoretical risks cannot be justified."[57] Yet no doctor can ever guarantee safety, and no practice is devoid of theoretical risks.[58] The Sears state that "there is no pain-relieving drug that has ever been proven to be totally safe for mother and baby" in childbirth.[59] But this is true, without exception, of every drug and consumer on the market; no medication has ever been shown to be completely safe for anyone. Likewise, as others have argued, pregnancy, and life in general, carry "an irreducible element of risk," which means that "pursuit of absolute zero risk to the fetus in clinical care or health policy is not only quixotic, it is disproportionate to how we think about risk elsewhere, including in the treatment of born children."[60] Sears and Sears selectively employ science in ways that exacerbate public misunderstanding of risk. They ignore costs and trade-offs, and they hold decision making in pregnancy to an impossible standard. In embracing the notion that mothers are responsible for eliminating all conceivable risks to their children, natural mothering furthers an ideology of total motherhood that is fundamentally similar to more mainstream approaches.

Whether they turn to science or nature or some combination of the two, what women internalize is a sense that proper attention to the mind and body will lead to conception, pregnancy, and a healthy child and that the inverse, the failure to cultivate mind and body, will inhibit a healthy outcome. Pregnancy in total motherhood literally embodies the essence of risk culture: the hyperawareness of potential danger, the illusion of control, and the conviction that proper planning can eliminate risk. It also reinforces neoliberal individualism in holding mothers uniquely responsible for protecting their fetuses from every imaginable danger. As Deborah Lupton, author of several books on risk, writes,

> More so than ever in the past pregnancy is portrayed as a series of events that are located within a sphere of rationalist control. Producing a "perfect" infant is seen to be at least partly a result of the woman's ability to exert control over the body, to seek and subscribe to expert advice and engage in self-sacrifice for the sake of her fetus.[61]

Whether practiced through science or nature, total motherhood denies mothers a subjectivity that is anything but maternally determined. If women are rational, they will devote themselves to creating the healthiest pregnancy; if women are naturally mothers, identity conflicts can develop only when women try to subvert nature. In both instances, the maternal and the personal are synonymous.

Maximizing Childhood

Negotiating conception, pregnancy, and childbirth is only the first stage of total motherhood. If good health in a risk culture is an indicator of a person's capacity to make wise choices, babies' physical and developmental well-being is a reflection of their mothers' discernment. Just as neoliberal individuals are expected to be healthy by engaging in constant self-surveillance, mothers are charged with monitoring virtually every dimension of their babies' and children's growth. Children no longer appear acceptable as they are or might develop on their own, and a recurring chorus—"that inattention to the needs of children leads to irreversible damage, and that lack of support leads to retarded development, if not under-achievement"—echoes throughout children's lives.[62] Like so many other institutions of authority in a risk culture, motherhood itself has become a less reliable guide. Experience, in other words, seems less valuable than it once was. Today's grandmothers, who put infants to sleep on their stomachs, left babies and toddlers in playpens, and allowed preschoolers to ride in the front seat, become less credible authorities as their daughters struggle to evaluate risks that their mothers could not have fathomed. What divides mothers across generations is not so much knowledge about child raising but expectations about what can be known. In a neoliberal culture, in which risk prevention is the moral obligation of individual citizens and the reach of science knows no bounds, babies and children must be continuously monitored, decisions constantly reevaluated in light of new information, and maternal identity perpetually remade. Mothering, therefore, is terminally reflexive, an ongoing process of warding off the potential shame of failing at total motherhood.

From birth, an infant is placed under medical observation. Each child has a unique trajectory that is compared with the development of others. Height, weight, and head circumference are measured, plotted, and evaluated in relation to "average" growth. Thus "even when the child is growing normally, the process of measurement simultaneously implies the possibilities of abnormality."[63] Although it is unclear when a single point on a growth chart, or a shift in development, is to be interpreted as problematic, every child is in constant danger of slipping further from the mean and closer to abnormal.[64] Babies, toddlers, and children undergo periodic "well checks" in which pediatricians survey their developmental progress in such areas as weight gain, head control, vocalizing, and muscle development. *What to Expect the First Year* advises that "all babies reach milestones on their own developmental time line" and assures each reader that "your baby's rate of development is normal for your baby." At the same time, the book offers a month-by-month guide to what each baby "should be able," "will probably be able," "may possibly be able," and "may even be able" to do, constantly reminding mothers of how their babies are progressing compared with others. For example, in the fifth month, a baby "should be able" to do the following: "hold head steady when upright; on stomach, raise chest, supported by arms; pay attention to an object as small as a raisin (but keep such objects out of baby's reach); squeal in delight; reach for an object; smile spontaneously; smile back when you smile; grasp a rattle held to backs or tips of fingers; [and] keep head level with body when pulled to sitting."[65] But what about a baby who does not perform one or more of these tasks? Is she normal or delayed? Does she have her "own developmental time line," or is she developmentally impaired? As during pregnancy, mothers must make sense of abundant and often contradictory information and be on the lookout for potential problems. *What to Expect the First Year* and other guides can help mothers identify problems early in their babies' lives, but they also promote the exaggerated sense of control and responsibility that is characteristic of life in a risk culture.

Total motherhood is marked by interminable decision making, and the number of choices and the volume of information required to make them are staggering. The retail business for baby products, for example, simultaneously creates and provides for a seemingly infinite set of baby needs. Marketers estimate that mothers spend $1.7 trillion a year and $700 million on toys for babies between birth and age two alone; books and advice abound on how to tap this "mom market."[66] As Susan J. Douglas and Meredith W. Michaels, authors of *The Mommy Myth*, write, "Conspicuous consumption has conquered childhood, motherhood, and the nursery, making just the normal acquisition of a plain old crib and stroller seem, well, negligent, or at the very least, withholding."[67] Created in 1996 to capitalize on the burgeoning market for baby products, Babies "R" Us offers a "New Parents' Checklist" with ninety-nine "essentials," some of which comprise multiple items, such as "toys for 0–12 months" and "Baby Boys'/Girls' Clothes."[68] Each purchase is fraught with implications for a baby's well-being, for a mother's sense of herself as a mother, and sometimes for politics. Should the baby wear cloth or disposable diapers? Which is more natural? Which will produce fewer rashes? Which is worse for the environment, the use of water to wash cloth diapers or the landfills required to contain disposables? What kind of pacifier will promote normal jaw development, latex or silicon, round tipped or orthodontic? Which mobile is best? The one that winds up and spins, or the one that is remotely controlled, plays Bach, Mozart, and Beethoven, and "combines 3 different movements and motions, not just the usual circular motion, to captivate and stimulate baby's developing senses [and keep] baby concentrated and interested at all times"?[69] No dimension of baby's existence is without the potential to be optimized through consumption, and no purchase is devoid of long-term implications.

"Be eternally vigilant," warns *What to Expect the First Year* in an admonition taken almost literally at one Babies "R" Us store.[70] On entering, shoppers immediately encounter a kiosk advertising "Baby Safety Events" taking place in the store and sponsored by various baby product companies. Patrons can attend a "Baby Safety Expo," participate in "Safe Home, Safe Baby" clinics, or register for a seminar on "Babies, Bellies, Booties . . . and Baby Safety," the last of which is available only to mothers who enroll in the gift registry. The first display in the infant section is for audio and video monitors that allow parents to keep tabs on what is happening in a baby's room from anywhere in the house. Some come equipped with motion sensors that sound an alarm if no movement, such as breathing, is detected. Also in the safety section are rail teethers that prevent babies who chew on their cribs from getting splinters; gates to confine babies to safe spaces; finger-pinch guards; locks for cabinets, refrigerators, drawers, and toilets; corner cushions and furniture bumpers; covers for stove and oven knobs and outlets; rear-view-mirror attachments that allow drivers to watch babies in the back seat; knee-protectors for crawling babies; and many other items. A large placard offers advice from Babies "R" Us identifying the features of various safety products and pointing out what consumers should consider.

Safety advice encapsulates many of the dilemmas of science in a risk culture. For example, it demonstrates reflexivity. For decades, mothers were told to put babies down for sleep on their stomachs to reduce the possibility that they would choke on their own vomit. In 1992, based on evidence of a correlation between prone sleeping and sudden infant death syndrome (SIDS), the American Academy of Pediatrics (AAP) issued a policy statement switching course and directing that healthy infants be positioned on their side or back.[71] In 1996, the AAP's Task Force on Infant Position and SIDS restated the risks of the prone position but stressed that the supine was superior to the side position. It also noted that no evidence existed for earlier concerns about aspiration.[72] By 2000, the AAP disavowed side sleeping altogether and credited the supine position with "dramatic decreases in the SIDS rates" in various countries.[73] Yet the "Back to Sleep Campaign," sponsored by the AAP, the Consumer Products Safety Commission, and the National Institute of Child Health and Human Development, took place at the same time as various diagnostic and behavioral shifts, and the precise impact of having babies sleep on their backs is difficult to determine. Fewer babies might be dying of SIDS, for example, at least partially because deaths that once were unexplainable now fall into other diagnostic categories. Indeed, in its 2005 policy statement, the AAP acknowledged that at least some of the decrease in the incidence of SIDS "may be a result of coding shifts to other causes of unexpected deaths."[74]

The effect of back sleeping on SIDS is ambiguous in other ways as well. As with much health advice in a risk culture, recommendations regarding sleep and SIDS are drawn from epidemiological studies designed to determine the probability that a particular behavior or exposure is associated with SIDS in the general population, with research finding that babies who died from SIDS—roughly one death per two thousand live births[75]—are more likely to have been prone than on their backs. Inferences drawn from this research are vulnerable to what social scientists call the ecological fallacy, a statistical error in which individuals are assumed to have all the characteristics of the group to which they belong. As the task force made clear—albeit in its report published in the AAP's professional journal, a venue unlikely to reach many lay people—the most recent recommendations

> were developed to reduce the risk of SIDS in the general population. . . . Scientifically identified associations between risk factors (e.g. socioeconomic characteristics, behaviors, or environmental exposures) and outcomes such as SIDS do not necessarily denote causality . . . [and] it is fundamentally misguided to focus on a single risk factor or to attempt to quantify risk for an individual infant.[76]

In fact, SIDS organizations report that as many as two-thirds of babies who die from SIDS have no known risk factors.[77] How, then, should mothers make sense of the task force's recommendations?

Putting babies to sleep on their backs creates both its own risks and increased monitoring responsibilities for mothers, thereby further demonstrating the reflexive nature of science in a risk culture. Many of the task force's recommendations are designed to reduce babies' arousal threshold, thereby making it more likely that they will awake if they are in distress. Yet the neurocognitive consequences of chronically reducing "slow-wave sleep" during the first year of brain development are unknown. It also is possible that a baby exhausted from waking frequently will eventually fall into a deeper sleep and develop a higher arousal threshold, which might mean an increase in the SIDS risk.[78] Babies who spend a large amount of time on their backs, furthermore, are more likely to develop positional plagiocephaly, or "flat head," which the task force recommends can be prevented by "placing the infant to sleep with the head to 1 side for a week or so and then changing to the other and periodically changing the orientation of the infant to outside activity (e.g. the door of the room)." Back sleepers are also more likely to develop an aversion to being on their stomachs, which can retard the development of the arm muscles necessary to crawl, so mothers need to make sure that babies get adequate "tummy time" when they are awake. Upright "cuddle time" is encouraged.[79] Reflexive mothers, in other words, reduce both risks and the risks that result from risk-reducing behavior. Babies "R" Us offers sleep positioners and monitors that purport to detect when an infant has stopped breathing. The AAP does not endorse these products, especially as a substitute for its explicit recommendations, but they are likely to make sense in a risk culture that expects comprehensive risk-reduction from mothers.

The monitoring imperative extends throughout childhood, when mothers are exhorted to watch for any sign of delayed development. The AAP has a formal policy advocating the "developmental surveillance and screening" of all children for potential disabilities,[80] and parenting magazines exhort mothers to pay close attention to developmental milestones. "Many children don't necessarily have autism, but they have 'almost autism,'" warns a magnified quotation from a psychologist, under a photo of a smiling toddler and his mother, in a popular parenting magazine.[81] While the symptoms of autism, particularly on the high-functioning end of the spectrum, can be ambiguous, signs of an "almost" autistic child no doubt will encompass a range of putatively normal behavior. Just as individuals in a risk culture wrestle with a constant state of "pre-illness," mothers must monitor their children for signs of being not quite sick. Is an inability to stack four blocks by the age of two a sign of cognitive or motor impairment? Does a failure to use prepositions by three years of age demonstrate a learning disability? Is taunting the family pet evidence of a mood disorder? In a risk culture, responsible motherhood demands attention even to potential pathology. Furthermore, when "invisible disabilities," such as psychological disorders, are diagnosed, the expectation of maternal surveillance can extend to children's adulthood; and even when these illnesses are deemed to be neurochemical in origin, neoliberal mothers can blame themselves for inadequately protecting or seeking out care for their special-needs children.[82]

Schools and the media treat raising children as a project of "concerted cultivation" to be carried out by mothers.[83] Sociologist Annette Lareau demonstrated that even children from lower-income families, in which parents seek less to encourage children's development than to enable their "natural growth," attend schools that are staffed by teachers and administrators whose expectations are based on concerted cultivation.[84] This strategy of constant and deliberate enrichment in child raising reveals the neoliberal orientation of American risk culture. As German sociologist Elisabeth Beck-Gernsheim describes it,

All possible flaws must be corrected (no more squinting, stuttering, bed-wetting), all possible talents must be stimulated (boom time for piano lessons, language holidays, tennis in summer and ski courses in winter). Countless guides to education and upbringing appear on the book and magazine market. As different as each one is, at bottom they all have a similar message: the success of the child is defined as the private duty and responsibility of the parents/the mother.[85]

Moreover, in Lareau's analysis of how different social classes approach child raising, it was mothers who most dramatically restructured their lives. Mothers were more likely than fathers to alter their career paths, manage information, and organize home labor. As Lareau described one set of parents, "He helped her."[86] Madeline Levine, author of the popular *The Price of Privilege: How Parental Pressure and Material Advantage Are Creating a Generation of Disconnected and Unhappy Kids*, suggests that middle-class children are suffering from a "maladaptive perfectionism."

> Between accelerated academic courses, multiple extracurricular activities, premature preparation for high school or college, special coaches and tutors engaged to wring the last bit of performance out of them, many kids find themselves scheduled to within an inch of their lives. Criticism and even rejection become commonplace as competitive parents continue to push their children toward higher levels of accomplishment.

Yet Levine, too, finds in mothers the antidote to this debilitating perfectionism. "It is emotional closeness, maternal warmth in particular, that is as close as we get to a silver bullet against psychological impairment."[87]

Breastfeeding and Total Motherhood

Total motherhood structures both the science and the practice of breastfeeding. In research comparing formula feeding and breastfeeding, studies almost always rely on maternal characteristics—such as mothers' BMI, IQ, or smoking history—to measure possible genetic influences on babies' health, a practice that ignores paternal genetic contributions and might well distort the effects of breastfeeding. Those studies that mention the possibility that behavior associated with breastfeeding is responsible for the benefits attributed to breastfeeding refer almost exclusively to maternal behavior, thereby reflecting and reinforcing assumptions about the unique responsibilities of mothers in child development. Moreover, as Jules Law observed, most studies of breastfeeding assume a normatively gendered division of domestic labor. Researchers and funding institutions typically believe that even small benefits to babies are worth pursuing because they assume that mothers should be primarily invested in child care and, therefore, that advantages to babies from this arrangement are without cost.[88]

However, it is worth considering whether a comparably reduced risk for obesity, diabetes, or infections would inspire the same scientific zeal if it required an equivalent commitment to domestic labor from fathers. Would such a risk reduction be as compelling to scientists if it demanded of fathers the comprehensive physical and emotional engagement that breastfeeding requires of mothers? If fathers, not mothers, could breastfeed, would the health benefits to babies appear to be as medically urgent? Science takes place in a social context, and the questions it asks reflect the dominant values of the culture in which it operates. Infant feeding research is structured in ways that reflect and reinforce the principles of total motherhood, but the veneer of scientific objectivity conceals this moral bias and makes maternal sacrifice appear less ideological than pragmatic. In this view, breastfeeding is the treatment that has the most health benefits for the child; it is simply good science, no more and no less.[89]

A research agenda not invested in total motherhood might measure nonmaternal dimensions of infant feeding, such as the relationship between fathers' engagement and various outcomes. How do variations in fathers' patterns of behavior, including bottle feeding, influence babies' social and cognitive development and their attachment to fathers? Are the results different for breast milk or formula? How does regulated formula feeding compare with regulated breast milk intake when measuring obesity, diabetes, and heart disease? Is consistent feeding with both mother and father—or with two mothers or fathers or a single parent—associated with outcomes different from exclusive feeding with either or one mother or father? Such studies would be limited by constraints similar to those in the existing infant-feeding research: reliable information on feeding practices is elusive, and interventions are difficult to isolate from confounding variables on the lengthy paths between intervention, or independent variables, and outcome, or dependent variables. But these problems have not prevented voluminous and ongoing research on breastfeeding, and researchers could easily formulate hypotheses, subject to the same methodological limitations, that do not assume maternal responsibility. Such questions would be no less *scientifically* viable, and if they appear to be, it is precisely because total motherhood is an ideologically implicit dimension of contemporary infant-feeding research. Whether it is inherently better for babies to attach more significantly to mothers instead of fathers or to one person instead of two or several are not abstract but social questions. That a father-baby attachment through feeding is rarely addressed in infant-feeding research simultaneously reveals and solidifies a long-standing pattern of social organization. It reifies a social arrangement, mother-infant attachment, as metaphysically normative.

Steeped in the self-monitoring, external surveillance, and attribution and internalization of responsibility that mark motherhood from before conception, the practice of breastfeeding also is integral to total motherhood. Good mothers consider their own physical and emotional health to the extent that it does not interfere with breastfeeding, which reduces risk to their babies. The recourse to "the natural," with all its attendant contradictions, is commonplace in breastfeeding advocacy, as are the failure to appreciate the moral dimension of risk, the ideological assumptions grounding what is conceptualized as risky, and the inevitability of risk. If risk disputes reveal value conflicts in a given society,[90] risk accords likewise can represent communal agreement. In the case of breastfeeding, the virtual unanimity surrounding its benefits amounts to a social consensus that risks to children are most important to address when they can be managed by mothers, and, by extension, that mothers are culturally responsible for reducing risks to their children. Indeed, mothers who bottle-feed often find themselves defending the practice in ways that demonstrate breastfeeding's power to signal commitment to total motherhood and responsible citizenship.

Women are instructed to think about how they intend to feed their babies early in pregnancy. "Read! Read! Read!" the La Leche League (LLL) advises women as they consider how to feed their newborns.[91] Just about all advice indicates that breastfeeding is the optimal form of nutrition. For example, *What to Expect When You're Expecting* and the ACOG state that infant feeding is every mother's choice, but they also stress unequivocally that breastfeeding is best. The former includes one and a half pages on "Why Breast Is Best" and one-half page on "Why Some Prefer the Bottle." Reasons for not breastfeeding are restricted to serious debilitating illness, severe infection, use of medication that is unsafe for babies, exposure to toxic chemicals in the workplace, AIDS, drug abuse, and "a deep-seated aversion to the idea of breastfeeding." Otherwise, in advice echoed by the ACOG, all new mothers should consider giving breastfeeding a try.[92] *Our Bodies, Ourselves*, the primer of the women's health movement and now in its twelfth edition, tells women that breastfeeding protects children against many short-term and chronic health problems and strengthens their resistance to infection and disease. The authors also claim that lactation has many benefits for mothers, including "a greatly reduced incidence of breast cancer," even though research has not consistently found that breastfeeding reduces this risk and has not distinguished the effects of breastfeeding from the behavior of women who breastfeed.[93]

The Sears, who are outspoken opponents of formula feeding, contend that breastfeeding is better for a baby's brain, eyes, ears, mouth, throat, kidneys, appendix, urinary tract, joints and muscles, skin, growth, and bowels, as well as its respiratory, heart, circulatory, digestive, immune, and endocrine system. They also suggest that breastfeeding has myriad incidental advantages. For instance, whereas the foul-smelling stools of formula-fed infants cause their mothers and fathers to cringe while changing diapers, the "not unpleasant, buttermilk-like odor" of breast milk stools are inoffensive. "When the baby looks at the face of the diaper-changing caregiver and sees happiness rather than disgust, he picks up a good message about himself—perhaps a perk for building self-esteem."[94] In a section of *The Baby Book*, the Sears advise pregnant women on how to ready themselves for breastfeeding. While the most recent edition no longer recommends a "prenatal nipple exam," it does offer clear advice on how to prepare the breasts for breastfeeding. Soap, which will cause nipples to dry out and crack during nursing, should be avoided. Concerns about inverted nipples may be taken up with a lactation consultant. Practicing breast massage during pregnancy will increase women's comfort handling their breasts and also will facilitate manual expression of breast milk after the baby is born. The Sears further advise pregnant women to enroll in a breastfeeding class, to learn the Sears-developed "right-start" techniques for proper positioning and latching on, and to join a breastfeeding support group.[95]

In public discourse, "breast or bottle" is an overdetermined opposition in which good mothers must opt for the former. Breastfeeding.com has a page entitled "Baby Formula Label, Want a Scare?" which lists the components of infant formula.[96] Some of these ingredients, the page points out, also exist in junk food. Whey, a by-product of cheese production, is mischaracterized as "waste" that has been added to formula. "Aren't you glad that the manufacturers now have a profitable way to dispose of their former waste products?" the page asks, suggesting that whey is more like toxic sludge than the family of common food by-products—including bran, germ, molasses, and gelatin—to which it belongs. It also neglects to mention that whey is a standard ingredient in such foods as bread and crackers and that whey protein is a regular dietary supplement. While the amount and composition of whey vary among infant formulas and between formula and breast milk, and scientists do disagree as to which is optimal, the consensus is that whey has nutritional value. The webpage ends by recounting the stories of two women whose decision to breast-feed might have saved their babies' lives. One had been stuck in a truck for five days during a snowstorm; another had been trapped without water for a week after Hurricane Andrew. The message to mothers is clear: it is your responsibility to feed your baby, under any circumstances. If you choose the bottle and your baby dies in a snowstorm—or, by implication, in any dire situation, regardless of its likelihood—it will be your fault. "Most people don't expect to have a disaster befall them. But acts of war, environmental accidents, and natural disasters are a part of life."[97]

For some proponents, breastfeeding confirms the virtues of nature and natural mothering. In this narrative, the "condensation of breast-feeding, maternal intuition, and maternal biology elevates 'nature' as the medium of a moral order in which mothers naturally (hormonally) fulfill their maternal potential."[98] Like hospitals, fetal monitors, and epidurals, here the bottle becomes a harmful intervention in the natural reproductive process, a substitute that can subvert nature's design and destabilize the hormonal underpinnings of good mothering. "Breastfeeding plays a critical role in nature's plan for ensuring that human babies survive and grow," writes the LLL in the most recent edition of *The Womanly Art of Breastfeeding*, the league's hallmark guide to breastfeeding. "Artificial feeding—formula feeding—is a substantial departure from nature's plan." Suckling stimulates the production of prolactin, the so-called mothering hormone that LLL and many other breastfeeding advocates contend enhances maternal intuition. "Nature intends for mothers to enjoy breastfeeding their babies, and the good feelings that come with breastfeeding help mothers become more attached to their babies."[99] According to anthropologist Katherine Dettwyler, a prominent breastfeeding advocate, millions of years of evolution indicate that the "natural" duration of breastfeeding for modern humans is somewhere between two and one-half and seven years and that humans, as mammals, are programmed to expect breast milk. Formula feeding is part of a pernicious culturalization in which women pit their own and their children's bodies against nature and, in the process, inhibit the natural attachment between mother and child.[100]

This "romance of the natural mother,"[101] however, is a partial story. It implies that what is natural is inherently superior, a premise that is not grounded in science. It ignores the myriad ways that scientific intervention has improved and prolonged life. It also conceals that breastfeeding and breast milk are "endorsed and managed by science," scoured by scientists from multiple disciplines and endlessly "analyzed and labeled scientifically" in a process of "recreating 'natural' on-demand feeding through expert intervention."[102] In fact, it is scientific authority, particularly the claim that research demonstrates breastfeeding's superiority, on which contemporary breastfeeding promotion largely depends, and this is true even for many advocates committed to a philosophy of natural mothering. Long wary of medicine's intervention in the "natural" process of mothering, for example, the LLL stresses "the unique importance of one mother helping another" and has as its mission to facilitate "mother-to-mother" support.[103] The league's position on the value of science, writes Bernice Hausman, is that "science should support and enhance nature"; that "all information needs the mediating presence of the breastfeeding mother"; and that "mother-to-mother support means that any scientific information is distilled and processed through the experience of a mother."[104] The league, in short, has been profoundly suspicious of medical authority.

In recent decades, however, as research has increasingly suggested that breastfeeding has health benefits for babies, the LLL has turned more to science to make its case. It also has promoted various artificial means to facilitate breastfeeding, such as tube-feeding systems for mothers having trouble establishing an adequate milk supply or persuading newborns to latch on properly to the breast. For example, it promotes the Medela Supplemental Nursing System, "two thin tubes, taped to each breast, [that] deliver a supplement to the nursing baby from a plastic container that hangs around the mother's neck." It also supports the Medela Hazelbaker FingerFeeder, in which milk comes through a tube attached to the mother's finger, which is then placed in the baby's mouth.[105] These devices challenge the conceptual boundaries of "the natural." As Hausman writes, they are part of

a de-naturalized repertoire of techniques and substitutions to correct the errancies of "natural" breastfeeding. . . . The League's representation of the mother who must learn to be natural and who uses science as the ideological evidentiary support for her natural mothering practices appears consistently throughout the six editions of *The Womanly Art of Breastfeeding.*

This judicious recourse to science "exerts a certain tension on the League philosophy of the mother as knowledgeable expert in her own domain."[106] It suggests that natural mothers do not reject science but rather invoke and deploy it selectively.

The promotion of breastfeeding as natural, moreover, wrongly implies both that nature is hermetically sealed from culture and that all mothers can choose to breastfeed and lead natural lives. Neither breast milk nor the process of feeding from the breast is immune to "unnatural" influences. Breastfeeding, like bottle feeding, is a cultured process, and no social context is without consequence for the breastfed baby. What mothers breathe and eat is transmitted to babies via breastfeeding, so their exposure to chemicals or pollutants and their consumption of genetically modified, organic, or processed food enmesh breastfed babies in a sprawling network of social processes. Often babies' exposures are heavily determined by mothers' socioeconomic status. Lower-income women, for example, are more likely to live in polluted areas and to consume cheaper and more calorie-dense foods, practices that affect the putatively natural composition of breast milk.[107] They also are more likely to work in environments in which frequent breaks for breast pumping are not possible, jobs that can make choosing to breastfeed and to live a more natural life nearly impossible.

Breastfeeding mothers, furthermore, can be as vulnerable to a socially imposed feeding schedule, one that accommodates the rhythms of different lives, as can those who bottle-feed. Indeed, not all breastfeeding societies produce the same feeding patterns, and not every breastfed baby feeds at the same intervals. Every baby is born into a culture, whether it is the often discussed !Kung San of southern Africa, in which mothers feed their babies semicontinuously, or middle-class American suburbia, in which babies feed in multiple discrete sessions at the breast or bottle. Hausman notes that "all patterns of infant feeding are cultural impositions on babies,"[108] and this is true whether these patterns are rooted in hunter-gatherer or industrial societies. Said differently, there is no unmediated space in which a baby is untouched by culture. The ubiquity of culture does not in itself preclude the possibility that one method of feeding might have advantages over another, but it does problematize the assertion that breastfeeding is superior *because* it is natural for mammals.

Finally, breastfeeding mothers are not immune to the current maternal culture of consumption that natural mothers vehemently criticize. For example, mothers can purchase a special nursing shirt that "incorporates the latest research in infant development by using patterns designed to stimulate babies' vision" and that provides "the equivalent of a visual workout for the baby."[109] Babies "R" Us lists 181 products for "bottle feeding," but it also carries 111 for "breastfeeding," including breast cream, nipple pads, nursing wraps, and reminder bracelets that indicate from which breast the baby last fed. A Medela Pump in Style breast pump costs around $275, and accessories—milk storage bags, "BPA-free" bottles, replacement parts—add additional expenses.[110] These products reveal a broad gulf between many middle-class women's fantasy of breastfeeding as a natural experience and the consumer project that it ultimately becomes.[111] They also expose the lie of many advocates' claims that breastfeeding is "free" and readily carried out even by low-income working mothers. Breastfeeding does not take place outside culture. Rather, it is a practice in which, as Linda Blum contends, "the cultural and corporeal merge, collide, twist, turn, and feed each other; they cannot be sorted into the truth and ultimate goodness of the 'natural' and the false, ultimately oppressive realm of the 'man-made.'"[112]

If a mother has chosen to breastfeed, according to most advice, both the practice and the surveillance of breastfeeding begin immediately after birth. A newborn should be placed on the mother's chest, skin to skin, and encouraged to feed immediately; most babies will find their way to the breast on their own, and the vast majority can be placed there within minutes of birth. Success in these early moments is crucial to continued breastfeeding. Moreover, mother and baby should be together in the hospital at all times, and efforts to separate them should be vigorously resisted. "There is *absolutely no medical reason* for healthy mothers and babies to be separated from each other, even for short periods," contends breastfeeding.com. Supplementary feeding with water, sugar water, or formula is rarely needed. Bottles are to be avoided, as milk flows more easily from latex and silicon nipples and might discourage babies from mastering the more difficult task of drawing milk from the breast.[113] "Lead mother not into temptation," warn Sears and Sears against the formula samples included in hospital discharge packs.[114] Here formula is sin, and exhausted mothers should not have it in their homes lest they succumb. In her twenty-four- to forty-eight-hour postpartum hospital stay, a new mother might have her breastfeeding monitored by a nursery nurse, a lactation specialist from her pediatrician's office, and a lactation consultant from the U.S. Department of Agriculture's Special Supplemental Nutrition Program for Women, Infants, and Children (WIC), each of whom may offer different and often contradictory technical advice. In 2008, vital statistics registrars reported that forty-two states and Puerto Rico collected, or would collect by 2010, breastfeeding data on birth certificates before mothers leave the hospital.[115]

As the focus of concern shifts from the fetus to the baby, from the womb as the "fetal environment" to the breast as milk machine, the mother is transformed from a fetal container to a milk producer. Like the fetus, conceptualized as a distinct entity vulnerable to the womb that sustains it, breast milk becomes the fetishized product of the breast that produces it. In both cases, women are disembodied, or reduced to wombs and breasts.[116] Women who monitored their lives with an eye toward conception, pregnancy, and birth now must track their behavior for its potential effects on the quantity and quality of their milk production. Having been told that a healthy diet would enhance fertility and optimize fetal development, breastfeeding mothers are now advised to monitor what they eat for evidence that particular foods are causing problems for their babies. Together, *What to Expect When You're Expecting* and *What to Expect the First Year* recommend increasing calories, calcium, and foods high in "brain-building DHA"; taking a vitamin formulated for pregnant or lactating women; limiting intake of foods containing preservatives, artificial colors and flavors, stabilizers, herbs, caffeine, and alcohol; avoiding residual pesticides by purchasing certified, organically grown produce and scrubbing other fruit and vegetable skins with produce wash; and minimizing exposure to mercury by limiting fish consumption.[117]

The LLL and other breastfeeding advocates recommend that mothers be particularly careful when they suspect colic, an unexplained condition in which babies cry uncontrollably for extended lengths of time. Infants with colic might be sensitive to particular foods in mothers' diets, and the Sears and breastfeeding.com recommend that mothers of colicky babies avoid an all-encompassing list of "colic-causing foods": dairy products, caffeine (coffee, tea, soda), soy products, peanuts, shellfish, chocolate, citrus fruits, wheat, chicken, beef, eggs, nuts, corn, the iron in prenatal vitamins, and gassy vegetables (broccoli, cauliflower, cabbage, onions, green peppers, tomatoes).[118] Colic, however, is loosely and variably defined. The AAP cautions that "if your baby cries and cries, no matter how you try to comfort her, the cause may be colic," and *What to Expect the First Year* suggests that 20 percent of babies have crying spells severe enough to be labeled colic.[119] The problem in identifying colic is that most babies cry, and "uncontrolled crying" is an ambiguous symptom; exhausted new mothers, whom the LLL, Sears, and others advise should breastfeed their babies for around an hour between eight and twelve times a day, might well interpret it broadly and assume colic. They are then likely to modify their diets or other routines because the principle that mothers can and should prevent any risk to babies, cost notwithstanding, tells them to behave in ways that have even the possibility of alleviating babies' distress.

Studies have suggested that stress, which women were cautioned could reduce fertility and put fetuses at risk, can also interfere with breastfeeding by preventing lactation or reducing the release of oxytocin, the hormone responsible for triggering women's milk-ejection reflex.[120] According to Sears and Sears, stress can also interfere with the hormones that make milk, and chronic, unresolved stress alters the biochemical equilibrium of the breastfeeding mother. Because only she can provide milk that is custom-made for her baby, they advise mother to relax and remember that "the milk you are giving your baby is going to raise his IQ and lower the risk of every major illness." The implication is that not breastfeeding will compromise baby's IQ and increase the risk of every major illness, advice that is at least as likely to exacerbate, rather than reduce, a mother's stress, which she otherwise has been instructed to control. "When you believe in your breasts, they will work for you. If you don't believe you can breastfeed, you set yourself up for all the problems that lead to failure. A doubt can become a self-fulfilling prophecy."[121] Breastfeeding failure, in this scenario, is personal, or the mother's fault; it results not from cultural or economic obstacles—poverty, a low-paying job, racism, sexism, or unreasonable expectations of mothers—but from a lack of confidence. In the late nineteenth and early twentieth century, doctors often recommended that mothers periodically give their babies bottles in order to relieve some of the strain of breastfeeding. Physicians argued that these bottles were necessary to keep mothers calm and happy so that their nerves would not interfere with the production of high-quality breast milk.[122] The concept of "relief bottles," as they were called, and the notion that the suffering of mothers themselves might be alleviated stand in stark contrast to current talk of "supplemental bottles." Whereas relief bottles at least implied attention to the mother—that she might be given some respite or reprieve—the current language of supplemental feeding shifts attention to the baby and concerns the mother largely as an inadequate breast.

A breastfeeding mother is often advised to consider her physical and emotional well-being in relation to the "needs" of her baby. The Sears' point of departure is babies' needs and the necessity of breastfeeding, both of which are predicated on an uninterrupted physical connection between mothers and babies. In a discussion of postpartum depression in *The Breast-feeding Book*, for example, they caution that independence is not good for mothers. "As you build your relationship with your baby, think of the two of you as *interdependent*. Each needs the other, and each has something to give to the other." "Respect your need to nest and nurse," they tell struggling women. "Do something every day just for yourself," but "choose something that does not require separation from your baby." Self-help measures for maternal depression are best for babies, and they require self-discipline, "but your desire to continue breastfeeding will be a powerful motivation." "Abrupt weaning can make depression worse," the Sears admonish. "Women who must wean quickly may feel devastated and may grieve for the end of their breastfeeding relationship with their baby. This feeling is more intense than when weaning was not the mother's choice."[123] On his website, Sears addresses depression only as it affects breast milk, in a discussion of antidepressants under the heading "Taking Medication While Breastfeeding." Here as well, he warns depressed mothers that discontinuing breastfeeding is harmful to babies.[124] In total motherhood, as Sears demonstrates, a mother cares for herself largely to the extent that she can simultaneously provide what is optimal for her baby, including breastfeeding.

The LLL underscores the need to breastfeed in the face of maternal depression. On its website, one woman described how breastfeeding became her reason to live. Another recounted how she breastfed her toddler and baby during a postpartum psychosis; still another mother, with bipolar disorder, explained how she managed breastfeeding in spite of her illness.[125] An LLL Internet article points to the risks to babies of untreated maternal depression:

> Research has shown that a mother who is struggling with depression will have trouble being a good mother to her baby. The baby's development depends on having a responsive caregiver. Babies' brains develop their many networks of nerves and information in response to the myriad daily interactions between the mother and baby. Babies learn social behavior, language, and a great deal more from eye-to-eye contact with mother, from her animated facial expressions, vocal responses, and the like. A mother who has no energy to get out of bed or to engage her baby in "conversation" is unable to meet these needs. At the same time, the depressed mother is robbed herself of the day-to-day happiness of mothering her baby and other children.[126]

If they are depressed, women can be neither effective nor happy mothers. Their needs *as individuals* are invisible.[127] The article goes on to describe the physical and emotional risks of early weaning, making clear both that mothers must be treated so they can provide for their babies and that any remedy must not interfere with breastfeeding.

Breastfeeding mothers are exhorted to watch for cues to babies' needs and to adhere to a standardized regimen of pediatrician visits. "The baby shows long before he starts crying that he is ready to feed," advises breastfeeding.com, and attentive mothers will recognize changes in breathing, vocalizing, or stretching as signs of hunger.[128] Products such as the Dunstan Baby Language Program or the WhyCry Baby Crying Analyzer claim to help mothers distinguish hunger cries from those expressing boredom, sleepiness, annoyance, or discomfort from gas.[129] The ultimate monitor, however, is the pediatrician's scale. A serious medical condition notwithstanding, a baby's health in the early weeks and months is measured largely by what she or he weighs. At every well check, a nurse places the baby on a scale that registers weight in ounces; pediatricians recommend that the same scale be used at every visit to ensure accuracy. Weight reflects consumption, and adequate weight gain demonstrates a mother's success as a milk producer. For a breastfeeding mother, therefore, responsibility is practically absolute, and a "failure to thrive" diagnosis is as much hers as her baby's.

Breastfeeding proponents who stress the putative risks of not breastfeeding tend to ignore both the social context in which risk decisions are made, including those about costs and trade-offs, and the moral dimension of risk analysis. As I discuss in the next chapter, even if the medical benefits to breastfeeding were compellingly demonstrated, the decision to breastfeed, or not to formula-feed, carries its own risks, and these trade-offs are largely rationalized or ignored in pro-breastfeeding discourse. One of the rare critics to challenge breastfeeding on both scientific and social grounds, Jules Law argues that risk analyses regarding infant feeding are based on the presumption of a gendered division of domestic labor and that breastfeeding advocacy reveals a "gendered double standard of risk assessment" in which the costs of breastfeeding for women are downplayed or ignored because their labor as mothers is normative.[130] While evidence suggests that in the aggregate, married fathers today spend more time with their children than fathers did in the past, married and single mothers still perform the overwhelming majority of routine and interactive child care.[131] Nonetheless, the problem with discussions of children's health in breastfeeding discourse is less that women are the presumptive maternal laborers than that as mothers they seem to lose their status as women, or as individuals, and therefore that they are not stakeholders in risk assessment. If mothers do not own their emotional, mental, and physical time, then the costs to them are not real. If they do not exist as subjects independent of their babies, then trade-offs need not be calculated. Total motherhood, as Douglas and Michaels argue in regard to the new momism, "is not about subservience to men. It is about *subservience to children*."[132] The double standard, in other words, is less about gender than it is about motherhood.

Breastfeeding in a Risk Culture

If breastfeeding reinforces long-standing notions of maternal obligation, it also serves in a risk culture to help manage anxiety about primary relationships that are no longer held together in traditional ways. The mother-child connection and the intimacy of breastfeeding provide something of an antidote to the tenuousness of what Anthony Giddens describes as "pure relationships," commitments that exist not because of biology, cultural obligation, or kinship criteria but only because they provide emotional satisfaction to the individuals involved.[133] As Ulrich Beck observes, the child today "is the source of the last *remaining, irrevocable, unexchangeable primary relationship*. Partners come and go. The child stays. Everything that is desired, but not realizable in the relationship, is directed to the child." He points to the "excessive affection for children, the 'staging of childhood' which is granted to them—the poor, overloved creatures" as evidence of widespread yearning for lasting relationships or for "an anachronistic social experience." In reflexive modernity,

> the child becomes the *final alternative to loneliness* that can be built up against the vanishing possibilities of love. It is the *private type of re-enchantment*, which arises with, and derives its meaning from, disenchantment. The number of births is declining, but the importance of the child is *rising*.[134]

In Beck's analysis, total motherhood represents the convergence of an unconscious mourning over the loss of irrevocable bonds and the assumption of maternal responsibility. In a risk culture, as faith in enduring human connection and allegiance to abiding affinity wane, anxiety about the disappearance of permanent relationships spurs renewed dedication to children, who are the last bastion of unconditional love and the sole remaining source of "enchantment." Here total motherhood is, in part, a reaction formation, an effort to sustain a simultaneously desired and rejected commitment, and breastfeeding is metonymic of an urgent nostalgia. Testimony to both the past and the continuing possibility of permanent relationships, breastfeeding serves as a talisman against mothers' and society's loneliness.

In a risk culture, identity is forged in negotiations within and between what Giddens calls abstract systems, the often highly specialized forms of knowledge that guide the interminable process of choosing. Maternal identity is continuously made and remade by drawing on this expertise—the advice of obstetricians, pediatricians, naturalists, herbalists, midwives, lactation specialists, psychologists, and others—in making choices designed to optimize the lives of fetuses, babies, and children. As choices multiply, mundane mistakes and momentary lapses in judgment inevitably increase. Not realizing a diaper needs changing, leaving a favorite toy at home, agreeing to a fast-food dinner—these can lead to guilt, and the cumulative effect of such "missteps" can be exhausting. Infant feeding, however, is a crossroad, a "fateful moment" in the construction of maternal identity. Fateful moments are turning points at which people must make highly consequential choices that speak to their identity, or who they are trying to be. Because they are character-defining junctures, they are opportunities less for guilt than for shame, which stems from the exposure of heretofore hidden or repressed traits clashing with the self-narrative that one is trying to write. It reflects an individual's fear that perhaps she is not up to the task of being the person she has purported to be.[135] For mothers, shame comes from violating the injunction that good mothers reduce all risks to babies, regardless of how small the risk or how costly it is to eliminate.

Shame is the consequence of not breastfeeding after having internalized the imperative of total motherhood. This sense of shame is revealed in the acrimonious accounts of formula-feeding mothers who simultaneously express regret and defend their decision. In these stories, mothers almost always attribute bottle feeding to circumstances beyond their control: insufficient milk, babies' failure to thrive or inability to breastfeed, or mothers' physical or mental illness. "I wanted desperately to breastfeed," wrote one mother to the *New York Times* in response to controversy over government-sponsored breastfeeding promotion. "Unfortunately, I had to stop after only one week because of illness." "When my son was born," wrote another, "I was intent on breast-feeding, regardless of the difficulties. But even with the help of my pediatrician and a lactation consultant, we needed to supplement with formula." "I cannot overstate how demoralized, confused and upset I felt" when my breastfed babies failed to gain sufficient weight, wrote still another mother who was unable to produce enough milk. All these women went on to defend themselves as mothers. "Let's not forget that healthy babies need mentally healthy mothers," stated a mother who did not breastfeed while suffering from postpartum depression. "Ultimately, my son has two parents who love him very much, and that's all that matters," wrote another.[136]

In these letters, as well as in myriad blog conversations, the desire and attempt to breastfeed become evidence of a dedication to total motherhood. Those who bottle-feed take great pains to demonstrate that they would have breastfed if it had been possible, that formula feeding was the result not of a partial commitment to motherhood but of a temporarily thwarted yet ongoing engagement with total motherhood.[137] In simultaneously expressing anguish at not breastfeeding and trying to narrate bottle feeding as consistent with total motherhood, they reveal a consciousness that formula feeding signals a failure to fulfill the responsibilities of maternal citizenship. What these mothers do not question is what British sociologist Elizabeth Murphy called the "fundamental assumption that their babies' welfare [is] paramount and that they should, in all circumstances, prioritize their babies' interests, whatever the personal costs."[138] Nor do they challenge the notion that breastfeeding is optimal for babies' health. Indeed, the superiority of breastfeeding is one of the rare "facts" about reproduction and child care that inspires widespread agreement among and between the medical community and the public, consensus that exists despite critical flaws in the scientific evidence and that has inspired dubious public health claims.

5

Scaring Mothers

The Government Campaign for Breastfeeding

IN 1984, THE U.S. Department of Health and Human Services (HHS) convened the Surgeon General's Workshop on Breastfeeding and Human Lactation. Although just two years earlier, the American Academy of Pediatrics (AAP) had warned against "ignoring the complexity" of infant feeding and had argued that "inherent" differences between mothers who bottle-fed and breastfed made the effects of either method "extremely difficult" to ascertain,[1] the workshop was devoted in large part to promoting breastfeeding. The two-day meeting included only two presentations on breastfeeding science, "Human Lactation as a Physiologic Process" and "The Unique Values of Human Milk." The latter, in repeatedly minimizing the shortcomings in breastfeeding research, revealed considerable distance between the clarity of advocates and the uncertainty of science about breastfeeding's benefits:

> Although the potential roles of specific antibodies, nonspecific immunologic factors, and other functional components may be extrapolated from laboratory studies, a definitive demonstration of their significance in free-living populations has been much more problematic. . . . Although most studies that compare morbidity among children fed human milk or synthetic formula have not controlled adequately for all of the confounding factors, most studies from developed and developing countries have reported significantly fewer illnesses in breastfed infants. . . . Whereas available data are not conclusive, they generally support the theory that human milk provides components that complement a developing immune system in the infant. Although it is not known whether these complementary components participate in the improved development of active immunoprotective abilities, they may serve as substitutes until the infant matures sufficiently to mount an active immune response. Whether or not the protective effects of human milk components are made real or potential by environmental conditions, such benefits are available only if the infant is breastfed.

The last sentence asserts "the protective effects of human milk" that the rest of the paragraph acknowledges are provisional.[2] Of the workshop's six working groups, five focused on how to increase the number of women breastfeeding. The last group made six recommendations regarding research, only two of which called for further investigation into the effects of different modes of feeding. The rest concerned research on promoting breastfeeding.

In the ensuing decades, HHS intensified its efforts to encourage breastfeeding. In 1985, it issued a follow-up report on the recommendations of the Surgeon General's Workshop, and in 1995, it supported the formation of the U.S. Breastfeeding Committee (USBC), an umbrella organization made up of governmental, educational, and nonprofit groups committed to advocating breastfeeding. HHS also sponsored the National Breastfeeding Policy Conference in 1998. In 2000, the HHS Office on Women's Health (OWH) issued the *Blueprint for Action on Breastfeeding*, in which Surgeon General David Satcher maintained that "breastfeeding is one of the most important contributors to infant health." The *Blueprint* deemed breastfeeding "a public health challenge" that required support from the health care system, the workplace, child care facilities, family, and community.[3] It reiterated the breastfeeding goals of *Healthy People 2010*, which outlined HHS's overall health objectives for the American population for the next decade: at least 75 percent of women should initiate breastfeeding; at least 50 percent should breastfeed exclusively through six months; and at least 25 percent should continue breastfeeding, supplemented with other foods, for the first year.[4] The *Blueprint* placed particular emphasis on the importance of persuading African American mothers to breastfeed.[5] At the same time, webpages for HHS and the Centers for Disease Control and Prevention (CDC) offered extensive information on a variety of topics: the health benefits of breastfeeding; the challenges of breastfeeding, including physical problems and work constraints; breastfeeding rights and legislation; data and statistics; promotion and support; and human milk banks, where women could donate or purchase breast milk. The National Women's Health Information Center, part of OWH, also instituted (and continues to operate) a breastfeeding help line with "La Leche League International trained Breastfeeding Peer Counselors" who speak both English and Spanish.[6]

In 2002, OWH announced that it would partner with the Advertising Council to promote breastfeeding in the United States. The result was the National Breastfeeding Awareness Campaign (NBAC), which ran from

June 2004 to April 2006 and was composed of television, radio, and print advertisements; pamphlets, posters, and billboards; and websites maintained by both OWH and the Ad Council. From the controversy surrounding its launch to the evaluation of its success, the NBAC revealed the workings of a risk culture marked by total motherhood. The campaign exploited the popular obsession with health and diet. It presented breastfeeding research as far more certain than it is and the risks of not breastfeeding as much more severe than they would be even if the science were compelling. It capitalized on the public's general confusion about risk, including ignorance of the ideological underpinnings of risk assessment and the inevitability of risk trade-offs. It embraced the principle that mothers have the unique capacity and obligation to protect their offspring from short- and long-term threats and that responsible mothers produce healthy babies. Moreover, it failed to consider meaningfully the needs and responsibilities of women apart from their obligations as mothers, and it was particularly insensitive to the structural and cultural significance of race and class. At best, the NBAC was misleading; at worst, it was an unethical effort to scare women into breastfeeding.

The NBAC and Public Health Ethics

Scheduled to be launched in fall 2003, the NBAC was postponed after the AAP leadership and the formula industry objected to proposed public service announcements (PSA) that had been leaked on the council's website. One, according to OWH senior science adviser Suzanne Haynes,[7] depicted a rubber nipple on top of an insulin bottle, suggesting that bottle feeding causes diabetes. Others portrayed pregnant women engaged in strenuous sports, such as roller derby and mechanical-bull riding. "You'd never take risks while you're pregnant. Why start when the baby's born?" asked the voice-over. The campaign also planned to advise that breastfeeding reduced babies' risk for ear infections, respiratory illnesses, diarrhea, and obesity; that babies who were exclusively breastfed for six months "have a better response to immunizations like polio, tetanus, diphtheria, and Haemophilus influenzae"; and that "results from some studies show that breastfed children have greater brain development than nonbreastfed children." On its website, the Ad Council stated that "babies who are not exclusively breastfed for at least 6 months will be more likely to contract asthma, allergies, diabetes and cancer; suffer more colds, flu and other respiratory illnesses; make more sick visits to the doctor; have inhibited potential IQ due to less infant neural development; [and] be obese adults."[8]

The leaked ads touched off a war of letters to Tommy Thompson, the secretary of HHS, with all the correspondents reiterating their support for promoting breastfeeding. The first came from Carden Johnston, newly elected president of the AAP, who had been approached about the campaign and the controversial PSAs by representatives of the formula industry at the AAP's annual convention in November 2003. Even though the AAP's Section on Breastfeeding had worked closely with the OWH and the Ad Council on the campaign, the AAP leadership did not learn that the NBAC was in the works, much less that it would be based on risk, until just before its scheduled launch.[9] While agreeing that breastfeeding was "the optimal source of nutrition for most infants in this country," Johnston expressed concern that the campaign's focus would be on "the risks incurred by not breastfeeding rather than . . . the benefits to be derived from breastfeeding." He counseled against this "negative approach" and stressed that the advertisements "must absolutely avoid making any claims that cannot be scientifically validated and thus undermine the credibility of the campaign."

On hearing of Johnston's letter, the Section on Breastfeeding sent Secretary Thompson a response. In it Lawrence Gartner, the section chair, asserted that all claims made in the ads were based on sound medical research and that "for the advertising campaign to be effective, it is essential that the message point out the risks of not breastfeeding." In a separate note to members of the AAP, Gartner complained that the formula companies, some of which were among the academy's top corporate donors, were exercising undue influence on the organization's leadership. Johnston and Joe Sanders, the AAP's executive director, denied that industry contributions had anything to do with their concerns.[10] "Some of the science behind these breastfeeding claims is shaky," argued Johnston, who also worried that mothers who did not breastfeed would feel guilty if their babies got sick.[11] At the same time, Marsha Walker, a member of the USBC, wrote Thompson that "there is no evidence that informing mothers regarding the differences in health outcomes of infants fed formula or breast milk makes them feel guilty if they formula feed."[12]

Meanwhile, the International Formula Council, which represented the formula manufacturers, hired Clayton Yeutter, the secretary of agriculture in President George H. W. Bush's administration, to lobby on its behalf. In a letter to Thompson, Yeutter stressed that the industry supported the idea of a breastfeeding campaign but opposed "scaring mothers into breastfeeding" as well as the ads' implication that feeding babies infant formula was dangerous.[13] At the same time, many breastfeeding advocates encouraged campaign supporters to write letters to both Thompson and their elected officials. The USBC, among whose members are the AAP, the American Academy of Family Physicians, and the American College of Obstetricians and Gynecologists, offered fax numbers, addresses, and a sample letter, as did *Mothering* magazine, the International Lactation Consultant Association, and a host of websites that promote breastfeeding. According to a USBC press release, HHS received more than one thousand communications supporting the NBAC.[14] In light of the controversy, HHS department officials met with members of the USBC and the formula industry and reviewed the campaign. Senior scientists at HHS determined that the evidence linking not breastfeeding to diabetes and leukemia was insufficient. In the final campaign, the broadcast and print ads focused on ear infections, respiratory illness, diarrhea, and obesity, although diabetes and leukemia remained on the Ad Council's campaign website. Specific risk ratios, or the statistical increases in risk associated with not breastfeeding, were omitted for fear that the public would misinterpret them. Because diabetes was withdrawn from the PSAs, the ad with the nipple-topped insulin bottle also was eliminated. The risk message, conveyed in ads featuring the mechanical bull and other extreme sports, such as logrolling, remained.

At the heart of the controversy over whether to frame the NBAC in terms of benefits or risks are perennial public health dilemmas that are particularly salient in contemporary risk culture: Is the scientific evidence strong enough to justify a public intervention, a government-funded attempt to alter the way that people live? Is it ethical to provoke extreme fear or anxiety, or to manipulate confusion about risk, in trying to persuade people to change their behavior? If so, how and under what circumstances? What role should the social context of the target population play in framing the campaign message? In short, what circumstances call for a risk-based public health campaign, such as the NBAC? Scientists, the American Public Health Association (APHA), and scholars have engaged in lengthy and ongoing debates about the ethical questions surrounding evidence quality, message design, and cultural sensitivity.[15] These conversations reveal an understanding that "while good science is essential, unassailable science is not possible."[16] Balancing the uncertainty inherent in observational research with the needs and rights of citizens, therefore, is a fundamental responsibility of public health decision makers. On one hand, they are reluctant to recommend lifestyle changes based on imperfectly understood associations, but on the other hand, they want to inform the public of findings that could improve health. Ethical quandaries arise at precisely these moments "when two valid concerns . . . come in conflict."[17]

If a consensus is reached that the evidence tips in favor of an intervention, a strategy must be developed that accurately portrays the science, including its ambiguities, and at the same time convinces people to adopt the recommended behavior. This is an especially delicate exercise in a risk- and health-consumed culture, in which the competition for public attention is fierce and health promoters might be inclined to exaggerate the urgency of a problem in order to "break through the clutter" of competing messages.[18] Psychoactive ads that cause a targeted group of people to feel intensely anxious or frightened are potentially more persuasive, but their success might rest on misleading or even deceitful portrayals of health risks. Indeed, because the information presented in any health intervention is inherently partial, a distillation of what is likely to be a vast body of research, "*one cannot not manipulate when communicating* about health and disease . . . [and] health communicators have a tremendous ethical responsibility to first determine what appropriate health messages are" and then to "develop strategies for the ethical use of manipulation techniques to promote health and prevent disease."[19] According to various professional codes, ethical campaigns are careful not to exaggerate, dramatize, or present evidence in misleading ways. They also are sensitive to the ways in which recommended behaviors might resonate in particular populations.[20]

Although the ethics of health communication is far from a settled matter, debates among scientists and scholars engaged in public health research provide good cause to question government-sponsored breastfeeding promotion and an even stronger reason to challenge a risk-based campaign. Current infant-feeding research is a weak justification for public health recommendations, and it is all the more so for a harm-focused message that generates and then profits from the anxieties of pregnant women and new mothers. Yet in its emphasis on the dangers of not breastfeeding, the NBAC consciously attempted to increase breastfeeding rates by manufacturing fear and exploiting the concerns of a risk culture. Moreover, it did so in ways that drew on the widespread popular misunderstanding of risk and deep-seated normative assumptions about *mothers'* responsibility to protect babies and children from harm. Finally, the campaign employed a crudely instrumental notion of cultural sensitivity and reduced difference to a matter of campaign strategy. From the emphasis on risk to the targeting of African American women, the NBAC demonstrated an awareness of the impediments to breastfeeding, of the obstacles to successful promotion, but not an appreciation of its costs or a sensitivity to the needs and values of different groups of women. In representing not breastfeeding as tantamount to mothers' endangerment of babies, the NBAC violated fundamental public health ethics and ignored the extent to which the politics of breastfeeding is enmeshed in the dynamics of a risk culture committed to total motherhood.

Science and Public Health

The results of breastfeeding research are inconsistent and fail to account for identifiable confounding variables, thereby providing a shaky foundation for the NBAC. This research also reveals the inevitable uncertainty involved in evaluating evidence for public health. As Alfred Sommer, former dean of the Johns Hopkins Bloomberg School of Public Health, lamented, epidemiologists "readily accept the fact that observational studies are inherently less conclusive than randomized trials, but to what degree? All else being equal, do 10 observational studies equal one controlled trial? . . . How many, and of what kind, do we require for conclusive evidence? What are our 'stopping rules'?"[21] Epidemiologists generally agree that compelling policy initiatives must be based on research demonstrating causal links that are strong, consistent, and highly plausible. Opinion varies about precisely what constitutes a "strong" association, but in a much-discussed article in *Science*, several prominent scholars indicated that they would be concerned about residual confounding in any study producing a risk ratio under three.[22] A risk ratio represents a comparison of the rate of risk in a "treated" or "exposed" group, such as babies who were breastfed, with the rate of risk in an untreated group, such as babies who were not breastfed. A risk ratio of three means that an identified risk is twice as high, or 200 percent greater, in the untreated than in the treated group. Research that finds breastfeeding to be protective, including the studies that the OWH lists as NBAC references, almost always calculates relative risks of well under two.[23] In investigations like these, in which the correlations are slight, "positive confounding or bias of a small magnitude may easily result in an observed weak association" that does not reflect the true level of effect.[24] The question then becomes at what point "a reported trivial increase in risk ratio, even if statistically significant, becomes a biologically important risk which merits public concern."[25]

To ascertain the real significance of correlations that are not powerful, epidemiologists employ various strategies. First, they look for consistency, a body of research with a uniform structure and findings. Made up largely of analyses of disparate independent and outcome variables, breastfeeding research is inconsistent in both design and result. What is more, if one study with critical methodological flaws is not convincing, one hundred or one thousand studies with the same weaknesses will be no more compelling. As Sir Richard Doll, the epidemiologist credited with first demonstrating the link between smoking and lung cancer, commented, "Bias times 12 is still bias."[26] A similar problem exists with meta-analysis, a statistical method of aggregating independent studies that is often employed to assess repeated small effects. "Meta-analyses can never be better than the primary studies included in them. If residual confounding is a problem of the observational studies there will also be potential residual confounding in the meta-analysis."[27] A meta-analysis that found breastfeeding to be associated with higher cognitive development,[28] for example, was discounted by critics for relying on methodologically flawed studies.[29]

Consistency of result, furthermore, does not take into account prepublication bias or establish plausibility. Several studies indicate that scientists believe journals, scientific societies, and funding agencies are prejudiced against null hypotheses, or research finding no statistical relationship between the variables being measured, and that this is especially true when an association is taken for granted.[30] Researchers, therefore, might cling to negligible risks and seize on very small associations. Or they might choose not to submit null findings for publication, known as "the file drawer problem."[31] While no analysis has been published regarding publication bias in infant-feeding research, belief in breastfeeding's superiority is so widespread that any bias, real or imagined, might result in both the publication of fewer negative studies and an association that appeared to be more consistent than it truly is. Consistent correlation, furthermore, does not demonstrate plausibility, or explain how the factor under examination could itself make a biological difference in outcome. In breastfeeding studies, however, plausibility is frequently not discussed,[32] minimally addressed,[33] or followed by the caveat that more research is needed to confirm the absence of confounding.[34] In considering plausibility, authors sometimes acknowledge that unaccounted-for behavioral differences could explain breastfeeding's protective effect.[35] In other cases, plausibility is not related to breastfeeding but to behavior—such as offering more frequent small feedings[36] or allowing for babies' self-regulation of intake[37]—that could be adopted by bottle-feeding caretakers.

Although HHS convened a panel of experts to evaluate the medical evidence for the NBAC, these scientists were constrained by what can be termed the "expert paradox": precisely what qualifies certain individuals to serve as advisers also can hinder their ability to assess the literature objectively. According to the OWH's Haynes, at least four of the six reviewers were either members of or government liaisons to the USBC, whose mission is "to improve the Nation's health by working collaboratively to protect, promote, and support breastfeeding."[38] These individuals' commitment to promoting breastfeeding made them strong choices for the NBAC, but it also might have impaired their ability either to critically evaluate the studies' systematic weaknesses or to assess the judiciousness of a public health campaign to promote breastfeeding. When epidemiologists and public health professionals address partiality or conflict of interest, they are largely concerned with researchers' ties to vested-interest groups, such as drug companies or employers, that favor certain results over others. However, they also stress that "all judgments are value driven in the sense that it is necessary to select from a myriad of detail in order to report what is important"[39] and that "partiality can arise through a scientist's own biases and preconceived notions about a problem being investigated."[40] For this reason, HHS's selection of advisers, all of whom were convinced of breastfeeding's health benefits, was unlikely to yield a critical, or fully balanced, evaluation of the literature. Had the panel included experts on obesity, ear infections, or diabetes—scientists invested not in breastfeeding but in the conditions for which breastfeeding is supposed to reduce risk—HHS might have received different recommendations.

Finally, the first tenet of the APHA Code of Ethics states that "public health should address principally the fundamental causes of disease and requirements for health" and explains that "this principle gives priority not only to prevention of disease or promotion of health but also at the most fundamental levels."[41] Drunk driving and smoking are underlying causes of traffic fatalities and lung cancer, and public health campaigns to reduce them would seem in keeping with the standard set by the APHA. But the evidence for breastfeeding is not nearly as powerful. Were breastfeeding research unassailable—the studies meticulously designed and carried out, confounding convincingly eliminated, and plausibility established—the associations still would not be strong enough to make the case that not breastfeeding is a *fundamental* cause of the health problems cited by the NBAC. By most measures, in fact, the campaign did not meet the evidentiary standards for ethical public health practice set by multiple institutions.

Framing Risk in Public Health

The controversy surrounding the breastfeeding campaign, however, did not concern weaknesses in the scientific evidence as such. Unlike debates about obesity, in which critics have challenged the claim that being overweight is itself a risk factor for illness and disease,[42] the NBAC conflict developed largely around "valence," or the framing of what all involved agreed was the worthy goal of increasing national breastfeeding rates.[43] In urging a more "positive" campaign, lobbyist Yeutter emphasized to HHS Secretary Thompson that the formula industry did not dispute breastfeeding's superiority.

> We all agree that breast feeding has advantages over any of the alternatives, and you'll hear no objections from us if HHS delivers that message regularly and with enthusiasm. Our objection is to the contemplated visuals, featuring pregnant women riding a mechanical bull or engaging in log-rolling. Those are catchy images, which obviously is what the advertising experts had in mind. But they are grossly misleading, and no department of our government should purposefully convey misleading information to the American public.[44]

The "misleading information" resulted from extensive consumer research. After announcing its cosponsorship of the NBAC in summer 2002, the Ad Council contracted with McKinney+Silver, an advertising agency, which then conducted research with thirty-six focus groups and determined that "many think breastfeeding is like supplementing a 'standard diet' with more vitamins. Formula, by default, is credited with the status of being the 'standard.'" Most people, the focus groups indicated, knew about the putative benefits of breastfeeding but did not perceive any disadvantage to choosing formula. The campaign strategy, therefore, would be one of "conversion," of suggesting not only that breastfed babies were healthier but that formula-fed babies were more likely to suffer from a variety of health problems, some of them serious. The idea, in other words, was not to persuade people that breastfeeding was better; most already believed that. Instead, the task was to convey that not breastfeeding was risky.[45]

The architects of the NBAC were not the first to determine that an anxiety-provoking message might persuade an otherwise complacent target group. Antitobacco messages frequently stress the health risks associated with smoking, and advertisements sponsored by the Partnership for a Drug-Free America—in the most notorious, an egg is cracked into a greasy frying pan while a voice intones, "This is your brain. This is your brain on drugs. Any questions?"—are deliberately designed to provoke discomfort.[46] In a risk culture preoccupied with health, the challenge for activists is "to convince others to understand the urgency implied in the tedious, quantitative language of the statistic," to convert boredom into a "statistical panic" in which "fraught decisions are reduced to no-brainers."[47] In choosing to emphasize the putative dangers of not breastfeeding, the NBAC sought to eliminate the complexity surrounding infant-feeding decisions and to locate formula in the same category as tobacco and illegal drugs. The risk-based ads were a form of public health communication known as "fear appeals," messages that try to provoke fear in order to persuade people determined to be "at risk" to adopt a recommended behavior.[48] These ads, commonly referred to as "loss frames," might have particular resonance in a risk culture, but they always have been controversial. While some scholars have suggested that fear can be an appropriate tool as long as the audience is offered viable behaviors by which risks can be reduced,[49] others contend that it is unethical to wittingly provoke fear in a targeted population[50] and that "wherever possible, people should be given the opportunity to participate *meaningfully* in medical decision-making."[51]

Conversations among practitioners as well as ethical codes established by epidemiologists almost always stipulate that great care should be taken to present research results honestly and without distortion and that this is part of the "implicit contract between epidemiologists and the members of society."[52] According to the Ethics Guidelines of the American College of Epidemiology, for example, "epidemiologists should strive to ensure that, at a minimum, research findings are interpreted and reported on accurately and appropriately. . . . The significance of the findings should neither be understated nor overstated. Epidemiologists should put the strengths and limitations of their research methods into proper perspective."[53] For researchers, this might mean foregrounding caveats that are normally found in the last paragraphs of published studies. For public health practitioners, it might require that campaign messages be carefully balanced and that those designed to scare people be limited to interventions for which the evidence is strong and the negative outcome serious and likely, conditions that do not obtain in formula feeding. In a risk culture, however, the desire not to be drowned out by the cacophony of information about health and the body can provoke even the most altruistic campaign planners to minimize methodological problems, overstate findings, and exaggerate danger. Once the NBAC framed infant feeding as a matter of sickness versus health, or danger versus safety, it was practically impossible to portray not breastfeeding as risky *and* to present the nuances of research findings. Whereas in ethical public health practice, a campaign is designed to represent the research, in the NBAC, the message subordinated the science.

Relative Risk in the NBAC

The NBAC was marked by overcharged rhetoric and disingenuous and morally dubious comparisons. In the Ad Council's news release announcing its partnership in the NBAC, the OWH's Haynes is quoted as saying, "I can't think of any campaign that will improve the health of children more than the National Breastfeeding Awareness Campaign."[54] Given the repeated correlation of poor child health with inadequate prenatal care, poverty, and lack of health insurance,[55] the assertion that increasing breastfeeding rates would most improve children's health seems excessive, at best. In addition, the campaign constructed a moral matrix in which mothers who do not breastfeed are positioned as the equivalent of pregnant women who engage in capricious recreation. Only a woman callous enough to compete in a logrolling competition when pregnant would feed formula to her baby, and bottle-feeders are like pregnant women who ride bulls (and presumably drink alcohol) in bars: they knowingly and needlessly put their babies at risk. This lent the ads a decidedly comic edge. Expectant mothers participating in extreme sports is absurd behavior and so, by implication, is formula feeding. The effects of deploying humor in anxiety frames have not been extensively explored, but some scholars have contended that the practice is unethical if it is based on a clever twist likely to trigger fear.[56] Moreover, while observers are likely to recognize the obvious exaggerations in the campaign imagery, the underlying message—that good mothers must protect their children from any imaginable risk—seems reasonable in a neoliberal and health-centered culture committed to total motherhood. The NBAC fused widespread anxiety about risk and an ethos of total motherhood, with the result that mothers' responsibility to protect babies from the dangers associated with bottle feeding became something of a moral absolute.

In the campaign, as in total motherhood, women *as women* were absent, or present only as mothers who functioned as vectors of risk for their babies. While the radio ads featured sons waxing sentimental about their mothers—"when it comes to disease resistance, that woman could breastfeed like nobody's business"—and men educating their partners about the benefits of breastfeeding—"Oooh, hello special lady. It's time for a one-on-one conversation . . . 'bout . . . recent scientific studies on lactation"—women's voices were conspicuously lacking. And while some women have written appreciatively of their breastfeeding experiences,[57] others describe it as physically and emotionally overwhelming;[58] as "mindblowingly tedious," "a devouring," and "a tactile overload";[59] and as feeling not natural and like a violation of their privacy.[60] Yet once breastfeeding became the object of a health campaign, the attention to the "competing needs" of different communities advocated in discussions of public health ethics[61] became secondary to the goal of promotion, and women's needs independent of their responsibilities as mothers receded.

Nowhere was the absence of women more striking than in the campaign's exclusive emphasis on babies, in its choice *not* to address breastfeeding's potential health advantages for mothers. While research on breastfeeding has concentrated overwhelmingly on the health of babies, a nascent literature has begun to examine whether breastfeeding is associated with various maternal outcomes, including reduced risk for breast cancer, heart disease, and diabetes. The campaign, however, failed to mention even the possibility of health benefits for lactating women. As Linda Blum pointed out more than a decade ago, women's health is often a peripheral matter in breastfeeding advocacy.[62] In the NBAC, *women's* bodies were absent, whereas *mothers'* bodies served as vehicles through which babies were exposed to risk.[63] The NBAC, as Jules Law wrote about breastfeeding promotion in general, was grounded in a notion of women and children as a single biological unit, a perspective that precluded the possibility of distinguishing mothers' from babies' needs.[64] Whereas some advocates contend that breastfeeding should be regarded as the final stage of reproduction, one at which mother and baby are inextricably bound,[65] others suggest that this kind of vision, which continues metaphorically throughout motherhood, is akin to mothers' "social exile" and likely to lead to "breakdown pathologies."[66] Law argued that considering women's needs separately is a precondition for "fully deliberated, ethical, and responsible caregiving,"[67] a position more consistent with the principles articulated by public health practitioners.

Yet the concerns of women *as women* or as individuals were largely absent from the NBAC. Despite acknowledging that women were well informed of breastfeeding's putative benefits, campaign spokespeople and supporters repeatedly stressed that their only intent was to provide women with accurate information. Indeed, they often expressed a certain incredulity that women could be told that "breast is best" and still choose formula, and they assumed that bottle-feeding mothers did not hear or understand the message.[68] While promoting the campaign, Surgeon General Richard Carmona argued that "very few situations" should "prevent a mom from breastfeeding."[69] According to the Ad Council's "Breastfeeding Awareness" web page, women "accept that breastfeeding is the 'best' option—and are generally aware of many specific advantages, but their fears and doubts about their ability and perceived inconvenience often outweigh for them what are perceived as the 'added benefits' of breastfeeding."[70]

In the NBAC, the reasons that women might choose not to breastfeed were understood as obstacles to be overcome rather than as considerations that might be weighed against the benefits attributed to breastfeeding. Women's needs—to work, sleep, control their bodies, or sustain an identity independent of their children—become, as Rebecca Kukla observed, "weaknesses in individual maternal character, to be corrected through educational messages."[71] This kind of reasoning, which implies that ignorance, cowardice, or selfishness is behind a mother's decision not to do what is best for her baby, "closes down any interrogation of *why* women might not behave as they are asked to, even if they hear and understand the request." The campaign slogan "'babies are born to be breastfed' . . . positions breastfeeding as easy and as natural, and even perhaps as a natural entitlement of infants; thus it suggests mothers are both failing at something simple and thwarting natural law if they don't manage to breastfeed."[72] Once the focus groups suggested that presenting breastfeeding as advantageous was unlikely to have much impact, women themselves became the obstacles to babies' good health. In that sense, the NBAC was not a matter of educating, supporting, or otherwise being sensitive to the concerns of women but an attempt to manufacture and exploit fear.

Directed at pregnant women, for whom "risk" is weighted with particular emotional freight, the NBAC also capitalized on the public misunderstanding of risk. Even if infant-feeding studies were more compelling, for example, the campaign drew questionable risk analogies. In the television spots, logrolling or riding a mechanical bull while pregnant and not breastfeeding were portrayed as similarly dangerous acts, or threats to a baby's safety. Yet if both bungee jumping and driving a car while pregnant create risks to a fetus, it does not follow that extreme sports and car riding are equally risky. Many of the campaign's most outspoken proponents, including the USBC's chair, Amy Spangler, likened bottle feeding to tobacco use. "We don't hesitate to tell parents what smoking does to themselves and their children," she said. "Why should we not tell people the consequences of not breastfeeding?"[73] Commenting on the NBAC, a pediatrician on ABC's 20/20 also contended that formula feeding and smoking carried similar risks.[74] Yet this kind of reasoning is specious. Compared with breastfeeding studies, the research linking various health problems with smoking consistently produces overwhelmingly strong statistical correlations. For example, whereas the much-lauded PROBIT study found that breastfed babies were 40 percent less likely to experience a gastrointestinal infection in the first year, the CDC and the American Cancer Society estimate that men who smoke are more than 2,000 percent more likely to develop lung cancer.[75] The rhetoric equating not breastfeeding with smoking, adopted by many of the campaign's proponents, both revealed and exacerbated widespread confusion about the meaning of risk.

Besides distorting the magnitude of the risks associated with formula feeding, the campaign also failed to present the risks and trade-offs of breastfeeding. For example, numerous studies have revealed that most lactating mothers have detectable and often elevated levels of environmental contaminants in their breast milk. The current evidence does not indicate that these pollutants—PCBs, DDT, PBDEs, dioxins, and heavy metals, among others—have dangerous short-term health effects or should discourage breastfeeding for most women. But largely because carefully designed longitudinal studies have not been conducted, the evidence also does not demonstrate that contaminated breast milk is safe and without long-term consequences for either lactating mothers or breastfed babies.[76] In fact, the research on and risk assessment of environmental contaminants in breast milk are marked by serious methodological problems:

studies examine a limited number of chemicals and are based mostly on small population samples in few locations; they lack consistent protocols and have no standardized methodology for collecting and analyzing milk samples; they provide little toxicokinetic evidence, or data on how women absorb, metabolize, and excrete these chemicals; they do not define clinically safe or dangerous levels of pollutants; and, except in cases in which mothers have become clinically ill, they offer no data on the health outcomes in breastfed infants. In addition, conventional risk assessment methods, based on adult body weights and food consumption data, do not consider the ways in which infants and children are uniquely susceptible to chemical exposures via mothers' milk.[77]

Walter Rogan, a scientist at the National Institute of Environmental Health Sciences, supports breastfeeding but also has argued that if breast milk were regulated in the same way as formula is, it "would commonly violate Food and Drug Administration action levels for poisonous or deleterious substances in food and could not be sold."[78] Yet breastfeeding advocates and even environmental activists have been reluctant to draw attention to pollutants for fear of discouraging women from breastfeeding.[79] Ruth Lawrence, a professor of pediatrics and obstetrics and gynecology and renowned breastfeeding advocate, told the *New York Times* in 2008: "When agencies like the E.P.A. decided to monitor the presence of toxins in the environment through breast milk, people like me said, 'Please don't do that—it will be misinterpreted.'"[80] Monitoring presumably would raise questions about the safety of breast milk and could reduce breastfeeding; knowing whether pollutants did compromise the safety of breast milk was less important than ensuring that women continued to breastfeed. Breastfeeding advocates who point only to the hazards of formula, such as that it can be contaminated in production, improperly prepared, and sold in cans and fed to babies in bottles containing Bisphenol A, neglect the fact that breastfeeding, too, has risks.[81]

Rarely, moreover, do choices involve a risk-versus-no-risk calculation; trade-offs are unavoidable, and ostensibly risk-reducing behavior is almost always accompanied by other risks or costs. Driving to avoid flying increases the risk of auto accidents; bottled water lacks fluoride; and using cloth instead of disposable diapers frees landfill space but requires more water for washing. Because risk is inevitable, the question for both policymakers and individual citizens is how to determine which risks should be avoided despite the costs. Or, phrased differently, which trade-offs are more manageable? For example, research indicates that a dietary supplement of 400 micrograms of folic acid before and during early pregnancy dramatically reduces the risk of having a baby with neural tube defects, such as spina bifida.[82] Some preliminary studies have suggested that the addition of folic acid to bread, pasta, and grain-based foods also is associated with an increase in colorectal cancer in the general population.[83] The science is far too rudimentary either to establish a causal relationship or to necessitate a reconsideration of folic acid supplementation. But should such a connection be demonstrated, this trade-off would have to be taken into account in any accurate risk assessment. In the meantime, unless research determines that folic acid supplementation has this or some hitherto unknown side effect, the benefits of taking it appears to far outweigh potential risks. The costs, moreover, are minor for most women. Folic acid is widely available, relatively inexpensive, and requires a few seconds of effort to take each day. The trade-offs do not appear to be prohibitive.[84]

Conversely, extensive research indicates that babies are at risk for a variety of developmental and health disorders in homes where mothers are psychologically depressed or impoverished.[85] For women who find the demands of breastfeeding overwhelming or who cannot reconcile breastfeeding with employment, bottle feeding might constitute the less risky option, *even* if breastfeeding's health benefits for babies were amply demonstrated. This cost, or trade-off, is almost never discussed in breastfeeding promotion. As William Arney argues in his history of the obstetrics profession, "Medicine does not present the choices it makes as ethical ones." Its autonomy and authority depend "on its ability to make ethical choices appear not to be ethical choices, on the ability to contain the ethical content of its work within its professional boundary." But "seeming 'good' done for the patient has 'bad' effects elsewhere, in the patient's family or the economy," so the ethical aspects of even so-called evidence-based recommendations "seep across this boundary."[86]

In other words, regardless of the degree to which infant-feeding research has demonstrated health advantages to breastfeeding, the choice to breastfeed or bottle-feed is necessarily about far more than any putative medical benefits to either baby or mother. Risk ratios concerning babies' health make sense only when they are compared with other risks that the mother, family, and child must negotiate, trade-offs that need to be assessed consciously and continuously. The problem is that advocates trying to draw attention to social problems tend to "present their claims in isolation. That is, they say, 'this is a big problem,' not 'this problem is bigger than other problems.'" They "highlight the benefits of a proposed change and ignore its costs."[87] They suffer from what critics of popular risk reasoning call "trade-off neglect," and they fail to grasp the ways in which their risk choices will affect other aspects of their lives.[88] In fact, as Law observed, "There is no risk-free way to raise a child. *Risk, benefit, advantage,* and *convenience* are all relative terms—relative both to one another and, more importantly, to a way of life."[89] What the NBAC offered, however, was a Hobson's choice: babies could be either safely breastfed or riskily formula fed.

The campaign's failure to consider the risks of breastfeeding is intimately connected to total motherhood. In risk management, trade-offs are more likely to be invisible when the person or institution paying the costs is not factored into the analysis. In most infant-feeding research, and in all the research cited by the NBAC, the putative benefits of breastfeeding for babies are calculated against the potential costs of formula feeding for babies, not the costs of breastfeeding for women who, as mothers, are presumed not to have needs that might diverge from those of their babies. "I'm not aware of any studies that have observed any health benefits of formula feeding," noted Michael Kramer, the lead author of the PROBIT investigation.[90] He might have added that such studies are nonexistent because the potential risks of breastfeeding for women have been largely ignored.

In epidemiological research, *who* is framed as potentially at risk is itself an ideological choice. One of public-health policymakers' most pressing tasks is to determine what makes a *statistically* significant finding *socially* significant, and this is an inherently value-driven process. "At the risk of restating the obvious," writes lactation scientist Judy Hopkinson about two studies of breastfeeding and ear infections, "a fifty percent reduction in risk of otitis media with effusion constitutes a significant public health benefit—not to mention a benefit for working mothers who will have a lower risk of missing work to care for a child with otitis media."[91] It is both illogical and demonstrably false, however, that risks are associated only with not breastfeeding and benefits only with breastfeeding. Women who breastfeed also might experience more stress and sleep less, both of which have been associated with more health problems and diminished performance in various activities. Exhaustion could lead to depression, which would lead to many health risks for both women and babies and also would detract from women's ability to be productive workers, attentive mothers, and good citizens.[92] A compellingly demonstrated 50 percent reduction in ear infections (or in any of the adverse outcomes associated with bottle feeding) would make breastfeeding an "obvious" public health matter only if women were not part of the risk calculation.

Even when research results are strong, consistent, and plausible, public health officials must explain statistical findings to the public and give them meaning in the social context. For example, as earlier argued, breastfeeding's advantages are most plausible in reducing gastrointestinal infections. PROBIT found a statistically significant relative risk reduction in a cohort of babies more likely to have breastfed longer and more exclusively. In the control group, 13.2 percent of babies experienced one or more episodes of GI infection, compared with 9.1 percent in the intervention group.[93] Assuming that the babies who were exposed to longer and more exclusive breastfeeding were, in fact, the ones who suffered fewer infections, and that caretaker behavior had no effect, breastfeeding reduced the risk by 40 percent. This does not mean that four in ten, or 40 percent of bottle-fed babies, will contract an infection, a common interpretive error among the public.[94]

Furthermore, this effect also could be described as a 4 percent drop in absolute risk. PROBIT demonstrated that for every one hundred breast-fed babies, four will be spared at least one infection; framed as the "number needed to treat"—that is, the number of people who would need to receive the intervention in order for one person to benefit—twenty-five babies must be breastfed to prevent one infection. Although both are correct, the statements that one in twenty-five bottle-fed babies will have an additional episode of diarrhea and that breastfed babies are 40 percent less likely to suffer an infection might resonate very differently among mothers. Both statistics are accurate, but in practical terms, the relative risk reduction is meaningful only when accompanied by the number needed to treat and the improvement in absolute risk. Both statistics, moreover, are useful only in the context of the particular outcome being studied. A 40 percent relative risk reduction in leukemia, for example, presumably would be more consequential than an equivalent risk reduction in GI infection, regardless of the magnitude of absolute risk. In short, the mathematical value of a statistic and its social significance are not equivalent. Only in a culture that subscribes to total motherhood, in which any diminishment in risk to babies is worth any cost paid by mothers, could the risk reduction provided by breastfeeding be "obviously" *socially* significant.

Total motherhood dictates that the wants and needs of mothers are necessarily congruent with what is "best" for babies. "Breastfeeding makes your life easier," the OWH tells mothers. "It saves time and money. You do not have to purchase, measure, and mix formula. There are no bottles to warm in the middle of the night!"[95] For many women, however, breastfeeding makes their lives harder, and the difficulties have little to do with the inconvenience of preparing formula. Rather, they are uncomfortable with spontaneous leakage from or changes in the appearance of their breasts; they prefer that their partners manage middle-of-the-night feedings and/or that they also have the opportunity to share the feeding experience; or they are frustrated with monitoring their diets, pumping their breasts, or otherwise having their bodies constantly in the service of their babies. In short, they desire the relative autonomy that comes with being a non-breastfeeding parent. But with respect to breastfeeding, the OWH assumes that women's wants and needs are largely confined to their capacity as mothers.

Of course, mothers (and fathers) frequently must honor needs and desires of their children that conflict with their own, but it also is true that parents sometimes choose to favor their own wants, and the debate about breastfeeding forces an examination of when such choices are socially acceptable. Some cars have better safety records than others. The air in congested cities and suburbs is more highly polluted and raises the risk of asthma and other illness. Yet parents are not the targets of concerted campaigns imploring them to trade their SUVs for safer minivans or to move to less populated areas for the sake of their developing babies. A sustained effort by interest groups, doctors, and the government to move every baby from urban areas in order to reduce the risk of asthma likely would be met with skepticism.[96] Parents would discuss trade-offs, or costs and benefits, and most probably would elect to stay in their relatively polluted neighborhoods. Riding in cars can be deadly. Although safety seats provide some protection, parents who drive with their babies and children routinely put them at risk.[97] Yet, it is difficult to imagine a cultivated campaign to keep families out of cars. Should such an effort materialize, it is liable to be met with resistance because driving is a cultural norm. The innumerable blog writers who are quick to blame mothers for bottle feeding when a baby is harmed by contaminated formula do not fault mothers for driving when a baby is hurt in a car accident. In public discourse, which is strongly informed by the principles of total motherhood, risks that can be alleviated by mothers appear inherently more important to address than those that require effort from others, including fathers, communities, and government. These risks are to be eliminated, regardless of the trade-offs for mothers. The ethic of total motherhood makes it impossible that when the risks are marginal, at best, mothers might morally choose to place their needs as individuals before those of their children. Even the suggestion is likely to promote significant discomfort. In erasing mothers' subjectivity as women, total motherhood makes breastfeeding the only, or "obvious," feeding choice.

When epidemiologists and public health practitioners discuss respecting cultural variations in values, they speak of "difficult choices" and "careful consideration,"[98] of the need to appreciate "cultural diversity,"[99] despite the strong tension between appreciation and manipulation of difference. In specifically targeting African American women, whose breastfeeding rates are well below those of white and Hispanic women, the campaign demonstrated less sensitivity than a tactical cultural awareness. Eighteen of McKinney+Silver's thirty-six focus groups were conducted with black women. The NBAC also sent breastfeeding materials with images of African Americans to local WIC offices, which offer nutritional counseling and supplementation to low-income women and infants. These posters and pamphlets included photos of supportive fathers, whom research has suggested are crucial to increasing breastfeeding among black women.[100] The woman riding the mechanical bull was African American, and a radio spot was set to soul music. The sense, according to Haynes, was that these approaches would "produce responses." But deploying black women and symbols likely to resonate among African Americans violates the spirit of what minority health advocates, including the HHS Office of Minority Health, term "cultural competence" in health care: "services that are respectful of and responsive to the health beliefs, practices and cultural and linguistic needs of diverse patients."[101] It represents a use, rather than an understanding, of cultural particularity,[102] and it was the outcome of market research (focus groups) that sought to determine how best to sell a product (breastfeeding) more than an effort to understand the "diverse values, beliefs, and cultures in the community."[103]

Others have determined that breastfeeding has particular meaning for many black women. In interviews with black and white working-class mothers, for example, Linda Blum found many of the same attitudes toward breastfeeding and motherhood but also noted that the latter was conceptualized as more of a collective undertaking for African Americans. "Good mothering was not defined by exclusivity, by the mother's singular, irreplaceable presence, as it was for so many of the white mothers."[104] Breastfeeding, moreover, was at odds with a notion of "kin-work" in black families.[105] African American women emphasized to Blum that bottle feeding allowed older children to be involved, which brought the family closer, and they stressed that it was more important to work to take care of their children than to be in an unsupportive marriage that might allow for a financial flexibility more conducive to breastfeeding. Their perspectives, moreover, were frequently "refracted through the distinct historical lens of slavery and race hatred, which casts particular meanings on women's bodies."[106] This lens reveals a landscape marked by the forced wet-nursing of white women's children—often to the detriment of their own—and charges of hypersexualization, animalism, and primitivism, a cultural legacy that makes the "naturalness" of breastfeeding reverberate in unappealing ways. Soul music and images of black women in campaign materials did not address any of these issues. As Mary Douglas observed in her classic study on risk and blame, "risk analysis that only allows the cautious, risk-averse behavior to be rational is convicted of crippling cultural bias."[107] Even if the risks associated with breastfeeding were compellingly proven, it is not clear that they would be strong enough to displace centuries of compounded cultural meaning.

Both total motherhood and the NBAC represent what Blum otherwise referred to as "a racialized class-enhancing project for white middle-class mothers."[108] Because data consistently show that these women have markedly higher breastfeeding rates than do African American and lower-income mothers, the campaign intentionally targeted the latter. Yet despite the presence of black actors and soul and country music in advertisements, as well as community demonstration projects in cities such as Birmingham, San Juan, Baltimore, and Knoxville, the campaign's message remained decidedly white and middle class. Advice about how to combine breastfeeding with work, for example, consisted largely of recommendations on how and when to use a breast pump, which can cost nearly $300, and assumed an idyllic work environment. "If you are having problems getting your milk to 'let-down' at the start of pumping," suggested the OWH webpage,

you may find it helpful to have a picture of your baby close-by. . . . Try to clear your head of stressful thoughts. Use a comfortable chair or pillows. Once you begin expressing your milk, think about your baby.

Let your employer know that you are breastfeeding and explain that, when you're away from your baby, you will need to take breaks throughout the day to pump your milk to give to your baby at a later time. Ask where you can pump at work, and make sure it is a private, clean, quiet area. Also make sure you have somewhere to store the milk. Discuss how you plan to fit pumping into your workday. You can offer to work out a different schedule, such as coming in earlier or leaving a little later each day to make up for any lost work time, if this comes up as an issue.[109]

Working-class mothers, and particularly shift workers—waitresses, retail associates, and factory workers—generally do not have enough cultural capital or job security to call attention to special circumstances, such as the need for time, private and relaxing space, and proper storage. Nor do these women, at least some of whom might prefer breastfeeding as a less expensive option, enjoy the flexibility in their schedules for frequent pumping breaks. For mothers paid by the hour or on a time clock, the NBAC did not make available a feasible strategy to alleviate the anxiety it deliberately provoked, which many scholars have argued is a requirement for fear appeals to be ethical and effective.[110]

Furthermore, for working-class women, "who are regularly perceived as harming their children through a host of other 'bad choices,'" including "making their children obese by feeding them cheap food,"[111] the NBAC offered yet another opportunity to fail the total motherhood ideal.[112] Since the campaign's motto was "babies were born to be breastfed," one critic remarked, working-class women might well ask, "What were *their* babies born to do?"[113] The NBAC's disregard for the social and economic constraints that many women face is apparent in other government programs, such as WIC, which provides fewer fruits and vegetables to bottle-feeding than to breastfeeding mothers.[114] Here the state promotes mothers' health to the extent that it benefits babies, and poor and lower-income mothers are penalized even when "breastfeeding is *not* in fact a livable choice."[115] As Pam Carter argues about breastfeeding in Britain, "it is not simply a fact that breastfeeding is better for babies. Rather, this needs to be explored, evaluated and its meaning deconstructed in relation to particular contexts . . . [and] race, class and ethnicity are highly significant in doing this."[116]

The Media and the NBAC

The NBAC misrepresented the research and risks associated with not breastfeeding and also functionalized the socioeconomic contexts in which feeding decisions are made, but the media offered little in the way of critical response. On the day the NBAC was launched, for example, ABC's *20/20* included a segment that was largely an indictment of those who had protested its risk-based approach.[117] Were the original advertisements canceled because they were wrong, asked John Stossel by way of introduction, "or was it money talking?" Reporter Brian Ross told viewers that statistics suggesting that babies who were not breastfed were 30 to 60 percent more likely to develop leukemia, ear infections, and diabetes had been eliminated "under pressure by the big companies that are in competition with breastfeeding, the companies that make infant formula. It's a controversy that some see as corporate power against mother's milk." Several times Ross referred to the original campaign as having been "killed" by the "three-billion-dollar-a-year formula industry" and its well-connected lobbyists. He confronted people who had challenged the original campaign and sympathetically interviewed those who had supported it.

Breastfeeding research was discussed twice: once, in a combative conversation between Ross and Cristine Beato, acting assistant secretary of health, that portrayed HHS as having been biased toward the formula industry; and again in a discussion with Lawrence Gartner, head of the AAP's Section on Breastfeeding, in which Gartner lamented the AAP leadership's failure to consult him before opposing the ads. Ross challenged Beato's contention that "there is no science to back up percentages" and no proof that bottle-fed babies are at higher risk of leukemia, but he accepted without question Gartner's claim that the early ads were "absolutely" backed by good research. As the segment ended, Jay Gordon, a pediatrician and a member of the La Leche League International Health Advisory Council, had the last word. Over a slowly fading image of a suckling baby, he stated: "The fact that [the formula industry] managed to get this campaign watered down is evidence that money can influence good medicine and that large amounts of money can influence even good doctors. And it's tragic, truly tragic. And it will hurt babies."

The 20/20 report also invoked a recent National Institutes of Health (NIH) study on breastfeeding and the risk of post neonatal death. That investigation is indeed noteworthy, although less for its findings than for its relative candidness. It is replete with qualifiers:

> "Studying the salutary effects of breastfeeding presents some widely recognized problems in inference."
> "Causality is difficult to demonstrate for any specific part of the interaction between the breastfeeding mother and her child. It may be that breastfeeding represents a package of skills, abilities, and emotional attachments that mark families whose infants survive and that it is these factors that produce the benefits seen, rather than breastfeeding or breast milk per se."
> Breastfeeding is not randomly assigned, and "reverse causality . . . might produce an artificial benefit of breastfeeding."

The authors openly questioned whether one of their own findings, that breastfed babies were 40 percent less likely to die of something other than an infectious disease, such as an accident, was "plausible." Whereas many have hypothesized that immunities transferred from mother to baby can prevent infection, "a satisfactory mechanism has not yet been proposed" to explain how breastfeeding itself might prevent a baby from dying, for example, from falling down a set of stairs. The NIH study was exceptional in that it mentioned problems in determining causality in the abstract conclusion, stating that "breastfeeding cannot be separated completely from other characteristics of the mother and child." But in the context of the broader literature on breastfeeding, the next sentence overshadowed the caution that preceded it: "Assuming causality, however, promoting breastfeeding has the potential to save or delay ~720 postneonatal deaths in the United States each year."[118] None of these caveats was mentioned in the *20/20* report. Ross referred to the study after a pediatrician asserted that bottle-fed babies are at higher risk of ear and upper respiratory infections and certain forms of cancer. "In fact," he said, "a study released just last month by the NIH found that babies who are not breastfed have a 20 percent higher risk of death in their first year."[119]

The media continued to stoke the controversy long after the campaign ended. In summer 2006, the *New York Times* ran a story entitled "Breast-Feed or Else," in which various advocates and detractors debated the relative merits of the NBAC's risk-based message. While readers responded with more than one hundred letters, many of which argued that women should not be made to feel guilty if they were unable to breastfeed, little critical attention was paid to infant-feeding research or to the possibility that HHS scientists had restricted the NBAC's claims because of valid reservations about the science.[120] The OWH's Haynes denied that the campaign was an effort to manipulate new mothers. "We're not trying to create guilt at all. What we're trying to do is reach the first-time moms who are out there, who are making the decision whether to breastfeed or not."[121] At the same time, salon.com's Lori Leibovich wrote that "it's hard to imagine a more guilt-inducing message" than the one offered by the NBAC.[122] The *Times* published an editorial a few weeks later claiming that "the science comes down hard on behalf of educating women about the clear advantages of breast-feeding. But that is no license to imply that mothers who cannot breast-feed or choose not to are putting their babies in grave danger."[123]

The following year, as the U.S. House of Representatives Committee on Oversight and Government Reform investigated allegations of political interference with health policy, the *Washington Post* ran a story entitled "HHS Toned Down Breast-Feeding Ads." The article gave considerable attention to HHS officials who said they had been pressured to "make sure we didn't somehow offend" in the NBAC and also to avoid publicizing a recent report by the department's Agency for Healthcare Research and Quality that confirmed an association between breastfeeding and lower rates of diabetes, leukemia, obesity, asthma, and sudden infant death syndrome (SIDS).[124] These officials did not mention the report's conclusion:

> Because almost all the data in this review were gathered from observational studies, one should not infer causality based on these findings. Also, there is a wide range of quality of the body of evidence across different health outcomes. For future studies, clear subject selection criteria and definition of "exclusive breastfeeding," reliable collection of feeding data, controlling for important confounders including child-specific factors, and blinded assessment of the outcome measures will help.[125]

The *Post* piece was followed by a series of headlines in other media essentially damning the formula industry and the White House for compromising babies' health. These stories—"Controversial Breastfeeding Ads Toned Down,"[126] "The White House vs. Mother's Milk,"[127] "More Meddling with Health,"[128] "Formula Industry Lobby Undermined Federal Breastfeeding Campaign"[129]—affirmed the dominant narrative that money had trumped science in the matter of infant feeding, an interpretation that resonated with other charges that President George W. Bush's administration had manipulated science for political ends. The removal of ads depicting a nipple on top of an insulin bottle and an inhaler were portrayed as the result of industry and political meddling.[130] The fact that a panel of senior scientists at HHS had recommended the changes did not provoke investigation of the research or of the received wisdom that breastfeeding is unparalleled as infant nutrition.

The Department of Health and Human Services, which tracked public attitudes before, during, and after the campaign, claimed on its website that the NBAC had enhanced public knowledge about breastfeeding. Awareness of messages about breastfeeding, the percentage of people who correctly identified at least six months as the recommended duration of exclusive breastfeeding, and the number of women who had ever breastfed all increased by around 10 percent.[131] Yet promotional efforts for breastfeeding have intensified in various institutions around the country, so the NBAC's role in altering attitudes or action is virtually impossible to measure. Shifts in awareness also are ambiguous indicators of behavior. The gap between public knowledge and observance of dietary and exercise guidelines provides a cautionary tale for those who would assume that awareness and practice are congruent.

"Ever breastfed," moreover, is a nebulous measure. According to the CDC's National Health and Nutrition Examination Surveys (NHANES), 77 percent of babies were breastfed at least once in 2005/2006, an increase from 60 percent in 1993/1994 and 67 percent in 2001/2002. The number was 80 percent for Mexican Americans, 79 percent for white Americans, and 65 percent for African Americans, up from 67 percent, 62 percent, and 36 percent, respectively, in 1993/1994. When the NHANES results were made public, various media announced that breastfeeding rates were at an all-time high. Yet "ever breastfed" does not indicate how many babies were breastfed twice, much less for weeks or months. The latest statistics on breastfeeding at six months, drawn from the 2003/2004 NHANES, indicated no significant change from 1993. No statistics on exclusivity were reported, so the percentage of infants still breastfed at six months included those who fed once a day at the breast while being supplemented with formula and/or solid foods and those who consumed nothing but breast milk. If duration and exclusivity of breastfeeding are important, as the NBAC stressed, the NHANES report reveals little even about the impact that the campaign *could* have had on babies' health.[132]

Furthermore, an association between the campaign and any increase in breastfeeding does not indicate a causal relationship. As the rate of "ever breastfed" babies has risen, so, too, has the incidence of childhood obesity.[133] No compelling evidence indicates that breastfeeding is a risk factor for obesity, but the correlation makes clear the imperative to carefully isolate direct links between feeding method and health measures before making causal claims. Indeed, a recent study demonstrated that expanded maternity-leave mandates in Canada led to a greater duration of both partial and exclusive breastfeeding but not to improved health outcomes.[134]

The NBAC and Public Health in a Risk Culture

Composed entirely of breastfeeding advocates, the review panel convened by HHS to evaluate the research for the NBAC was unlikely to find fundamental problems in the literature. Extensive research has demonstrated that when like-minded individuals deliberate, they usually arrive at a more radical version of their initial views. Through a process of group polarization, people surrounded by others who share their opinions are likely to become even more certain and to adopt more extreme positions.[135] This polarization might have been diminished in the NBAC with the addition of experts in the outcome variables, or the conditions that breastfeeding is said to ameliorate. A respected scientist in oncology or endocrinology, for example, could have commented intelligently on the research concerning infant feeding and cancer or diabetes as well as on the merits of framing breastfeeding as risk-reducing behavior. In addition, a medical ethicist could have helped make moral issues explicit and to construct a campaign message consistent with both the science and the particular concerns of the mothers and families that constituted the campaign's target population. *Ethical* manipulation might be genuinely possible only in such a deliberative context, one consciously designed to maximize diversity, uncertainty, and sensitivity.

Both the NBAC and breastfeeding promotion in general demonstrate how health scientists, health officials, and activists can become "scientific partisans,"[136] often well-meaning advocates who offer hyperbole and inconsistent reasoning in defense of claims they believe to be incontrovertible. During the campaign, for example, the AAP issued a policy statement indicating that babies should be offered pacifiers after the first month to decrease the risk for SIDS,[137] a recommendation that drew the ire of breastfeeding partisans who maintained that the use of pacifiers interfered with breastfeeding. The USBC responded with a press release stating that the pacifier protocol lacked "a clear scientific basis," constrained parental choice, complicated "the potentially challenging process of putting infants to sleep," and impaired breastfeeding.[138] Yet, with the exception of the last, all the USBC's objections to the pacifier protocol also are true for the AAP's breastfeeding guidelines, which the USBC supports. Gartner told *Newsweek* that the evidence for pacifiers' protective effect against SIDS was suspect because it was based on retrospective research and relied on parents' recall about past pacifier use.[139] These, too, are problems with much of the research suggesting benefits to breastfeeding. Dr. Melissa Bartick, chair of the Massachusetts Breastfeeding Coalition, wrote a provocative letter in *Pediatrics*, the AAP's journal, in which she implied that the task force responsible for the pacifier recommendations had "financial conflicts of interest," a charge that she did not substantiate and that the task force called "absurd."[140] The claim by some NBAC proponents that nicotine and formula are analogous, another example of partisan rhetoric, was an effort not to refute specific challenges to the campaign but to deny the legitimacy of posing questions altogether. For health partisans, including many breastfeeding proponents, the merits of the cause are no longer subject to debate. They are common sense.

The NBAC also revealed how public health campaigns can hinder informed decision making by "instrumentalizing anxiety"[141] and effectively limiting viable options. In a neoliberal risk culture, a veneer of choice exists, but proscribed behaviors are clear. Dutiful individuals internalize surveillance, self-regulate, and are normalized as good citizens; others eat too many carbohydrates, fail to exercise, and bottle-feed. Risk analysts David Gray and George Ropeik suggest that "most risk communication fails because it tells people only what the communicators want them to know, to get them to behave 'rationally'—that is, the way the communicator wants them to behave."[142] Because risk advice tends to reflect the values of the institution offering it, the target audience can find it impractical or even irrational. Gray and Ropeik further argue that "risk communication is more likely to succeed if it sets the more realistic goal of helping people understand the facts, in ways that are relevant to their own lives, feelings, and values, so they are empowered to put the risk in perspective and make more informed choices."[143]

Public health, in this analysis, should devote itself to providing accurate risk information about probabilities and trade-offs in order to enable informed decision making. Rather than provoke or manipulate fear, productive messages should address two questions: "How big is my risk, and how does this risk compare with other risks?"[144] The answers should vary according to every individual's cultural and socioeconomic context. At least one critic contends that "nearly all public health issues can be explained satisfactorily to almost every adult,"[145] and the focus groups conducted by McKinney+Silver revealed that most women understand why breastfeeding is recommended. If "there is no ultimate deterrent . . . no mother of all health warnings,"[146] educating people about how to make informed decisions might be the only ethical mission for public health. The NBAC, however, decontextualized risk and became something of a crusade. Grounded in science that is not nearly as settled as its partisans suggest, the NBAC was a moral campaign as much about maternal responsibility in a risk culture as it was about the health benefits of breastfeeding per se.

Health campaigns establish codes for ethical personhood and responsible citizenship. Their impact, therefore, is measured not solely by how many people adopt recommended behaviors but also by the degree to which they make individuals feel virtuous or shamed. In issues surrounding motherhood, "their power lies not in their ability to make women do what they would otherwise not have done, but in their authority to define the standards by which mothers' feeding activities are to be judged, by others and indeed by the women themselves."[147] In the aftermath of the campaign, the number of women who expressed self-reproach or debated whether mothers *should* feel guilty for not breastfeeding challenges the almost parodic neoliberal contention of the USBC's Marsha Walker that breastfeeding promotion does not make women feel guilty because "guilt, like any other emotion, is something one *chooses* to feel."[148] Regardless of why they bottle-feed, many mothers frame their use of formula as a dereliction of maternal obligation. One woman, whose baby was hospitalized for dehydration, said using formula made her feel "like a failure." Another, who produced insufficient milk, said, "I was terrified I was hurting my baby."[149] "Notwithstanding the fact that it was physically impossible for me to breast-feed," said still another woman, "there were moments when I felt like an utter failure as a mother."[150] These stories reflect formula feeding as an experience of maternal delinquency. Rooted in the overwrought rhetoric of breastfeeding promotion, they are narratives of shame. The NBAC told mothers that not breastfeeding was risky, a message that encapsulated the terms of maternal citizenship and the central principle of total motherhood: that good mothers incur any cost to reduce any risk to babies. Bottle feeding challenges mothers' integrity as citizens and their virtue as mothers; in maligning those who turn to formula, the NBAC made not breastfeeding shameful.

Indeed, both the campaign and breastfeeding policy in general reveal what historian Charles Rosenberg has called the "drama of contested moral choice and social commitment" that is health in a neoliberal risk culture. "What is the role of the state in a just . . . society? How does one balance individual responsibility against the need for social intervention? How much does the entirely rational attempt to reduce risk through individual suasion serve to blame victims and avoid the necessity of dealing with structural inequalities?"[151] These ethical dilemmas are also apparent in New York City's 2007 decision to ban baby formula samples, coupons, and other promotional materials in its eleven public hospitals. Is discontinuing formula giveaways and coupons an ethical way to try to raise breastfeeding rates? If so, what are the costs, and who will bear them? Is a potential increase in breastfeeding among middle-class babies worth the hardship that it might cause economically distressed families? Is a possible increase in breastfeeding among lower-income babies worth the burdens it could impose on poor women and their families? What kinds of risk biases are reflected when New York eliminates a program that reduces the cost of formula at the same time that it fails to provide adequate health care to many of the city's pregnant women, new mothers, and children? Should the national government be spending scarce public health resources on promoting a single regimen of breastfeeding, a process whose benefits to babies (or mothers) have not been rigorously defined or demonstrated? Will the benefits of breastfeeding ever be strong and generalizable enough to justify a comprehensive state recommendation that mothers assume the kind of responsibility for babies' health implied by the NBAC? If so, how would the risks, or costs, be distributed? When health, risk, and individual and maternal responsibility collide, public policy on breastfeeding is a microcosm of life in contemporary neoliberal risk culture.

6

Conclusion

Whither Breastfeeding?

FEW PEOPLE ARE against health. Or freedom. Or compassion. But when one person's freedom to drive her car at any speed infringes on another's freedom to travel safely, or when compassion for others leads to a loss of self, the merits of restriction and selfishness begin to emerge. Ostensibly unobjectionable ideals become controversial when advocates become myopic and lobby for their cause with a single-minded zeal that borders on monomania.

Likewise, preventing risk, promoting health behavior, and providing for babies are, in theory, not terribly contentious agendas. They become problematic when proponents do not adequately consider the complex social environments in which they are pursued, as if their desirability could be challenged only by the ignorant or nefarious. Reducing risks to the environment raises manufacturing costs, which makes consumer goods more expensive and decreases buying power. For low-income families, marginal cost increases can wreak havoc on finances, so helping the environment might be virtuous but unaffordable. Advocating healthy choices can create social ostracization by exaggerating personal control and understating the influence of socioeconomic structures on well-being. Nurturing babies and children can lead to a loss of self, particularly when the burden for that care falls disproportionately on one family member. The problem, therefore, is not risk aversion, health promotion, or concern for children but the insular and unidimensional zealotry they often inspire.

Science and Public Health

In the United States, a veritable health mania has led to moral agendas predicated on limited science and to prescriptions for behavior that reflect a crucial misunderstanding of the methods with which scientific evidence is constructed.[1] Among the most common practices across the sciences is the computation of statistical significance, which determines whether a relationship between two variables exists. For example, if the correlation between body fat and coronary disease, or breastfeeding and better health, is statistically significant, this means that an individual who is overweight runs a higher risk of developing heart disease and that children who are breastfed are more likely to be healthier. What statistical significance cannot determine is whether adipose tissue or breastfeeding causes particular outcomes. It is a useful calculation that can help scientists orient future research, but it cannot answer fundamental questions about what leads to better health.

In an extended critique of contemporary science, Stephen Ziliak and Deidre McCloskey lament that a "cult of statistical significance" has "metastasized" throughout various sciences. "Existence, the question of whether, is interesting," they contend, "but it is not scientific." Rather, scientific questions ask about causal relationships, about "salience, adequacy, nonnegligibility, real error, an oomph that measures the practical difference something makes."[2] Because statistical significance cannot demonstrate how or why an association exists and whether or how much it matters, by itself it is a weak scientific tool. Scientists who answer the metaphysical question—is there a relationship?—but fail to tackle the scientific question—what does the relationship mean?—elide the difference between the statistical and social meaning of the word "significant" and can end up "causing damage with a broken statistical instrument."[3]

Such damage results today when people change their behavior in response to the almost daily release of new research on how lifestyle affects health. If the practical meaning of a statistically significant association is limited, the medicalization of life has made clear that the conceptual terrain on which such relationships can be established is virtually limitless. Almost every dimension of a person's life—from what she breathes, eats, and drives to her family and social networks—can somehow be quantified and measured in relation to various health outcomes, and the results of these analyses are often inconsistent. According to Barry Kramer, associate director for disease prevention at the National Institutes of Health, much of health research today amounts to "the cure of the week or the killer of the week, the danger of the week." He likened it to treating people to "an endless regiment of whiplash." Stan Young, a statistician at the National Institute of Statistical Sciences, stated that epidemiological research is so often wrong that it approaches "worthless." "We spend a lot of money and we could make claims just as valid as a random number generator."[4]

If not all scientists are quite so disparaging, many nonetheless recognize that the proliferation of epidemiological health studies has produced much confusion among and between scientists and the public. The primary problem with this research is that statistical significance measures only chance, not the presence of selection bias or confounding variables. Even when multiple studies do demonstrate a correlation between two variables, the existence of this relationship proves neither that one causes the other nor that the association has social value. Ostensibly, controlling for confounding variables should help isolate causality, but this is true only if the measures employed are valid: that is, if the proxy really is an effective measure of the variable that one is trying to assess. Is the frequency of a family dinner an appropriate measure of family cohesion? Do education and social class reliably convey health behavior? Are moderate drinkers healthier because they drink moderately or because people who drink moderately tend to behave more healthily?

Breastfeeding advocacy is but one example of the limits of statistical significance; the ongoing campaign against America's "obesity epidemic," intended to persuade Americans to lose weight, is another. Indeed, an increasing number of scholars are questioning the widespread belief that obesity causes health problems. They point to the weakness of body mass index (BMI) as a measure of healthy body weight and to the absence of evidence showing that weight loss itself produces better health.[5] Eric Oliver, for example, points out that "heavier people may have a higher mortality rate but this does not necessarily mean that it is their body fat that is killing them. . . . It must be verified that the trait in question is the direct source of the problem and not simply a proxy for other causes."[6] What is unclear in both obesity and infant-feeding research is whether the variable being measured, excess body fat or bottle feeding, is itself the problem or is a stand-in for some other determinant.

Oliver contends that body weight cannot be considered independent of diet, exercise, family history, and genetics; that no convincing theory demonstrates how extra fat tissue causes heart disease, cancer, or other ailments; and that altering the metabolic processes that are behind the various maladies associated with obesity makes more scientific sense than targeting weight per se. "There is little evidence that obesity itself is a primary cause of our health woes," he writes, and "telling most Americans they need to worry about their weight is like telling someone dying of pneumonia that they need to worry about how much they are coughing; it conflates the real source of our health problems with a relatively benign symptom."[7] Much the same might be said about breastfeeding. Infant feeding research often acknowledges but never eliminates the possibility that breastfeeding is an indicator, a sign of parents' general commitment to well-being that in itself has little impact. No compelling evidence establishes how breastfeeding reduces the risk of diabetes, obesity, or respiratory disease, and equally plausible theories for these risks could be cited that have nothing to do with breastfeeding. Warning mothers that not breastfeeding creates health risks for their babies, therefore, might be like telling them that not having family dinners puts their children's academic success at risk: it conflates a proxy with a cause.

In examining existing survey data, Oliver found that the best predictor of obesity in middle- and high school students, besides genetics, was toothbrushing.

> Now obviously, the act of brushing one's teeth plays little direct role in a child's weight, but it is a good indicator of something else—in what type of household that child lives. Children who brush their teeth more often are more likely to come from homes where health and hygiene are a priority.

These children, he argues, are also more likely to eat fresh fruits and vegetables, drink milk instead of soda, and spend less time playing video games or watching television.[8] As toothbrushing is to obesity, breastfeeding might well be to the various ailments associated with bottle feeding: a sign of a much more comprehensive commitment to healthy living that is itself responsible for salutary outcomes. And while toothbrushing has been proven to promote healthy teeth and gums, the independent effects of breast milk are largely undemonstrated. Increasing breastfeeding rates, in other words, might have little to do with improving babies' health. What Oliver argues about promoting weight loss—"Public health officials and doctors need to stop making weight a barometer of health and issuing so many alarmist claims about the obesity epidemic"[9]—might also be true of advocating breastfeeding. Those who suggest that not breastfeeding constitutes a public health threat today comparable to the early twentieth century (before pasteurization, refrigeration, and the production of reliable breast milk substitutes),[10] or that no public health effort would contribute more to improving children's health than a breastfeeding campaign,[11] or that increased breastfeeding could "blunt the worldwide epidemic of obesity,"[12] are using hyperbole to transmit a message that the science does not warrant.

Nonetheless, in the general population and much of the public health community, the health dangers of obesity and infant formula take the form of received wisdom. Various experts point to a large body of evidence indicating a statistically significant relationship between obesity or formula feeding and various health problems, and they infer that the relationship is causal. They offer provisional explanations for the connection, and the public assumes that these hypotheses are correct because they make sense or are logical. Breast milk, for example, must reduce infection because it contains maternal antibodies. That science has not demonstrated that these antibodies have any real effect outside the gastrointestinal tract is interpreted by many professionals and lay people not as a challenge to the theory but as the slowness of science to establish what everyone knows is true.[13] History, however, certainly does not lack for cautionary tales about unproven assumptions. For most of the twentieth century, for example, scientists and physicians believed that stomach ulcers were caused by stress and lifestyle. Pharmaceuticals, psychiatry, gastroenterology, and a self-help industry all developed around this theory. When two Australian researchers discovered that the bacterium Helicobacter pylori was actually the cause, the belief that bacteria could not survive in the stomach and that ulcers were induced by stress was so entrenched in the scientific community that few were willing to take them seriously. In 1982, one of the scientists, Barry Marshall, swallowed a cocktail of the bacteria, gave himself an ulcer, and successfully treated it with an antibiotic. In 2005, he and his colleague, Robin Warren, were awarded the Nobel Prize in medicine for their discovery. Today, between 80 and 90 percent of ulcers are attributed to Helicobacter pylori.[14]

As Gina Kolata illustrates in her history of obesity research, the most elegantly crafted scientific logic has little value if it cannot be empirically demonstrated.[15] The dilemma for both public health officials and citizens is what to do with the seemingly daily discovery of statistically significant relationships and the behavior changes they inevitably inspire. At one extreme of thinking are the "risk averse" who advocate some version of the Precautionary Principle: "Avoid steps that will create a risk of harm. Until safety is established, be cautious; do not require unambiguous evidence. In a catchphrase: Better safe than sorry."[16] If breastfeeding and losing weight are not dangerous, then what is the harm of either? Why not pursue both, especially since evidence of an association between the two and better health does exist? This perspective ignores that breastfeeding and weight loss are undertaken in social contexts in which trade-offs are inescapable and harm need not be biological. At the other extreme are those who demand that scientists be absolutely certain about causality before making recommendations. This "radical skepticism" or "immoderate doubt"[17] is tantamount to a nihilism that refuses to recognize that even compelling science confronts an unavoidable degree of uncertainty. By such a standard, all science would be futile. Between these two poles is a gray zone of interpretation in which both scientists and the public make choices that necessarily reflect personal, social, cultural, political, and professional values. For their part, the media tend to report on the latest findings and never visit them again. An ever expanding catalog of statistically significant relationships then confronts a public with limited knowledge of how to make sense of them.

What is more, in a neoliberal risk culture, a veritable "cult of personal responsibility"[18] makes it seem as if virtuous citizens are wholly accountable for their health. When the path to health is presented as certain, as in the injunctions to be thin and to breastfeed, social disparities recede from view, and exercising personal responsibility becomes nearly compulsory. Failure to maintain a "healthy" weight or to breastfeed becomes irresponsible behavior, despite extensive evidence that weight control and infant feeding are often biologically and/or socioeconomically circumscribed and therefore not entirely under personal control. When such prescriptions are built on weak science, people find themselves in the absurd position of being held accountable for illness when they have not adopted behaviors that might have little to do with health, anyway.

The conviction with which breastfeeding and dieting are embraced as keys to good health is, in part, a response to the ambiguity of a risk culture in which information is constantly produced and revised and truth is fleeting. The certainty that fat and bottle feeding are unhealthy provides some cognitive rootedness and, for those who have sufficient resources, a blueprint for responsible living.[19] Certitude, however, clouds judgment. It conceals the relationship between social structures, such as gender, class, and race, and health. It also blinds people to the reality that risk is omnipresent, that values shape which risks are made visible, and that risk-reducing behaviors have inevitable costs whose discernability often depends on who is shouldering them.

In light of the current discourse on health, replete with incipient associations, scientists interested in breastfeeding must begin to assess the benefits and costs of further epidemiological research, or what Ziliak and McCloskey call "the opportunity cost of specializing in [statistical significance] excessively."[20] Will such study shed light on crucial unanswered questions in the current literature? The present offers little cause for optimism. The risk-factor model does not allow for an analysis of causal links and cannot establish that breastfeeding is, in itself, medically advantageous. New approaches to this research, moreover, are unlikely. As Dr. Otis W. Brawley, chief medical officer at the American Cancer Society, observed, "The problem in science is that the way you get ahead is by staying within narrow parameters and doing what other people are doing. No one wants to fund wild new ideas." Researchers who need grants to keep their laboratories operating or even to keep their positions tend to be cautious when submitting proposals, and review committees are wary of awarding scarce money to newfangled projects.[21]

In addition, the current literature is already rife with unexamined hypotheses about how breastfeeding might contribute to better health. No doubt, lactation scientists have made significant inroads in understanding how breast milk might affect the progression of such illnesses as necrotizing enterocolitis and gastrointestinal infections.[22] Nonetheless, countless hypotheses about breastfeeding and heart disease, intelligence, diabetes, obesity, asthma, and other health outcomes have not been tested, much less demonstrated, in biological science. This research, which is essential to determine whether breastfeeding causes better outcomes, promises a far greater knowledge yield than do additional epidemiological studies. But scientists studying the relationship between mode of infant feeding and ear infections or obesity do not generally compete for funding with scientists conducting biological research. A decrease in support for the former will not lead necessarily to an increase in the latter. In the short term, therefore, continued epidemiological research is likely to further entrench the public health message that breastfeeding provides myriad health benefits for babies, thereby making causality seem even more probable than the evidence indicates. One recent example of this is the National Academies Institute of Medicine report recommending the promotion of breastfeeding as one of seven strategies local governments should adopt to combat obesity.[23]

Perhaps the best hope for breastfeeding research lies in randomized controlled trials (RCT) in which mothers and babies are randomly assigned to breastfeeding or bottle feeding. If a reasonable hypothesis is that women who choose to breastfeed are also more able and likely to encourage health-promoting behaviors, then eliminating the choice by randomly allocating mothers to breast and bottle feeding also should nullify its effects. In a well-constructed RCT with a sufficiently large subject population, therefore, the problem of confounding would be less salient. RCTs, however, are unlikely. As earlier noted, because the health benefits of breastfeeding are so widely accepted, scientists consider it unethical to assign mothers and babies to formula feeding. Women also are likely to be reluctant to volunteer for such studies, either because the costs of formula or breastfeeding are too high or because they have been persuaded by the public health message that not breastfeeding is risky.

In fact, it is the consensus that breast is best that is the greatest obstacle to determining whether, or under what circumstances, breast is best. As Michael Kramer, the lead author of the PROBIT investigation and an advocate of breastfeeding, has argued, it is unclear "why it is less ethical to randomize individuals to a control group in evaluating a potentially effective public health intervention than it is with drugs, surgery, or other clinical interventions," for which randomization is common. "Nor is it clear why it is considered ethical to institute a useless or perhaps even harmful program whose efficacy and safety have not been established by rigorous scientific standards."[24] Indeed, one might ask why it is ethical to tell women to choose breastfeeding, most of whose health benefits have not been demonstrated and whose costs can be exorbitant, but it is unethical to randomly assign mothers to formula feeding, whose harms also have not been established, especially when RCTs could provide critical information. The answer lies partially in researchers' certainty that breastfeeding is medically superior, but it also is rooted in total motherhood, or the relative willingness in American risk culture to assume that mothers will bear the cost, no matter how high, of reducing any risk, no matter how small, to children.

At present, the public health message about breastfeeding is out of sync with both the infant-feeding science and the realities of many women's lives. Even if the evidence were stronger, if the results of the best research were more compelling, the notion that not breastfeeding is risky would fail to convey that every feeding choice involves trade-offs and produces new risks. Breastfeeding makes extraordinary demands on women's emotional and physical energy; for every woman who enjoys it, another finds it intolerable. Breastfeeding places mothers at the center of babies' existence; for every mother who desires exclusivity, another is committed to equal parenting with her partner. Breastfeeding requires flexibility in the workday; for every woman who can combine employment and breastfeeding, another cannot reconcile her job with the demands of breastfeeding.

The neoliberal message of the National Breastfeeding Awareness Campaign (NBAC) and other public health efforts is especially insensitive to many mothers' socioeconomic constraints. Indeed, emphasizing mothers' putatively unique capacity to contribute to babies' health also is politically self-serving. If healthy babies can be produced by individual mothers who choose to behave responsibly, then poverty, unemployment, and other intractable social problems decline in significance, despite their persistent correlation with poor health, and public institutions are relieved of obligation. By targeting mothers with low breastfeeding rates, such as poor and African American women, the government is offering what amounts to symbolic assistance for marginalized populations at little cost. In Eric Oliver's terms, the promotion of breastfeeding addresses a "relatively benign symptom," not breastfeeding, with a "real cause" of poor health, socioeconomic marginalization.[25] As structural problems, which are far more complicated and expensive than failures of individual will to address, recede from view, not breastfeeding is judged as a poor choice, and each mother, regardless of her resources, is held personally accountable for its presumptive consequences.[26]

Breastfeeding and Maternal Responsibility

I opened this book with a broad question: Why, when the science is not compelling, have so many experts and the public come to be persuaded of a breastfeeding imperative? Much of the answer, I have argued, can be found in the workings of a risk culture. Breastfeeding sits at the intersection of public discourse on science, health, and personal responsibility. It is grounded in social dynamics that are at work in matters stretching far beyond either infant feeding or motherhood, and it reveals that the inevitable biases of a risk culture—including the risks scientists pursue and the choices they and the public make about which risks are most significant to families—are today often based on presumptions about maternal responsibility.

In fact, as I also have contended, the research on and practice of breastfeeding are a microcosm of total motherhood. From before pregnancy and throughout children's lives, girls and then women are taught to think of themselves in relation to a normative motherhood. They are instructed by various experts to contemplate and make choices that minimize all risks to their future offspring, regardless of how serious or likely these risks are or what the cost might be. The recommendation to breastfeed reflects this project, and it is based on scientific research that also is grounded in the principles of total motherhood, or the assumption that no risk is too small and no cost too great when it comes to mother's obligation to optimize children's health. Contrary to what Bernice Hausman maintains, therefore, deconstructing the scientific discourse on breastfeeding is neither a simple "rhetorical strategy" that feminists employ in order to criticize "domestic femininity" nor "a side show that should be set aside" by feminists who instead ought to focus on removing the obstacles confronted by women who want to breastfeed.[27] Rather, questioning breastfeeding science is an integral part of any feminist engagement that seeks to demonstrate how choices are enabled and constrained by gender. It is not a foundation for or peripheral to feminist critique. It is feminist critique.

For their part, feminists have waged innumerable internecine battles over the antinomies of body politics. For some, pornography and prostitution epitomize the objectification of women's bodies and are a source of violence against women; for others, they represent women's right to control their bodies and to embrace their sexual desire. Some argue that pain medication during childbirth provides relief from unnecessary suffering, while others contend that it separates women from their bodies and transfers control over birth to doctors and machines. In fact, pornography, prostitution, epidurals—in addition to abortion, assisted reproduction, and so many other issues surrounding women's bodies—are unavoidably feminist and antifeminist. Efforts to stake out a universal feminist position on these issues necessarily fail because feminism does not exist outside the myriad social contexts it analyzes, and what appears to be feminist in one time or place might seem decidedly antifeminist in others.

Breastfeeding presents similar contradictions. On one hand, it is a celebration of women's bodies and their ability to sustain life; it wrests control over babies from doctors, formula manufacturers, and men and gives it to women. On the other hand, breastfeeding reinforces traditional notions of women, their bodies, and their "natural" orientation toward caregiving; it keeps women tethered to their babies and creates risks for them in a market that demands total commitment from "ideal workers."[28] The breast pump is equally confounding. It frees women to separate themselves physically from their babies, for either work or pleasure, and to share responsibility for child care; it also represents a fetishization of breasts that can transform women into virtual machines whose primary function is milk production. Breastfeeding advocates, including those who demand that work environments and other public spaces be more accommodating, have broadened the spectrum of choices for women by normalizing breastfeeding; they also have circumscribed the feeding decision by exploiting the fears and concerns of women who continue to be told that they are mothers above all and that their bodies exist first for their offspring. Breastfeeding, in short, can be inserted into multiple narratives, some oppressive and some empowering. Given the infinite variety of women and mothers and the ongoing power of social location to frame choices, no perfect feminist world exists in which either breastfeeding or bottle feeding is intrinsically preferable. Both take place in complex personal, political, and cultural environments that, as Linda Blum and Pam Carter pointed out long ago, preclude the possibility of a normative prescription.[29]

As Blum and Carter also demonstrated, breastfeeding, like so many putatively healthy behaviors in a neoliberal culture, is not even an option for many poor and low-income women, at least some of whom might prefer it to purchasing formula. Educated and middle-class women are more likely to breastfeed, to be able to purchase a breast pump, and to work in environments in which breastfeeding is possible.[30] To the extent that feminism seeks to break down barriers that restrict women's choices, therefore, advocating social change that would make the public sphere more hospitable to breastfeeding is a logical feminist goal. Such developments, in fact, would likely have beneficial effects on babies independent of any increase in breastfeeding rates. Today, labor markets that require workers to be available in ways that preclude caretaking, miserly family-leave policies, and limited access to quality child care severely limit families' choices once a child is born. Mandated, subsidized, and regulated child care would facilitate breastfeeding for more working women, but it would also provide the babies of working parents with safe, hygienic, and engaging environments likely to stimulate physical, intellectual, and emotional development. Flexible work schedules, including the demarginalization of so-called family-friendly policies and part-time employment, might enable more women to breastfeed, but they also would make it easier for parents to schedule babies' doctor appointments and coordinate home care and would allow for more interactive time between parents and children. Paid and extended family leave policies that do not penalize workers whose futures depend on seniority might promote breastfeeding, but they also could enhance parent-infant bonding, reduce the need for early child care, and therefore limit the number of people, and germs, to which babies are exposed. In other words, structural changes that would further breastfeeding would create other possibilities as well, opportunities that themselves are likely to lead to healthier babies across class divides.

By expanding families' viable choices, moreover, these changes would promote the decentralization of responsibility for children.[31] Policies that target children but do not assume that mothers are singularly responsible for their well-being—those that recognize that children are public goods for which the responsibility rests with all those who benefit, including fathers, communities, and government—are likely to have payoffs that include but extend far beyond babies' health. If behavior associated with breastfeeding can explain many of the benefits attributed to breastfeeding, then democratizing access to those behaviors is a matter for public health advocates and feminists alike.

In the meantime, infant formula is a remarkable example of human ingenuity. That it cannot exactly replicate breast milk is clear; that this makes much of a difference in the health of most babies in the developed world is far less certain. For some women, the choice is limited: they are medically unable to breastfeed or financially unable to formula-feed. But many women and their families struggle to balance multiple considerations. While some mothers enjoy the kind of intimacy that breastfeeding makes possible, others choose not to have their bodies constantly available. Some manage easily with a breast pump; others find onerous the mental and physical demands of pumping or combining work with breastfeeding. Some women belong to families and social networks in which breastfeeding is welcome, but others live in personal, social, or political communities where breastfeeding is not encouraged. Race, class, and other social locations, as well as personal preferences, are likely to exert powerful influence over how the feeding decision is made, and in the absence of either a strong case for benefits to breastfeeding or a comprehensive analysis demonstrating that its risks outweigh its benefits, these are not necessarily obstacles that good mothers need to overcome for the sake of their babies.

Ultimately, women might choose to breastfeed for various reasons: they find breastfeeding more convenient than bottle feeding; they do not want to support formula manufacturers; they believe, for religious or cultural reasons, that mothers have a unique obligation to their babies, which includes breastfeeding; or they want to shrink their "carbon footprint" and help the environment by reducing the production of formula. These all are legitimate motivations, but they should not be cloaked in language about the medical dangers of infant formula. More women might well choose to breastfeed if public spaces, including workplaces, were more favorable.

More women might also choose to formula-feed if they knew that the putative medical benefits of breastfeeding were largely undemonstrated. Everyone concerned about mothers and babies should work toward ensuring that mothers are well informed of the advantages and disadvantages of different feeding methods. But such an effort will fail if it is driven by the assumption that any woman who cares about her baby will breastfeed.

The science today indicates that if breastfeeding has health advantages, they are, for most babies in the developed world, marginal. If, however, science should demonstrate in the future that breastfeeding's benefits are extensive, then public health officials, women, and their families will have to determine whether the advantages of breastfeeding override its costs. For the time being, the "Call to Action" to increase breastfeeding that the Centers for Disease Control and Prevention and the U.S. Department of Health and Human Services' Office on Women's Health were to issue in 2010, a project they defined as "an urgent public health priority," seems at least slightly overwrought.[32] In the overwhelming majority of cases, either breastfeeding or formula feeding is a healthy option.

Notes

Preface

1. Jules Law, "The Politics of Breastfeeding: Assessing Risk, Dividing Labor," *Signs: Journal of Women in Culture and Society* 25, no. 2 (2000): 407.

2. Bernice L. Hausman, *Mother's Milk: Breastfeeding Controversies in American Culture* (New York: Routledge, 2003), 223.

3. Katherine A. Dettwyler, "Formula Is Bad for Babies," *Chicago Parent,* January 2004.

4. Maloney proposed the breastfeeding promotion act in 2001 and has reintroduced the bill in every succeeding House session. Jeff Merkley of Oregon became the first Senate sponsor of the bill in 2009, when it was presented in both chambers.

5. Among the organizations and institutions officially recommending breastfeeding are the American Academy of Family Physicians, "AAFP Policy Statement on Breastfeeding," 2001; the American College of Obstetricians and Gynecologists, "Breastfeeding: Maternal and Infant Aspects," 2001; the American Dietetic Association, "Position of the American Dietetic Association: Promoting and Supporting Breastfeeding," 2009; the American Association of Health Plans, "Advancing Women's Health: Health Plans'

Innovative Programs in Breastfeeding Promotion," 2001; the American Public Health Association (www.apha.org/advocacy/policy/policysearch/default.htm?id=1360); the Centers for Disease Control and Prevention (www.cdc.gov/breastfeeding/); and the U.S. Department of Health and Human Services (www.4woman.gov/breastfeeding/).

6. AAP, Section on Breastfeeding, "Policy Statement: Breastfeeding and the Use of Human Milk," *Pediatrics* 115, no. 2 (2005): 496.

7. Jodi R. Godfrey and David Meyers, "Toward Optimal Health: Maternal Benefits of Breastfeeding," *Journal of Women's Health* 18, no. 9 (2009): 2.

8. The one clear exception is gastrointestinal infections, which I address in chapter 2.

9. Because breastfeeding promotion has been primarily a discourse about babies, my analysis of the science focuses exclusively on breastfeeding's health effects on babies.

10. AAP, "Policy Statement: Breastfeeding," 499; www.llli.org/FAQ/frequency.html (accessed August 4, 2009).

11. I did discover pioneering works by Pam Carter and Linda Blum, which were followed by

thoughtful analyses from Jules Law, Glenda Wall, Bernice Hausman, and others, scholarship that I address in chapter 1. But I remained struck by the absence of a sustained feminist conversation about breastfeeding comparable to ongoing feminist debates about such matters as pregnancy and childbirth.

12. Some of my analysis, particularly the discussion of breastfeeding research, poses important questions about feeding in any context. But to unpack the international dimension of breastfeeding, particularly the politics of breastfeeding in the developing world, is well beyond the scope of this book. While other scholars have taken up this issue, I concentrate on the United States.

13. Gloria Steinem, "If Men Could Menstruate," *Ms.,* October 1978.

14. Male lactation in mammals has been observed in two species of bats, flying foxes and Dayak fruit bats, and increased levels of the hormone prolactin can cause spontaneous lactation in human males. However, extensive research on male lactation or breastfeeding has not been conducted. See Thomas H. Kunz and David J. Hosken,

"Male Lactation: Why, Why Not and Is It Care?" *Trends in Ecology and Evolution* 24, no. 2 (2009): 80–85; Nikhil Swaminathan, "Strange but True: Males Can Lactate," *Scientific American*, September 6, 2007; and Charles M. Francis et al., "Lactation in Male Fruit Bats," *Nature* 367 (1994): 1691–92.

15. Linda M. Blum, *At the Breast: Ideologies of Breastfeeding and Motherhood in the Contemporary United States* (Boston: Beacon Press, 1999); Sharon Hays, *The Cultural Contradictions of Motherhood* (New Haven, CT:

Yale University Press, 1996); Susan J. Douglas and Meredith W. Michaels, *The Mommy Myth: The Idealization of Motherhood and How It Has Undermined Women* (Boston: Free Press, 2004).

16. Douglas and Michaels, *The Mommy Myth*, 6.

17. Stevi Jackson and Sue Scott, "Risk Anxiety and the Social Construction of Childhood," in *Risk and Sociocultural Theory: New Directions and Perspective*, ed. Deborah Lupton (Cambridge: Cambridge University Press, 1999), 89.

18. On the need to situate gender in other contexts, see Joan W. Scott, "Gender: A Useful Category of Historical Analysis," *American Historical Review* 91, no. 5 (1986): esp. 1065–70; and Joan W. Scott, "Deconstructing Equality-Versus-Difference: Or, the Use of Poststructuralist Theory for Feminism," *Feminist Studies* 14, no. 1 (1988): 33–50. On race, see William Julius Wilson, *The Bridge over the Racial Divide: Rising Inequality and Coalition Politics* (Berkeley: University of California Press, 2001).

Chapter 1

1. Janet Golden, *A Social History of Wet Nursing in America: From Breast to Bottle* (Cambridge: Cambridge University Press, 1996), 11–50.

2. Ibid., 53.

3. C. Becket Mahnke, "The Growth and Development of a Specialty: The History of Pediatrics," *Clinical Pediatrics* 39 (2000): 709. If infant mortality had continued at this rate, more than 500,000 babies would have died at the end of the twentieth century. The actual number was just over 28,000. See CDC, *Morbidity and Mortality Weekly Report* 48, no. 38 (October 1999).

4. My discussion of the twentieth century draws heavily on Rima D. Apple, *Mothers and Medicine: A Social History of Infant Feeding, 1890–1950* (Madison: University of Wisconsin Press, 1987). I have included page numbers for direct citations, but unless otherwise noted, the ideas expressed in this brief history of breastfeeding are based on this text.

5. Jeffrey P. Brosco, "Weight Charts and Well-Child Care: How the Pediatrician Became the Expert in Child Health," *Archives of Pediatric and Adolescent Medicine* 155 (2001): 1388.

6. Apple, *Mothers and Medicine*, 87, 56.

7. Charles Rosenberg, *No Other Gods: On Science and American Social Thought* (Baltimore: Johns Hopkins University Press, 1997), 3.

8. Barbara Ehrenreich and Deirdre English, *For Her Own Good: Two Centuries of the Experts' Advice to Women* (New York: Anchor Books, 2005), 33 (italics in original).

9. Apple, *Mothers and Medicine*, passim.

10. Rima D. Apple, *Perfect Motherhood: Science and Childrearing in America* (New Brunswick, NJ: Rutgers University Press, 2006), 56–61, 72.

11. Benjamin Spock, *The Common Sense Book of Baby and Child Care* (New York: Duell, Sloan and Pearce, 1946), 3.

12. Dorothy Pawluch, *The New Pediatrics: A Profession in Transition* (New York: Aldine de Gruyter, 1996), 32–33, 41.

13. Ibid., 37–43.

14. In a 2005 survey, most pediatricians expressed satisfaction with the current system of well-care provision. At the same time, more than half those surveyed believed that many dimensions of well-child care did not require a physician and could be more efficiently provided by nurse practitioners, physicians' assistants, registered nurses, and medical assistants. See Tumaini Coker et al., "Should Our Well-Child Care System Be Redesigned? A National Survey of Pediatricians," *Pediatrics* 118, no. 5 (2006). In 2009, the AAP issued a policy statement on the prevention of youth violence in which it urged pediatricians to "incorporate preventative education, screening for risk, and linkages to community-based counseling and treatment

resources" into routine practice, indicating the continual expansion of well-child care. See AAP, "Policy Statement—Role of the Pediatrician in Youth Violence Prevention," *Pediatrics* 124, no. 1 (2009): 393–402.

15. See David Armstrong, "The Invention of Infant Mortality," *Sociology of Health and Illness* 8, no. 3 (1986): 211–32.

16. Barbara Duden, *Disembodying Women: Perspectives on Pregnancy and the Unborn* (Cambridge, MA: Harvard University Press, 1993), 50–51.

17. William G. Rothstein, *Public Health and the Risk Factor: A History of an Uneven Medical Revolution* (Rochester, NY: University of Rochester Press, 2003), 137.

18. Lorna Weir, *Pregnancy, Risk and Biopolitics: On the Threshold of the Living Subject* (London: Routledge, 2006), 2, 3.

19. William Ray Arney, *Power and the Profession of Obstetrics* (Chicago: University of Chicago Press, 1982), 54, 90, 89.

20. Diane Eyer, *Mother-Infant Bonding: A Scientific Fiction* (New Haven, CT: Yale University Press, 1992), 142–43; Arney, *Power and the Profession of Obstetrics*, 54.

21. Weir, *Pregnancy, Risk and Biopolitics*, 29.

22. Critics argue that most prenatal care is routine and could be provided more economically and efficiently by midwives or trained assistants. But the public believes that obstetricians provide superior treatment, and prenatal care sustains many obstetrical practices. See Thomas H. Strong, *Expecting Trouble: The Myth of Prenatal*

Care in America (New York: New York University Press, 2000), 83–91; and Ann Oakley, *Social Support and Motherhood: The Natural History of a Research Project* (Oxford: Blackwell, 1992), 10–11.

23. Boston Women's Health Book Collective, *Our Bodies, Ourselves: A Book by and for Women*, 1st ed. (New York: Simon & Schuster, 1973), 1; Sandra Morgen, *Into Our Own Hands: The Women's Health Movement in the United States, 1969–1990* (New Brunswick, NJ: Rutgers University Press, 2002), 120.

24. Boston Women's Health Book Collective, *Our Bodies, Ourselves: A Book by and for Women*, 2nd ed. (New York: Touchstone, 1976), 248.

25. Morgen, *Into Our Own Hands*, 120–52.

26. Arney, *Power and the Profession of Obstetrics*, 136.

27. Ibid., 123.

28. Ibid., 54–58, 123–38.

29. Jule DeJager Ward, *La Leche League: At the Crossroads of Medicine, Feminism, and Religion* (Chapel Hill: University of North Carolina Press, 2000), 4.

30. La Leche League International, *The Womanly Art of Breastfeeding*, 2nd ed. (Franklin Park, IL: La Leche League International, 1963), 5–6, 20, 53, 132–33, italics in original.

31. The authors of *Our Bodies, Ourselves*, for example, embraced breastfeeding to help build babies' immunities and recommended *The Womanly Art of Breastfeeding* for guidance. The book "will answer any specific questions you might have," they wrote, "but its philosophy is different from ours. We do

not believe that breast-feeding has to dominate your life to the extent that you have the sole responsibility for your new baby" (Boston Women's Health Collective, *Our Bodies, Ourselves*, 1973, 225).

32. Mike Muller, *The Baby Killer: A War on Want Investigation into the Promotion and Sale of Powdered Baby Milks in the Third World* (London: War on Want, 1974).

33. See Andrew Chetley, *The Politics of Baby Foods: Successful Challenges to an International Marketing Strategy* (New York: St. Martin's Press, 1986). The United States voted against the code in 1981, during Ronald Reagan's presidency, but endorsed it in 1994, when Bill Clinton was president. Adherence to the code is voluntary, and enforcement has been largely absent.

34. AAP, "Policy Statement Based on Task Force Report: The Promotion of Breastfeeding," *Pediatrics* 69, no. 5 (1982): 654–55, 661.

35. Search conducted on PubMed, a database of medical literature maintained by the National Library of Medicine, November 21, 2008.

36. AAP, Section on Breastfeeding, "Policy Statement: Breastfeeding and the Use of Human Milk," *Pediatrics* 115, no. 2 (2005): 1036.

37. Pediatricians do continue to monitor feeding by keeping tabs on babies' weight at well checks.

38. See, for example, Lori B. Feldman-Winter et al., "Pediatricians and the Promotion and Support of Breastfeeding," *Archives of Pediatric and Adolescent*

Medicine 162, no. 12 (2008): 1142–49. For a discussion of a public health campaign in which the AAP's relationship with the formula industry came under intense scrutiny, see also chapter 5.

39. AAP, Section on Breastfeeding, "Policy Statement: Breastfeeding and the Use of Human Milk," *Pediatrics* 115, no. 2 (2005): 496–506.

40. Linda M. Blum, *At the Breast: Ideologies of Breastfeeding and Motherhood in the Contemporary United States* (Boston: Beacon Press, 1999), 200.

41. Jules Law, "The Politics of Breastfeeding: Assessing Risk, Dividing Labor," *Signs: Journal of Women in Culture and Society* 25, no. 2 (2000): 407–8, passim.

42. Glenda Wall, "Moral Constructions of Motherhood in Breastfeeding Discourse," *Gender & Society* 15, no. 4 (2001): 592–610. Wall's discussion of the value of personal responsibility in the Canadian context helped frame my analysis of neoliberalism in American risk culture.

43. Ellie J. Lee, "Living with Risk in the Age of 'Intensive Motherhood': Maternal Identity and Infant Feeding," *Health, Risk, and Society* 10, no. 5 (2008): 467–77; Ellie Lee and Jennie Bristow, "Rules for Feeding Babies," in *Regulating Autonomy: Sex, Reproduction, and Family*, ed. Shelley Day Sclater et al. (Oxford: Hart Publishing, 2009), 73–91; Joyce L. Marshall, Mary Godfrey, and Mary J. Renfrew, "Being a 'Good Mother': Managing Breastfeeding and Merging Identities," *Social Science & Medicine* 65 (2007): 2147–59; Fiona Dykes, "'Supply' and 'Demand': Breastfeeding as Labour," *Social Sciences & Medicine* 60 (2005): 2283–93; Renée Flacking, Uwe Ewald, and Bengt Starrin, "'I Wanted to Do a Good Job': Experiences of 'Becoming a Mother' and Breastfeeding in Mothers of Very Preterm Infants after Discharge from a Neonatal Unit," *Social Science & Medicine* 64 (2007): 2405–16; Virginia Schmied and Deborah Lupton, "Blurring the Boundaries: Breastfeeding and Maternal Subjectivity," *Sociology of Health and Illness* 23, no. 2 (2001): 234–50; Alison Bartlett, "Breastfeeding as Headwork: Corporeal Feminism and Meanings for Breastfeeding," *Women's Studies International Forum* 25, no. 3 (2002): 373–82.

44. Elizabeth Murphy, "'Breast Is Best': Infant Feeding Decisions and Maternal Deviance," *Sociology of Health and Illness* 21, no. 2 (1999): 187–208; Elizabeth Murphy, "Risk, Responsibility, and Rhetoric in Infant Feeding," *Journal of Contemporary Ethnography* 29, no. 3 (2000): 291–325; Orit Avishai, "Managing the Lactating Body: The Breastfeeding Project and Privileged Motherhood," *Qualitative Sociology* 30 (2007): 135–52.

45. Bernice L. Hausman, *Mother's Milk: Breastfeeding Controversies in American Culture* (New York: Routledge, 2003), 6.

46. Ibid., 198, 199, 208, 204, 199.

47. Blum points out that scientists have only a minimal understanding of how the protective mechanisms of breastfeeding might operate and that they have expressed concern that the benefits attributed to breastfeeding could be spurious (*At the Breast*, 49–50). Law identifies basic mistakes in the medical literature and argues that public health policy and popular advice literature depend on "assertions that were either significantly qualified or hypothetically postulated in the medical literature" ("The Politics of Breastfeeding," 409).

48. Hausman, *Mother's Milk*, 15.

49. Scot D. Yoder, "Individual Responsibility for Health: Decision, Not Discovery," *Hastings Center Report* 32, no. 2 (2002): 25 (italics in original).

50. See Donna Haraway, "Situated Knowledges: The Science Question in Feminism and the Privilege of Partial Perspective," *Feminist Studies* 14, no. 3 (1988): 575–99. Haraway argues that "the alternative to relativism is not totalization and single vision [but] partial, locatable, critical knowledges sustaining the possibility of webs of connections called solidarity in politics and shared conversations in epistemology" (584). All forms of knowledge, all facts, can be located in various networks of meaning, and it is only in the collection of partial perspectives that a compelling concept of objectivity can be developed.

51. Judy M. Hopkinson, "Response to 'Is Breast Really Best? Risk and Total Motherhood in the National Breast-Feeding Awareness Campaign,'" *Journal of Health Politics, Policy and Law* 32, no. 4 (2007): 645.

52. Jacqueline H. Wolf, "Low Breastfeeding Rates and Public Health in the United States," *American Journal of Public Health* 93, no. 12 (2003): 12.

53. Eyer, *Mother-Infant Bonding*, 13.

Chapter 2

1. AAP, Work Group on Breastfeeding, "Policy Statement: Breastfeeding and the Use of Human Milk," *Pediatrics* 100, no. 6 (1997): 1035.

2. ISI Journal Citation Reports, 2000–2008 (http://isi9.isiknowledge.com/portal.cgi/jcr); Catherine S. Birken and Patricia C. Parkin, "In Which Journals Will Pediatricians Find the Best Evidence for Clinical Practice?" *Pediatrics* 103, no. 5 (1999): 941. The value of the impact-factor rating in determining the significance of any particular article has been hotly contested (see, for example, the debate in the May 2008 issue of *Epidemiology*). At the same time, the National Institutes of Health suggests that a journal's impact factor indicates its importance compared with others in the same field (http://nihlibrary.nih.gov), and some research has demonstrated a strong correlation between a publication's impact-factor rating and how it is evaluated by clinical practitioners and scientists. See Somnath Saha, Sanjay Saint, and Dimitri A. Christakis, "Impact Factor: A Valid Measure of Journal Quality?" *Journal of the Medical Library Association* 91, no. 1 (2003): 42–46. This chapter focuses on the most commonly cited studies in particular research areas, such as asthma or obesity. While most of these appear in journals with relatively high impact factors, others, including many cited by the 2004–2006 National Breastfeeding Awareness Campaign (NBAC), do not. I discuss the NBAC in chapter 5.

3. These journals assume, in other words, that breastfeeding is superior. *Breastfeeding Medicine*, for example, is the journal of the American Academy of Breastfeeding Medicine, "a worldwide organization of physicians dedicated to the promotion, protection and support of breastfeeding and human lactation" (www.bfmed.org, accessed December 5, 2008). The publisher's homepage indicates that the journal publishes articles on the "epidemiologic, physiologic, and psychologic benefits of breastfeeding" and the "health consequences of artificial feeding" (www.liebertpub.com/Products/Product.aspx?pid=173, accessed December 5, 2008). The *International Breastfeeding Journal* publishes articles on "all aspects of breastfeeding," including "identifying women who are at increased risk of not breastfeeding; the impediments to breastfeeding and the health effects of not breastfeeding for infants and their mothers; interventions to increase breastfeeding initiation and duration; and the management of breastfeeding problems" (www.internationalbreastfeedingjournal.com/info/about/, accessed December 5, 2008). The *Journal of Human Lactation*, the official publication of the International Lactation Consultant Association, presents itself as "strongly advocating and supporting breastfeeding" but just as committed to publishing "a balanced view of many of the issues." In practice, these "issues" do not include *whether* breastfeeding is medically superior

to formula feeding (www.sagepub.com/journalsProdDesc.nav?prodId=Journal201341, accessed December 5, 2008).

4. Hans-Olov Adami and Dimitrios Trichopoulos, "Epidemiology, Medicine and Public Health," *International Journal of Epidemiology* 28 (1999): S1005.

5. Mervyn Susser, "Does Risk Factor Epidemiology Put Epidemiology at Risk? Peering into the Future," *Journal of Epidemiology and Community Health* 52 (1998): 608.

6. S. Schwartz, E. Susser, and M. Susser, "A Future for Epidemiology?" *Annual Review of Public Health* 20 (1999): 24.

7. "The Limits of Epidemiology," STATS, June 1, 2000, available at www.stats.org/record.jsp?type=news&ID=352.

8. John B. McKinlay and Lisa D. Marceau, "To Boldly Go . . . ," *American Journal of Public Health* 90, no. 1 (2000): 26; Neil Pearce, "Traditional Epidemiology, Modern Epidemiology, and Public Health," *American Journal of Public Health* 86 (1996): 682.

9. John P. A. Ioannidis, "Contradicted and Initially Stronger Effects in Highly Cited Clinical Research," *Journal of the American Medical Association* 294, no. 2 (2005): 223–25.

10. Moyses Szklo, "The Evaluation of Epidemiologic Evidence for Policy-Making," *American Journal of Epidemiology* 154, no. 12 (2001): S13; Cesar G. Victora, Jean-Pierre Habicht, and Jennifer Bryce, "Evidence-Based Public Health: Moving beyond Randomized Trials," *American Journal of Public Health* 94, no. 3 (2004): 401.

11. Eirik Evenhouse and Siobhan Reilly, "Improved Estimates of the Benefits of Breastfeeding Using Sibling Comparisons to Reduce Selection Bias," *Health Sciences Research* 40, no. 6, part I (2005): 1781, 1797.

12. Melissa C. Nelson, Perry Gordon-Larsen, and Linda S. Adair, "Are Adolescents Who Were Breast-fed Less Likely to Be Overweight?" *Epidemiology* 16, no. 2 (2005): 252; Matthew W. Gillman et al., "Breast-Feeding and Overweight in Adolescence," *Epidemiology* 17, no. 1 (2006): 114.

13. K. B. Michels et al., "A Longitudinal Study of Infant Feeding and Obesity throughout the Life Course," *International Journal of Obesity* 31 (2007): 1078–95.

14. Man Ki Kwok et al., "Does Breastfeeding Protect against Childhood Overweight? Hong Kong's 'Children of 1997' Birth Cohort," *International Journal of Epidemiology*, electronic publication (2009): 1–9; N. Al-Qaoud and P. Prakash, "Can Breastfeeding and Its Duration Determine the Overweight Status of Kuwaiti Children at the Age of 3–6 Years?" *European Journal of Clinical Medicine* 63 (2009): 1041–43; Karina Huus et al., "Exclusive Breastfeeding of Swedish Children and Its Possible Influence on Development of Obesity: A Prospective Cohort Study," *BMC Pediatrics* 8, no. 42 (2008): 106; Jaimie N. Davis et al., "Influence of Breastfeeding on Obesity and Type 2 Diabetes Risk Factors in Latino Youth with a Family History of Type 2 Diabetes," *Diabetes Care* 30, no. 4 (2007): 784–89; Michels et al., "A Longitudinal

Study"; Salome Scholtens et al., "Breast Feeding, Parental Allergy and Asthma in Children Followed for 8 Years: The PIAMA Birth Cohort Study," *American Journal of Epidemiology* 165 (2007): 919–26; Pamela J. Salsberry and Patricia B. Reagan, "Dynamics of Early Childhood Overweight," *Pediatrics* 116, no. 6 (2005): 1329–38; L. Li, T. J. Parsons, and C. Power, "Breast Feeding and Obesity in Childhood: Cross Sectional Study," *British Medical Journal* 327 (2003): 904–5; Cesar G. Victora et al., "Anthropometry and Body Composition of 18 Year Old Men according to Duration of Breast Feeding: Birth Cohort Study from Brazil," *British Medical Journal* 327 (2003): 904.

15. Sandra B. Proctor and Carol Ann Holcomb, "Breastfeeding Duration and Childhood Overweight among Low-Income Children in Kansas, 1998–2002," *American Journal of Public Health* 98, no. 1 (2008): 106–10; Valerie Burke et al., "Breastfeeding and Overweight: Longitudinal Analysis in an Australian Birth Cohort," *Journal of Pediatrics* 147 (2005); K. E. Bergmann et al., "Early Determinants of Childhood Overweight and Adiposity in a Birth Cohort Study: Role of Breastfeeding," *International Journal of Obesity* 27 (2003): 162–72; Kristen G. Elliott et al., "Duration of Breastfeeding Associated with Obesity during Adolescence," *Obesity Research* 5, no. 6 (1997): 538–41; Gillman et al., "Breastfeeding and Overweight in Adolescence"; Matthew W. Gillman, "Breast-Feeding and Obesity," *Journal of Pediatrics* 141, no. 6 (2002): 749–50; Matthew W. Gillman et al., "Risk of

Overweight among Adolescents Who Were Breastfed as Infants," *Journal of the American Medical Association* 285, no. 19 (2001): 2461–67; Mary L. Hediger et al., "Association between Infant Breastfeeding and Overweight in Young Children," *Journal of the American Medical Association* 285, no. 19 (2001): 2453–60; Nelson, Gordon-Larsen, and Adair, "Are Adolescents Who Were Breast-fed"; Richard Strauss, "Breast Milk and Childhood Obesity: The Czechs Weigh In," *Journal of Pediatric Gastroenterology and Nutrition* 37, no. 2 (2003): 210–11. Other studies fail to address these problems. See, for example, Anette E. Buyken et al., "Effects of Breastfeeding on Trajectories of Body Fat and BMI throughout Childhood," *Obesity* 16, no. 2 (2008): 389–95; Rüdiger von Kries et al., "Breast Feeding and Obesity: Cross Sectional Study," *British Medical Journal* 319 (1999): 147–50; Jessica G. Woo et al., "Breastfeeding Helps Explain Racial and Socioeconomic Status Disparities in Adolescent Adiposity," *Pediatrics* 121, no. 3 (2008): e458–65; Julie Armstrong, John J. Reilly, and the Child Health Information Team, "Breastfeeding and Lowering the Risk of Childhood Obesity," *The Lancet* 359 (2002): 2003–4.

16. Nancy F. Butte, "The Role of Breastfeeding in Obesity," *Pediatric Clinics of North America* 48, no. 1 (2001): 196.

17. Alan S. Ryan, "Breastfeeding and the Risk of Childhood Obesity," *Collegium Antropologicum* 31 (2007): 19–28. Ryan is employed by Abbott Laboratories, a producer of infant formula, and his work is widely cited in breastfeeding research.

See also Stephan Arenz and Rüdiger von Kries, "Protective Effect of Breastfeeding against Obesity in Childhood: Can a Meta-Analysis of Observational Studies Help to Validate the Hypothesis?" *Advances in Experimental Medicine and Biology* 569 (2005): 40–48; Christopher G. Owen et al., "The Effect of Breastfeeding on Mean Body Mass Index throughout Life: A Quantitative Review of Published and Unpublished Observational Evidence," *American Journal of Clinical Nutrition* 82 (2005): 1298–1307; Laurence M. Grummer-Strawn and Zuguo Mei, "Does Breastfeeding Protect against Pediatric Overweight? Analysis of Longitudinal Data from the Centers for Disease Control and Prevention Pediatric Nutrition Surveillance System," *Pediatrics* 113, no. 2 (2004): e81–e86; S. Arenz et al., "Breast-Feeding and Childhood Obesity—A Systematic Review," *International Journal of Obesity* 28 (2004): 1247–56. Thomas Harder et al., "Duration of Breastfeeding and Risk of Overweight: A Meta-Analysis," *American Journal of Epidemiology* 162 (2005): 397–403, acknowledge that confounding cannot be ruled out but also argue that evidence of a dose-response relationship, in which longer breastfeeding increases benefits, reduces the likelihood of confounding. For how maternal behavior might affect a dose-response relationship, see my later discussion of PROBIT.

18. Nancy F. Butte, "Impact of Infant Feeding Practices on Childhood Obesity," *Journal of Nutrition* 139, no. 2 (2009): 412S–16S; Mark Bradley Cope and David B. Allison, "Critical Review of the World Health Organization's (WHO) 2007 Report on 'Evidence of the Long-Term Effects of Breast-feeding': Systematic Reviews and Meta-Analysis with Respect to Obesity," *Obesity Reviews* 9, no. 6 (2008): 594–605; Tammy J. Clifford, "Breast Feeding and Obesity," *British Medical Journal* 327 (2003): 879–80.

19. Owen et al., "The Effect of Breastfeeding," 1298. For a discussion of publication bias, see chapter 5.

20. Hediger et al., "Association between Infant Breastfeeding and Overweight in Young Children," 2453; Gillman et al., "Risk of Overweight," 2461.

21. Hediger et al., "Association between Infant Breastfeeding and Overweight," 2458; Gillman et al., "Risk of Overweight," 2462.

22. Tim Byers, Barbara Lyle, and Workshop Participants, "Summary Statement," *American Journal of Clinical Nutrition* 69 (1999): 1365S–66S; Alan Petersen and Deborah Lupton, *The New Public Health: Health and Self in the Age of Risk* (London: Sage, 1996), 42.

23. von Kries et al., "Breast Feeding and Obesity," 149.

24. Kelley E. Borradaile et al., "Associations between the Youth/Adolescent Questionnaire, the Youth/Adolescent Activity Questionnaire, and Body Mass Index z Score in Low-Income Inner-City Fourth through Sixth Grade Children," *American Journal of Clinical Nutrition* 87 (2008): 1650; Elizabeth Goodman, Beth R. Hinden, and Seema Khandelwal, "Accuracy of Teen and Parental Reports of Obesity and Body Mass Index," *Pediatrics* 106, no. 1 (2000): 56.

25. Gillman et al., "Risk of Overweight," 2466.

26. Research on breastfeeding and obesity also inconsistently evaluates the role of genetic factors, which have been highly correlated with overweight and obesity. For a brief discussion of key studies, see Gina Kolata, *Rethinking Thin: The New Science of Weight Loss—And the Myths and Realities of Dieting* (New York: Farrar, Strauss & Giroux, 2007), 119–24. While maternal body mass index (BMI) at childbirth or at the time of the study is sometimes considered, paternal weight is virtually never assessed.

27. M. Bartels, C. E. M. van Beijsterveldt, and D. I. Boomsma, "Breastfeeding, Maternal Education and Cognitive Function: A Prospective Study in Twins," *Behavior Genetics* 39 (2009): 616–22; Wendy H. Oddy et al., "The Long-Term Effects of Breastfeeding on Child and Adolescent Mental Health: A Pregnancy Cohort Study Followed for 14 Years" (2009), electronic publication, 1–7; Emily Oken et al., "Associations of Maternal Fish Intake during Pregnancy and Breastfeeding Duration with Attainment of Developmental Milestones in Early Childhood: A Study from the Danish National Birth Cohort," *American Journal of Clinical Nutrition* 88 (2009): 789–96; Daniel I. Rees and Joseph A. Sabia, "The Effect of Breast Feeding on Educational Attainment: Evidence from Sibling Data," *Journal of Human Capital*

3, no. 1 (2009): 43–72; Avshalom Caspi et al., "Moderation of Breastfeeding Effects on the IQ by Genetic Variation in Fatty Acid Metabolism," *Proceedings of the National Academy of Sciences* 104, no. 47 (2007): 18860–65; Jordi Julvez et al., "Attention Behaviour and Hyperactivity at Age 4 and Duration of Breast-Feeding," *Acta Paediatrica* 96 (2007): 842–47; Evenhouse and Reilly, "Improved Estimates of the Benefits of Breastfeeding"; R. F. Slykerman et al., "Breastfeeding and Intelligence of Preschool Children," *Acta Paediatrica* 94 (2005): 832–37; Wendy H. Oddy et al., "Breast Feeding and Cognitive Development in Childhood: A Prospective Birth Cohort," *Paediatric and Perinatal Epidemiology* 17 (2003): 81–90; Erik Lykke Mortensen et al., "The Association between Duration of Breastfeeding and Adult Intelligence," *Journal of the American Medical Association* 287, no. 18 (2002): 2365–72; N. K. Angelsen et al., "Breast Feeding and Cognitive Development at Age 1 and 5 Years," *Archives of Disease in Childhood* 85 (2001): 183–88; James W. Anderson, Bryan M. Johnstone, and Daniel T. Remley, "Breastfeeding and Cognitive Development: A Meta-Analysis," *American Journal of Clinical Nutrition* 70 (1999): 525–35; L. John Horwood and David Fergusson, "Breastfeeding and Later Cognitive and Academic Outcomes," *Pediatrics* 101, no. 1 (1998): e9–e15; A. Lucas et al., "Breast Milk and Subsequent Intelligence Quotient in Children Born Preterm," *The Lancet* 339 (1992): 261–64.

28. Extensive evidence indicates that IQ and other standardized tests are poor measures of intelligence. Sociologists have demonstrated that performance on these tests can be affected by altering the context in which they are given. For example, see Dana Gresky et al., "Effects of Salient Multiple Identities on Women's Performance under Mathematics Stereotype Threat," *Sex Roles* 53, nos. 9/10 (2005): 703–16; and Michael Lovaglia et al., "Status Processes and Mental Ability Test Scores," *American Journal of Sociology* 104 (1998): 195–228. Other research suggests that proportions of the variance in IQ in poor and affluent families vary nonlinearly with socioeconomic status. In poor families, the contribution of genes to IQ is close to zero, and shared environment explains more than half the variance. In wealthy families, the explanation is almost exactly the reverse. See Eric Turkheimer et al., "Socioeconomic Status Modifies Heritability of IQ in Young Children," *Psychological Science* 14, no. 6 (2003): 623–28.

29. Scott Krugman et al., "Breastfeeding and IQ," *Pediatrics* 103 (1999): 193. See also A. G. Gordon, "Breast-Feeding, Breast-Milk Feeding, and Intelligence Quotient," *American Journal of Clinical Nutrition* 72 (2000): 1063–64; and Myrna Weissman et al., "Breastfeeding and Later Intelligence," *Journal of the American Medical Association* 288, no. 7 (2002): 828–30.

30. Mortensen et al., "The Association between Duration of Breastfeeding and Adult Intelligence," 2371.

31. Sandra W. Jacobson, Lisa M. Chiodo, and Joseph L. Jacobson, "Breastfeeding Effects on Intelligence Quotient in 4- and 11-Year-Old Children," *Pediatrics* 103, no. 5 (1999): e71.

32. Catharine Gale et al., "Breastfeeding, the Use of Docosahexaenoic Acid-Fortified Formulas in Infancy and Neuropsychological Function in Childhood," *Archives of Disease in Childhood*, electronic publication (2009): 1–6; Christina M. Gibson-Davis and Jeanne Brooks-Gunn, "Breastfeeding and Verbal Ability of 3-Year-Olds in a Multicity Sample," *Pediatrics* 118, no. 5 (2006): e1444–51.

33. Denise L. Drane and Jeri A. Logemann, "A Critical Evaluation of the Evidence on the Association between Type of Infant Feeding and Cognitive Development," *Paediatric and Perinatal Epidemiology* 14 (2000): 349–56; Anjali Jain, John Concato, and John M. Leventhal, "How Good Is the Evidence Linking Breastfeeding and Intelligence?" *Pediatrics* 109, no. 6 (2002): 1052.

34. Linda C. Duffy et al., "Exclusive Breastfeeding Protects against Day Care Exposure to Otitis Media," *Pediatrics* 100, no. 4 (1997): e7–e15; and Burris Duncan et al., "Exclusive Breast-Feeding for at Least 4 Months Protects against Otitis Media," *Pediatrics* 91, no. 5 (1993): 867–72, found that breastfeeding, particularly exclusive breastfeeding, had a protective effect against acute infection. Michael S. Kramer et al., "Promotion of Breastfeeding Intervention Trial (PROBIT): A Randomized Trial in the Republic of Belarus," *Journal of the American Medical Association* 285 (2001): 413–20, found no effect. See my later discussion of PROBIT.

35. Stanley Ip et al., *Breast-feeding and Maternal and Infant Health Outcomes in Developed Countries*, Evidence Report / Technology Assessment no. 153, prepared by Tufts–New England Medical Center, Evidence-Based Practice Center, under contract no. 290-02-0022, AHRQ publication no. 07-E007 (Rockville, MD: Agency for Healthcare Research and Quality, April 2007), 158.

36. AAP and American Academy of Family Physicians, Subcommittee on Management of Acute Otitis Media, "Diagnosis and Management of Acute Otitis Media," *Pediatrics* 113, no. 5 (2004): 1459.

37. Kathleen A. Daly and G. Scott Giebink, "Clinical Epidemiology of Otitis Media," *Pediatric Infectious Disease Journal* 19, no. 5 (2000): S31–36; and Jack L. Paradise et al., "Otitis Media in 2253 Pittsburgh-Area Infants: Prevalence and Risk Factors during the First Two Years of Life," *Pediatrics* 99, no. 3 (1997): 229–30.

38. Paradise et al., "Otitis Media in 2253 Pittsburgh-Area Infants," 330–31 (italics in original).

39. Suvi M. Virtanen and Mikael Knip, "Nutritional Risk Predictors of ß Cell Autoimmunity and Type 1 Diabetes at a Young Age," *American Journal of Clinical Nutrition* 78 (2003): 1053; Jill M. Norris and Fraser W. Scott, "A Meta-Analysis of Infant Diet and Insulin-Dependent Diabetes Mellitus: Do Biases Play a Role?" *Epidemiology* 7 (1996): 87–92.

40. David J. Pettitt et al., "Breastfeeding and Incidence of Non-Insulin-Dependent Diabetes Mellitus in Pima Indians," *The Lancet* 350 (1997): 166–68; David Simmons, "NIDDM and Breastfeeding," *The Lancet* 350 (1997): 157–58.

41. Elizabeth Mayer-Davis et al., "Breast-Feeding and Type 2 Diabetes in the Youth of Three Ethnic Groups," *Diabetes Care* 31 (2008): 470–758; T. Kue Young et al., "Type 2 Diabetes Mellitus in Children: Prenatal and Early Infancy Risk Factors among Native Canadians," *Archives of Pediatric Adolescent Medicine* 156, no. 7 (2002): 651–55.

42. S. Scholtens et al., "Breast Feeding, Parental Allergy and Asthma in Children Followed for 8 Years: The PIAMA Birth Cohort Study," *Thorax* 64, no. 7 (2009): 604–9; Inger Kull et al., "Breast-Feeding Reduces the Risk of Asthma during the First 4 Years of Life," *Journal of Allergy and Clinical Immunology* 114 (2004): 755–60; Wendy H. Oddy et al., "The Relation of Breastfeeding and Body Mass Index to Asthma and Atopy in Children: A Prospective Cohort Study to Age 6 Years," *American Journal of Public Health* 94, no. 9 (2004): 1531–37.

43. Michael S. Kramer et al., "Effect of Prolonged and Exclusive Breast Feeding on Risk of Allergy and Asthma: Cluster Randomized Trial," *British Medical Journal* 335 (2007): 385–90; Rosângela da Costa Lima et al., "Do Risk Factors for Childhood Infections and Malnutrition Protect against Asthma? A Study of Brazilian Male Adolescents," *American Journal of Public Health* 93, no. 11 (2003): 1858–64; Malcolm R. Sears et al., "A Longitudinal,

Population-Based, Cohort Study of Childhood Asthma Followed to Adulthood," *New England Journal of Medicine* 349, no. 15 (2003): 1414–22; Claire Infante-Rivard et al., "Family Size, Day-Care Attendance, and Breastfeeding in Relation to the Incidence of Childhood Asthma," *American Journal of Epidemiology* 153 (2001): 653–58. See also Joanne M. Duncan and Malcolm R. Sears, "Breastfeeding and Allergies: Time for a Change in Paradigm?" *Current Opinion in Allergy and Clinical Immunology* 8, no. 5 (2008): 398–405; and Richard J. Morris, "Are Breastfeeding and Diet Strategies Overrated for the Prevention of Atopy?" *American Journal of Clinical Nutrition* 101 (2008): 113.

44. G. Nagel et al., "Effect of Breastfeeding on Asthma, Lung Function and Bronchial Hyperreactivity in ISAAC Phase II," *European Respiratory Journal* 33, no. 5 (2009): 993–1002; I. U. Ogbuano et al., "Effect of Breastfeeding Duration on Lung Function at Age 10 Years: A Prospective Birth Cohort Study," *Thorax* 64 (2009): 62–66; Xiaohui Xu et al., "The Effects of Birthweight and Breastfeeding on Asthma among Children Aged 1–5 Years," *Journal of Paediatrics and Child Health* 45 (2009): 646–51; Leslie Elliott et al., "Prospective Study of Breast-Feeding in Relation to Wheeze, Atopy, and Bronchial Hyperresponsiveness in the Avon Longitudinal Study of Parents and Children (ALSPAC)," *Journal of Allergy and Clinical Immunology* 122, no. 1 (2008): 49–54; Frank R. Greer et al., "Effects of Early Nutritional Interventions

on the Development of Atopic Disease in Infants and Children: The Role of Maternal Dietary Restriction, Breastfeeding, Timing of Introduction of Complementary Foods, and Hydrolyzed Formulas," *Pediatrics* 121, no. 1 (2008): 183–91; Theresa W. Guilbert et al., "Effect of Breastfeeding on Lung Function in Childhood and Modulation by Maternal Asthma and Atopy," *American Journal of Respiratory and Critical Care Medicine* 176 (2007): 843–48; Xiao-Mei Mai et al., "The Relationship of Breastfeeding, Overweight, and Asthma in Preadolescents," *Journal of Allergy and Clinical Immunology* 120 (2007): 551–56; Piush J. Mandhane, Justina M. Greene, and Malcolm R. Sears, "Interactions between Breast-Feeding, Specific Parental Atopy, and Sex on Development of Asthma and Atopy," *Journal of Allergy and Clinical Immunology* 119, no. 6 (2007): 1359–66; Melanie Claire Matheson et al., "Breastfeeding and Atopic Disease: A Cohort Study from Childhood to Middle Age," *Journal of Allergy and Clinical Immunology* 120 (2007): 1051–57; S. Mihrshahi et al., "The Association between Infant Feeding Practices and Subsequent Atopy Among Children with a Family History of Asthma," *Clinical and Experimental Allergy* 37 (2007): 671–79; Bianca E. P. Snijders et al., "Breast-Feeding Duration and Infant Atopic Manifestations, by Maternal Allergic Status, in the First 2 Years of Life (KOALA Study)," *Journal of Pediatrics* 151 (2007): 347–51.

45. Romina Libster et al., "Breastfeeding Prevents Severe Disease in Full Term Infants with Acute Respiratory Infection," *Pediatric Infectious Disease Journal* 28, no. 2 (2009): 131–34; M. Inès Klein et al., "Differential Gender Response to Respiratory Infections and to the Protective Effect of Breast Milk in Preterm Infants," *Pediatrics* 121 (2008): 1510–16; Maria A. Quigley, Yvonne J. Kelly, and Amanda Sacker, "Breastfeeding and Hospitalization for Diarrheal and Respiratory Infection in the United Kingdom Millennium Cohort Study," *Pediatrics* 119, no. 4 (2007): 837–42; Caroline J. Chantry, Cynthia R. Howard, and Peggy Auinger, "Full Breastfeeding Duration and Associated Decrease in Respiratory Tract Infection in US Children," *Pediatrics* 117, no. 2 (2006): 425–32; Virginia R. Bachrach et al., "Long-Term Follow-up of Asthma," *New England Journal of Medicine* 350, no. 3 (2004): 304; Anusha Sinha et al., "Reduced Risk of Neonatal Respiratory Infections among Breastfed Girls but Not Boys," *Pediatrics* 112, no. 4 (2003); Virginia R. Galton Bachrach, Eleanor Schwarz, and Lela Rose Bachrach, "Breastfeeding and the Risk of Hospitalization for Respiratory Disease in Infancy," *Archives of Pediatric and Adolescent Medicine* 157 (2003): 237–43; Wendy H. Oddy et al., "Breast Feeding and Respiratory Morbidity in Infancy: A Birth Cohort Study," *Archives of Disease in Childhood* 88 (2003): 224–28; W. H. Oddy et al., "Association between Breast Feeding and Asthma in 6 Year Old Children: Findings of a Prospective Birth Cohort Study," *British Medical Journal* 319 (1999): 815–19; Alice Cushing et al.,

"Breastfeeding Reduces Risk of Respiratory Illness in Infants," *American Journal of Epidemiology* 147, no. 9 (1998): 863–70; Per Nafsted et al., "Breastfeeding, Maternal Smoking and Lower Respiratory Tract Infections," *European Respiratory Journal* 9 (1996): 2623–29; Micheline Beaudry, Renee Dufour, and Sylvie Marcoux, "Relation between Infant Feeding and Infections during the First Six Months of Life," *Journal of Pediatrics* 126, no. 2 (1995): 191–97; Peter W. Howie et al., "Protective Effect of Breast Feeding Against Infection," *British Medical Journal* 300 (1990): 11–16.

46. Quigley, Kelly, and Sacker, "Breastfeeding and Hospitalization"; Chantry, Howard, and Auinger, "Full Breastfeeding Duration"; Bachrach, Schwarz, and Bachrach, "Breastfeeding and the Risk of Hospitalization."

47. Kramer et al., "Promotion of Breastfeeding Intervention Trial (PROBIT)." See my later discussion of the PROBIT investigation. See also Kathryn G. Dewey, M. Jane Heinig, and Laurie A. Nommsen-Rivers, "Differences in Morbidity between Breast-Fed and Formula-Fed Infants," *Journal of Pediatrics* 126, no. 5 (1995): 696–702.

48. Eric A. F. Simoes, "Environmental and Demographic Risk Factors for Respiratory Syncytial Virus Lower Respiratory Tract Disease," *Journal of Pediatrics* 143 (2003): S118–26; Catherine J. Holberg et al., "Risk Factors for Respiratory Syncytial Virus-Associated Lower Respiratory Illnesses in the First Year of Life," *American Journal of Epidemiology* 133, no. 11 (1991): 1135–51.

49. Michael S. Kramer et al., "Effects of Prolonged and Exclusive Breastfeeding on Child Behavior and Maternal Adjustment: Evidence from a Large, Randomized Trial," *Pediatrics* 121, no. 3 (2008): 436.

50. Laurence M. Grummer-Strawn et al., "Infant Feeding and Feeding Transitions during the First Year of Life," *Pediatrics* 122 (2008): S36–S42; CDC, *Morbidity and Mortality Weekly Report* 56, no. 30 (August 3, 2007); Indu B. Ahluwalia et al., "Who Is Breast-Feeding? Recent Trends from the Pregnancy Risk Assessment and Monitoring System," *Journal of Pediatrics* 142 (2003): 486–93; Ruowei Li et al., "Breastfeeding Rates in the United States by Characteristics of the Child, Mother, or Family: The 2002 National Immunization Survey," *Pediatrics* 115, no. 1 (2005): e31–e37; Renata Forste, Jessica Weiss, and Emily Lippincott, "The Decision to Breastfeed in the United States: Does Race Matter?" *Pediatrics* 108, no. 1 (2001): 291–96.

51. Mary Jean Owen et al., "Relation of Infant Feeding Practices, Cigarette Smoke Exposure, and Group Child Care to the Onset and Duration of Otitis Media with Effusion in the First Two Years of Life," *Journal of Pediatrics* 123 (1993): 707.

52. Thomas M. Ball and Anne L. Wright, "Health Care Costs of Formula-Feeding in the First Year of Life," *Pediatrics* 103, no. 4 (1999): 870.

53. Nurit Guttman and Deena R. Zimmerman, "Low-Income Mothers' Views on Breastfeeding," *Social Science & Medicine* 50 (2000): 1462.

54. Belarus was selected because basic health services and sanitary conditions were similar to those in North America and Western Europe. An uncontaminated water supply was ensured and monitored, and hospital services were available and accessible, even in rural areas. Moreover, standard maternity hospital practices in Belarus were similar to those in Western developed countries twenty to thirty years earlier, which provided a greater potential contrast between the control and experimental study groups. Cultural differences were not considered. See Kramer et al., "Promotion of Breastfeeding Intervention Trial (PROBIT)," 414.

55. Kramer et al., "Promotion of Breastfeeding Intervention Trial (PROBIT)"; Ruth A. Lawrence, "Breastfeeding in Belarus," *Journal of the American Medical Association* 285, no. 4 (2001): 463.

56. Kramer et al., "Promotion of Breastfeeding Intervention Trial (PROBIT)," 419.

57. Kramer et al., "Effect of Prolonged and Exclusive Breastfeeding on Risk of Allergy and Asthma."

58. Michael S. Kramer et al., "Effects of Prolonged and Exclusive Breastfeeding on Child Height, Weight, Adiposity, and Blood Pressure at Age 6.5 Y: Evidence from a Large Randomized Trial," *American Journal of Clinical Nutrition* 86 (2007): 1717–21.

59. Michael S. Kramer et al., "The Effect of Prolonged and Exclusive Breast-Feeding on Dental Caries in Early School-Age Children: New Evidence from a Large Randomized Trial," *Caries Research* 41 (2007): 484–88.

60. Michael S. Kramer et al., "Breastfeeding and Child Cognitive Development: New Evidence from a Large Randomized Trial," *Archives of General Psychiatry* 65, no. 5 (2008): 578.

61. Women describe similar difficulties in England, Australia, and Canada. See Joyce L. Marshall, Mary Godfrey, and Mary J. Renfrew, "Being a 'Good Mother': Managing Breastfeeding and Merging Identities," *Social Science & Medicine* 65 (2007): 2147–59; Virginia Schmied and Deborah Lupton, "Blurring the Boundaries: Breastfeeding and Maternal Subjectivity," *Sociology of Health and Illness* 23, no. 2 (2001): 234–50; and Christa M. Kelleher, "The Physical Challenges of Early Breastfeeding," *Social Science & Medicine* 63 (2006): 2727–38.

62. See www.cdc.gov/breastfeeding/data/NIS_data/index.htm (accessed August 12, 2008).

63. See, for example, Shannon L. Kelleher and Bo Lönnerdal, "Immunological Activities Associated with Milk," in *Advances in Nutritional Research*, ed. B. Woodward and H. Draper (New York: Plenum Press, 2001), 39–65.

64. International public health organizations strongly promote breastfeeding in developing countries that do not always have access to a continuous supply of uncontaminated water, necessary to mix formula powder. In these countries, mothers are often economically disadvantaged and undernourished compared with men. Whether and how they ought to be encouraged to breastfeed is a complicated political and moral question that is beyond the scope of this book.

On breastfeeding in developing countries, see Naomi Baumslag and Dia L. Michels, *Milk, Money, and Madness: The Culture and Politics of Breastfeeding* (Westport, CT: Bergin & Garvey, 1995); Linda Blum, *At the Breast: Breastfeeding and Motherhood in the Contemporary United States* (Boston: Beacon Press, 1999), 45–47; Bernice L. Hausman, *Mother's Milk: Breastfeeding Controversies in American Culture* (New York: Routledge, 2003), 202–3, 208; Vanessa Maher, "Breast-Feeding in Cross-Cultural Perspective" and "Breast-Feeding and Maternal Depletion: Natural Law or Cultural Arrangements?" in *The Anthropology of Breast-Feeding: Natural Law or Social Construct?* ed. Vanessa Maher (Oxford: Berg, 1992), 1–36, 151–80; and Penny van Esterik, *Beyond the Breast-Bottle Controversy* (New Brunswick, NJ: Rutgers University Press, 1989).

65. Whether protection against GI distress is a sufficient basis on which to recommend exclusive breastfeeding for the first six months of a baby's life is addressed in chapter 5.

66. Breast milk has higher concentrations of docosahexaenoic acid (DHA), a fatty acid that contributes to brain development, and infant formulas are now fortified with DHA. At least one study suggests that fortified formula might be better for brain growth: adolescents born prematurely and fed enriched formula, rather than breast milk or standard formula, had higher verbal scores, and males had higher caudate volumes, or greater growth in regional gray matter. See Elizabeth B. Isaacs et al., "The Effect

of Early Human Diet on Caudate Volumes and IQ," *Pediatric Research* 63 (2008): 308–14. But the process by which either breastfeeding or formula feeding would enhance intelligence has not been demonstrated.

67. Yoon K. Loke and Sheena Derry, "Does Anybody Read 'Evidence-Based' Articles?" *BMC Medical Research Methodology* 3 (2003): 14.

68. Paula A. Rochon et al., "Comparison of Review Articles Published in Peer-Reviewed and Throwaway Journals," *Journal of the American Medical Association* 287, no. 21 (2002): 2853.

69. Donna M. Windish, Stephen J. Huot, and Michael L. Green, "Medicine Residents' Understanding of the Biostatistics and Results in the Medical Literature," *Journal of the American Medical Society* 298, no. 9 (2007): 1014–16.

70. Sanjay Saint et al., "Journal Reading Habits of Internists," *Journal of General Internal Medicine* 15 (2000): 883.

71. David T. Burke et al., "Reading Habits of Practicing Physiatrists," *American Journal of Physical Medicine & Rehabilitation* 81, no. 10 (2002): 779, 786. Pediatricians spend an average of only twenty minutes on each article they read. See Carol Tenepoir et al., "Journal Reading Patterns and Preferences of Pediatricians," *Journal of the American Medical Association* 95, no. 1 (2007): 59.

72. Roy M. Pitkin, Mary Ann Branagan, and Leon F. Burmeister, "Accuracy of Data in Abstracts of Published Research Articles," *Journal of the American Medical Association* 281, no. 12 (1999): 1111.

73. Jules Law, "The Politics of Breastfeeding: Assessing Risk, Dividing Labor," *Signs: Journal of Women in Culture and Society* 25, no. 2 (2000): 413n. The study in question was Walter J. Rogan et al., "Should the Presence of Carcinogens in Breast Milk Discourage Breastfeeding?" *Regulatory Toxicology and Pharmacology* 13, no. 3 (1991): 228–40.

74. Grummer-Strawn and Mei, "Does Breastfeeding Protect against Pediatric Overweight?" e81.

75. Mortensen et al., "The Association between Duration of Breastfeeding and Adult Intelligence," 2371.

76. William H. Dietz, "Breastfeeding May Help Prevent Childhood Overweight," *Journal of the American Medical Association* 285, no. 19 (2001): 2506–7; Hediger et al., "Association between Infant Breastfeeding and Overweight in Young Children," 2459.

77. Maria Weyermann, Herman Brenner, and Dietrich Rothenbacher, "Adipokines in Human Milk and Risk of Overweight in Early Childhood," *Epidemiology* 18, no. 6 (2007): 722–29.

78. Matthew W. Gillman and Christos S. Mantzoros, "Breast-Feeding, Adipokines, and Childhood Obesity," *Epidemiology* 18, no. 6 (2007): 730.

79. Janet Pinelli, Saroj Saigal, and Stephanie A. Atkinson, "Effect of Breastmilk Consumption on Neurodevelopmental Outcomes at 6 and 12 Months of Age in VLBW Infants," *Advances in Neonatal Care* 3, no. 2 (2003): 76. By contrast, a systematic review of the evidence regarding breast milk and infection in

preterm babies found "serious methodological flaws" in all the studies, including "poor study design, inadequate sample sizes, neglecting to account for some confounders, failure to eliminate the effects associated with maternal choice of feeding method and other maternal sociodemographic variables." See A. de Silva, P. W. Jones, and S. A. Spencer, "Does Human Milk Reduce Infection Rates in Preterm Infants? A Systematic Review," *Archives of Disease in Childhood, Fetal Neonatal Edition* 89 (2004): F512.

80. Ricardo Uauy and Patricio Peirano, "Breast Is Best: Human Milk Is the Optimal Food for the Brain," *American Journal of Clinical Nutrition* 70 (1999): 433–34.

81. Law, "The Politics of Breastfeeding," 412.

82. AAP, "Policy Statement Based on Task Force Report: The Promotion of Breastfeeding," *Pediatrics* 69, no. 5 (1982): 655.

83. AAP, Work Group on Breastfeeding, "Policy Statement: Breastfeeding and the Use of Human Milk," (1997): 1035.

84. See www.ncbi.nlm.nih.gov/pubmed/. Search conducted May 22, 2009.

85. David Hirshleifer, "The Blind Leading the Blind: Social Influence, Fads, and Informational Cascades," in *The New Economics of Human Behavior*, ed. Mariano Tommasi and Kathryn Ierulli (Cambridge: Cambridge University Press, 1995), 188–215.

86. Brian S. Alper et al., "How Much Effort Is Needed to Keep up with the Literature Relevant for Primary Care?" *Journal of the*

American Medical Association 92, no. 4 (2004): 433.

87. G. S. Rust et al., "Does Breastfeeding Protect Children from Asthma? Analysis of NHANES III Survey Data," *Journal of the National Medical Association* 93, no. 4 (2001): 139.

88. Paradise et al., "Otitis Media in 2253 Pittsburgh-Area Infants," 329–30.

89. Hediger et al., "Association between Infant Breastfeeding and Overweight in Young Children," 2459.

90. Michels et al., "A Longitudinal Study of Infant Feeding," 1085. As evidence, it cited one investigation, conducted by two of the same authors, suggesting an association between duration of breastfeeding and diabetes in mothers.

91. National Institutes of Health, "Breastfeeding Has Minor Effect in Reducing Risk of Childhood Overweight," NIH News Release, May 15, 2001.

92. Gillman et al., "Breast-Feeding and Obesity," 750.

93. Susan Yadlon notes a similar tendency of scientists to assume that limiting dietary fat reduces the risk for breast cancer and also to acknowledge that no direct evidence exists. See Susan Yadlon, "Skinny Women and Good Mothers: The Rhetoric of Risk, Control, and Culpability in the Production of Knowledge about Breast Cancer," *Feminist Studies* 23, no. 3 (1997): 657.

94. See, for example, Amanda R. Cooklin, Susan M. Donath, and Lisa H. Amir, "Maternal Employment and Breastfeeding: Results from the Longitudinal Study of Australian Children,"

Acta Paediatrica 97 (2008): 620–23; Fani Ladomenou, Anthony Kafatos, and Emmanouil Galanakis, "Risk Factors Related to Intention to Breastfeed, Early Weaning and Suboptimal Duration of Breastfeeding," *Acta Paediatrica* 96 (2007): 1441–44; and Elsie M. Taveras et al., "Clinician Support and Psychosocial Risk Factors Associated with Breastfeeding Discontinuation," *Pediatrics* 112, no. 1 (2003): 108–15.

95. Cass R. Sunstein, *Laws of Fear: Beyond the Precautionary Principle* (Cambridge: Cambridge University Press, 2005), 95.

96. Daniel Glick, "Rooting for Intelligence," *Newsweek*, March 1, 1997.

97. Atul Singhal et al., "Breastmilk Feeding and Lipoprotein Profile in Adolescents Born Preterm: Follow-up of a Prospective Randomized Study," *The Lancet* 363 (2004): 1571–78; Patricia Reaney, "Breastfeeding Cuts Cardiovascular Risk—Study," Reuters, May 13, 2004.

98. *The Early Show*, September 4, 2004, www.cbsnews.com.

99. Mike Stobbe, "Breastfeeding Won't Deter Obesity," *Associated Press*, April 24, 2007.

100. Krugman et al., "Breastfeeding and IQ," 193.

101. "Breast-Feeding While on Seizure Meds Doesn't Harm Babies," Yahoo! News, April 17, 2008.

102. Miles Little, "Assignments of Meaning in Epidemiology," *Social Science and Medicine* 47, no. 9 (1998): 1144.

103. Eunice Kua, Michael Reder, and Martha J. Grossel, "Science in the News: A Study

of Reporting Genomics," *Public Understanding of Science* 13 (2004): 319.

104. Diane Eyer, *Mother-Infant Bonding: A Scientific Fiction* (New Haven, CT: Yale University Press, 1992), 198.

105. Cornelia Dean, "New Complications in Reporting on Science," *Nieman Reports* 56, no. 3 (2002): 25–26.

106. Robert Lee Hotz, "The Difficulty of Finding Impartial Sources in Science," *Nieman Reports* 56, no. 3 (2002): 6; Miriam Shuchman and Michael S. Wilkes, "Medical Scientists and Health News Reporting: A Case of Miscommunication," *Annals of Internal Medicine* 126, no. 12 (1997): 976–82; Michael F. Weigold, "Communicating Science: A Review of the Literature," *Science Communication* 23, no. 2 (2001): 169, 183; Melinda Voss, "Checking the Pulse: Midwestern Reporters' Opinions on Their Ability to Report Health Care News," *American Journal of Public Health* 92, no. 7 (2002): 1158–59; Jim Willis, *Reporting on Risks: The Practice and Ethics of Health and Safety Communication* (Westport, CT: Praeger, 1997), 6, 11–12.

107. Andrea H. Tanner, "Agenda Building, Source Selection, and Health News at Local Television Stations," *Science Communication* 25, no. 4 (2004): 355–59.

108. Robert Steinbrook, "Medical Journals and Medical Reporting," *New England Journal of Medicine* 342, no. 22 (2000): 1670.

109. Jon Franklin, "The Extraordinary Adventure That Is Science Writing," *Nieman Reports* 56, no. 3 (2002): 8.

110. Timothy Johnson, "Shattuck Lecture—Medicine and the Media," *New England Journal of Medicine* 339, no. 2 (1998): 88; Eleanor Singer and Phyllis M. Endreny, *Reporting on Risk: How the Mass Media Portray Accidents, Diseases, Disasters, and Other Hazards* (New York: Russell Sage Foundation, 1993), 151; Michael S. Wilkes, "The Public Dissemination of Medical Research: Problems and Solutions," *Journal of Health Communication* 2, no. 1 (1997): 3–15; Shuchman and Wilkes, "Medical Scientists and Health News Reporting"; Willis, *Reporting on Risks*, 14.

111. Steven Woloshin and Lisa M. Schwarz, "Press Releases: Translating Research into News," *Journal of the American Medical Association* 287, no. 21 (2002): 2858.

112. Tanner, "Agenda Building," 360.

113. Lisa M. Schwartz, Steven Woloshin, and Linda Baczek, "Media Coverage of Scientific Meetings: Too Much, Too Soon?" *Journal of the American Medical Association* 287, no. 21 (2002): 2862.

114. Johnson, "Shattuck Lecture," 91–92.

115. National Science Foundation, *Science and Engineering Indicators 2008* (Arlington, VA: NSB 08-01; NSB 08-01A, June 2008), chap. 7.

116. Stephen P. Norris, Linda M. Phillips, and Connie A. Korpan, "University Students' Interpretation of Media Reports of Science and Its Relationship to Background Knowledge, Interest, and Reading Difficulty," *Public Understanding of Science* 12, no. 2 (2003): 138–39.

Similarly, 78 percent of patients in one study demonstrated a deficient grasp of their emergency care and discharge instructions, but only 20 percent of those perceived difficulty with comprehension. See Kirsten G. Engel et al., "Patient Comprehension of Emergency Department Care and Instructions: Are Patients Aware of When They Do Not Understand?" *Annals of Emergency Medicine* 53, no. 4 (2008): 454–61.

117. Jon D. Miller, "Public Understanding of, and Attitudes toward, Scientific Research: What We Know and What We Need to Know," *Public Understanding of Science* 13 (2004): 275–82.

118. Mark Kutner et al., *The Health Literacy of America's Adults: Results from the 2003 National Assessment of Adult Literacy* (NCES-483) (Washington, DC: National Center for Education Statistics, U.S. Department of Education, 2006), 10; Lynn Nielsen-Bohlman, Allison M. Panzer, and David A. Kindig, eds., *Health Literacy: A Prescription to End Confusion* (Washington, DC: National Academies Press, 2004), 66.

119. Approximately 10 million women, or half of all women who have undergone a hysterectomy, are estimated to be screened annually and unnecessarily for cervical cancer, or cancer in an organ they no longer have. These women receive vaginal smears, which screen for vaginal cancer, a rare malignancy that is less common than cancer of the tongue or small intestine. Vaginal cells, moreover, are much more likely to produce false positives than they are to

find cancers. Healthy women with positive screens then undergo treatment and are labeled as cancer patients. Pressure from patients who are anxious about cancer and do not understand precisely what the test screens for, the ease and relatively low cost of the procedure, and doctors' concerns about litigation are among the reasons that unnecessary Pap tests continue to be administered. See Brenda E. Sirovich and H. Gilbert Welch, "Cervical Cancer Screening among Women without a Cervix," *Journal of the American Medical Association* 291, no. 24 (2004): 2990; and Gina Kolata, "10 Million Women Who Lack Cervices Still Get Pap Tests," *New York Times*, June 23, 2004.

120. Ruth M. Parker, Michael S. Wolf, and Irwin Kirsch, "Preparing for an Epidemic of Limited Health Literacy: Weathering the Perfect Storm," *Journal of General Internal Medicine* 23, no. 8 (2008): 1273–76; Kutner et al., *The Health Literacy of*

America's Adults; Nielsen-Bohlman, Panzer, and Kindig, *Health Literacy*, 218; Barry D. Weiss, "Outside the Clinician-Patient Relationship: A Call to Action for Health Literacy," in *Health Literacy: A Prescription to End Confusion*, ed. Lynn Nielsen-Bohlman, Allison M. Panzer, and David A. Kindig (Washington, DC: National Academies Press, 2004), 285–99.

121. For example, that epitopes, which stimulate immune responses, are present in breast milk does not demonstrate that they have any biological effect on babies. See Nicole L. Wilson et al., "Glycoproteomics of Milk: Differences in Sugar Epitopes on Human and Bovine Milk Fat Globule Membranes," *Journal of Proteome Research* 7, no. 9 (2008): 3687–96.

122. In his own research, Abraham Bergman was struck by "the lack of risk factors in the vast majority of the SIDS victims we studied." He estimated that "over 80% of

published papers about SIDS contain conclusions that have not been substantiated," and he cited the "lack of appropriate controls" and a focus on "the relationship of epidemiologic risk factors to SIDS" as major reasons. Both SIDS and breastfeeding investigation are constrained by risk-factor epidemiology. See Abraham B. Bergman, "Wrong Turns in Sudden Infant Death Syndrome Research," *Pediatrics* 99, no. 1 (1997): 120, 119.

123. For an analysis of how low social status leads to poor health, see Donald A. Barr, *Health Disparities in the United States: Social Class, Race, Ethnicity, and Health* (Baltimore: Johns Hopkins University Press, 2008), 73–103.

124. Mark Atkinson and Edwin A. M. Gale, "Infant Diets and Type I Diabetes: Too Early, Too Late, or Just Too Complicated?" *Journal of the American Medical Association* 290, no. 13 (2003): 1771–72.

Chapter 3

1. Karen Karbo, "Goodbye, Moon," *New York Times*, December 4, 2005.

2. Deborah Lupton, *Risk* (New York: Routledge, 1999), 13.

3. David Ropeik and George Gray, *Risk: A Practical Guide for Deciding What's Really Safe and What's Really Dangerous in the World around You* (Boston: Houghton Mifflin, 2002).

4. See www.ers.usda.gov/briefing/organic/demand.htm (accessed June 16, 2009).

5. Darshak Sanghavi, "Why Do We Focus on the Least

Important Causes of Cancer?" www.slate.com, April 25, 2008.

6. Michael Power, "The Nature of Risk: The Risk Management of Everything," *Balance Sheet* 12, no. 5 (2004): 20, 24.

7. Howard Kunreuther and Paul Slovic, "Coping with Stigma: Challenges and Opportunities," in *Risk, Media, and Stigma: Understanding Public Challenges to Modern Science and Technology*, ed. James Flynn, Paul Slovic, and Howard Kunreuther (London: Earthscan, 2001), 343.

8. For a discussion of realist and constructionist perspectives, see Lupton, *Risk*, 17–35.

9. Ulrich Beck, *Risk Society: Towards a New Modernity* (London: Sage, 1992).

10. Anthony Giddens, *Modernity and Self-Identity: Self and Society in the Late Modern Age* (Stanford, CA: Stanford University Press, 1991), 19, 3, 111, 119. Giddens is more centrally concerned with the construction of self-identity in high modernity, and I return to his work later in this chapter.

11. Beck, *Risk Society*, 20 (italics in original).

12. Ibid., 35–41.

13. Ibid., 36 (italics in original).

14. Alan Scott, "Risk Society or Angst Society," in *The Risk Society and Beyond: Critical Issues for Social Theory*, ed. Barbara Adam, Ulrich Beck, and Joost Van Loon (London: Sage, 2000), 42.

15. John Tulloch and Deborah Lupton, "Consuming Risk, Consuming Science: The Case of GM Foods," *Journal of Consumer Culture* 2, no. 3 (2002): 382.

16. Mick Smith, "Sociology and Ethical Responsibility," *Sociology* 39, no. 3 (2005): 544.

17. As Ruth Levitas stresses, a broad divide separates "a discourse of risk," which has to do with the uncertainty, anxiety, and insecurity that many people confront in thinking about risk, and "a discourse of risk *society* . . . a theoretical discourse of sociologists" with systemic implications. A risk discourse "appeals quite separately from the substance of Beck's argument." See Ruth Levitas, "Discourses of Risk and Utopia," in *The Risk Society and Beyond: Critical Issues for Social Theory*, ed. Barbara Adam, Ulrich Beck, and Joost Van Loon (London: Sage, 2000), 200.

18. Sewell describes culture as "relatively autonomous." In that spirit, I understand risk culture as an analytically distinct dimension of social practice that simultaneously shapes and is shaped by other practices, such as class, gender, or geography. See William H. Sewell Jr., *Logics of History: Social Theory and Social Transformation* (Chicago:

University of Chicago Press, 2005), 164.

19. Giddens, *Modernity and Self-Identity*, 111; Robert Castel, "From Dangerousness to Risk," in *The Foucault Effect: Studies in Governmentality* (Chicago: University of Chicago Press, 1991), 289.

20. Elizabeth Beck-Gernsheim, "Life as a Planning Project," in *Risk, Environment, and Modernity: Towards a New Ecology*, ed. Scott Lash, Bronislaw Szerszynski, and Brian Wynne (London: Sage, 1996), 139.

21. Beck, *Risk Society*, 33; and Ulrich Beck, "Politics of Risk Society," in *The Politics of Risk Society*, ed. Jane Franklin (Cambridge: Polity Press, 1998), 11.

22. Niklas Luhmann, *Risk: A Sociological Theory* (New York: Aldine de Gruyter, 1993), 37.

23. Beck, *Risk Society*, 162 (italics in original).

24. Giddens, *Modernity and Self-Identity*, 20.

25. Beck, *Risk Society*, 158.

26. Donna Haraway, "Situated Knowledges: The Science Question in Feminism and the Privilege of Partial Perspective," *Feminist Studies* 14, no. 3 (1988): 590, 581 (italics added).

27. David Denney, *Risk and Society* (London: Sage, 2005), 30.

28. Richard V. Ericson and Kevin D. Haggerty, *Policing the Risk Society* (Toronto: University of Toronto Press, 1997), 98.

29. Beck, *Risk Society*, 166 (italics in original).

30. Cass R. Sunstein, *Laws of Fear: Beyond the Precautionary Principle* (Cambridge: Cambridge University Press, 2005), 34.

31. David Hirshleifer, "The Blind Leading the Blind: Social Influence, Fads, and Informational Cascades," in *The New Economics of Human Behavior*, ed. Mariano Tommasi and Kathryn Ierulli (Cambridge: Cambridge University Press, 1995), 204 (italics in original).

32. Ericson and Haggerty, *Policing the Risk Society*, 101; Beck, *Risk Society*, 173.

33. The practical meaning of this is revealed in one study in which more than 25 percent of academic scientists reported feeling deterred by both explicit and informal constraints from pursuing "sensitive" topics and compelled to investigate others. See Joanna Kempner, Clifford S. Perlis, and Jon F. Merz, "Forbidden Knowledge," *Science* 307 (2005): 854.

34. Beck, *Risk Society*, 176.

35. Ibid., 168–69 (italics in original).

36. Roger E. Kasperson, Nayna Jhaveri, and Jeanne X. Kasperson, "Stigma and the Social Amplification of Risk: Toward a Framework of Analysis," in *Risk, Media, and Stigma: Understanding Public Challenges to Modern Science and Technology*, ed. James Flynn, Paul Slovic, and Howard Kunreuther (London: Earthscan, 2001), 18.

37. Ericson and Haggerty, *Policing the Risk Society*, 102.

38. Sunstein, *Laws of Fear*, 36–37, 81, 64–65, 89. See also Maia Szalavitz, "10 Ways We Get the Odds Wrong," *Psychology Today*, January/February 2008.

39. Sunstein, *Laws of Fear*, 83, 65.

40. Beck, *Risk Society*, 157, 169 (italics in original).

41. Jerome Kagan, *Three Seductive Ideas* (Cambridge, MA: Harvard University Press, 1998), 98.

42. William Cronon, "Introduction: In Search of Nature," in *Uncommon Ground: Toward Reinventing Nature*, ed. William Cronon (New York: Norton, 1995), 36, 25.

43. Beck, *Risk Society*, 80.

44. Sunstein, *Laws of Fear*, 44; Ropeik and Gray, *Risk*, 16. See also James P. Collman, *Naturally Dangerous: Surprising Facts about Food, Health, and the Environment* (Sausalito, CA: University Science Books, 2001), 61–85, 107–13; and Sanghavi, "Why Do We Focus on the Least Important Causes of Cancer?"

45. On the ways in which both the production and consumption of "organic" food are inextricably bound up in class and gender politics, see Julie Guthman, "Fast Food / Organic Food: Reflexive Tastes and the Making of 'Yuppie Chow,'" *Social and Cultural Geography* 4, no. 1 (2003): 45–58.

46. Giddens, *Modernity and Self-Identity*, 5.

47. Kathleen Woodward, "Statistical Panic," *differences* 11, no. 2 (1999): 194, 180.

48. Beck, *Risk Society*, 136, 137 (italics in original). Relationships, too, are reflexively organized. Structural and cultural imperatives, such as class status or religious doctrines, recede in importance, and individuals increasingly choose relationships less for ascriptive compatibility than for emotional satisfaction. These are what Giddens terms "pure relationships," connections

that lack external anchors and are valued for their own sake or for the satisfaction they bring to the people involved. Pure relationships require constant examination, an ongoing process of determining whether the relationship is meeting the emotional needs of each partner. "How am I" becomes "how are we," and "the self-examination inherent in the pure relationship clearly connects very closely to the reflexive project of the self" (Giddens, *Modernity and Self-Identity*, 89–91).

49. Giddens, *Modernity and Self-Identity*, 65–69, 186.

50. Beck, *Risk Society*, 28, 72.

51. Giddens, *Modernity and Self-Identity*, 3.

52. Ibid., 23.

53. The concept of neoliberalism has generated voluminous scholarship, much of which centers on markets, the world economy, and the promotion of government partnership with private industry to stimulate democratic development. Neoliberalism is a global phenomenon with varying social, political, and economic implications in different national and international contexts. Most of this lies well beyond the scope of this chapter, which is concerned largely with the relationship between neoliberalism and notions of responsibility. My discussion here draws heavily on Colin Gordon, "Governmental Rationality: An Introduction," in *The Foucault Effect: Studies in Governmentality*, ed. Graham Burchell, Colin Gordon, and Peter Miller (Chicago: University of Chicago Press, 1991), esp. 43–45.

54. Michel Foucault, "Governmentality," in *The Foucault Effect: Studies in Governmentality*, ed. Graham Burchell, Colin Gordon, and Peter Miller (Chicago: University of Chicago Press, 1991), esp. 102–3.

55. Alan R. Petersen, "Risk and the Regulated Self: The Discourse of Health Promotion as Politics of Uncertainty," *Australian & New Zealand Journal of Sociology* 32, no. 1 (1996): 48.

56. Ibid.

57. Mitchell Dean, *Governmentality: Power and Rule in Modern Society* (Thousand Oaks, CA: Sage, 1999), 167.

58. Nikolas Rose, "The Politics of Life Itself," *Theory, Culture & Society* 18, no. 6 (2001): 7.

59. Joel Best, "Social Progress and Social Problems: Toward a Sociology of Doom," *Sociological Quarterly* 42, no. 1 (2001): 4. See also Peter Berger, "Towards a Religion of Health Activism," in *Health, Lifestyle and Environment: Countering the Panic*, ed. Social Affairs Unit / Manhattan Institute (London: SAU/MI, 1991), 25.

60. Rose, "The Politics of Life Itself," 16.

61. Petersen and Lupton, *The New Public Health*, 49.

62. Michael Fitzpatrick, *The Tyranny of Health: Doctors and the Regulation of Lifestyle* (New York: Routledge, 2001), 6.

63. On how health advice about breast cancer highlights risk factors that emphasize choice and personal control, see Susan Yadlon, "Skinny Women and Good Mothers: The Rhetoric of Risk, Control, and Culpability in the Production of Knowledge about Breast Cancer," *Feminist Studies* 23, no. 3 (1997): 645–77.

64. David Armstrong, "The Rise of Surveillance Medicine," *Sociology of Health and Illness* 17, no. 3 (1995): 400.

65. Thomas Lemke, "Disposition and Determinism—Genetic Diagnostics in Risk Society," *Sociological Review* (2004): 556.

66. Lisa M. Schwartz and Steven Woloshin, "The Case for Letting Information Speak for Itself," *Effective Clinical Practice* 4 (2001): 76–79.

67. Woodward, "Statistical Panic," 196.

68. Armstrong, "The Rise of Surveillance Medicine," 401.

69. H. Gilbert Welch, Lisa Schwartz, and Steven Woloshin, "What's Making Us Sick Is an Epidemic of Diagnoses," *New York Times*, January 2, 2007.

70. The concept of "health citizenship" is discussed in Patricia Geist-Martin, Eileen Berlin Ray, and Barbara F. Sharf, *Communicating Health: Personal, Cultural, and Political Complexities* (Belmont, CA: Wadsworth / Thomson Learning, 2003).

71. Petersen, "Risk and the Regulated Self," 52.

72. William G. Kirkwood and Dan Brown, "Public Communication about the Causes of Disease: The Rhetoric of Responsibility," *Journal of Communication* 45, no. 1 (1995): 58–60.

73. Lemke, "Disposition and Determinism," 556.

74. Beck, *Risk Society*, 135.

75. See www.cdc.gov/nccdphp/dnpa/obesity/index.htm (accessed June 18, 2007). U.S. Department of Health and Human Services, "Statistics Related to Overweight and Obesity," available at win.niddk.nih.gov/statistics/index.htm (accessed June 18, 2007).

76. CDC, available at www.cdc.gov/nccdphp/dnpa/obesity/economic_consequences.htm (accessed June 18, 2007).

77. While few health experts deny the association between obesity and various health problems, an increasing number question the extent to which individuals can control their weight and the health benefits of weight loss per se. See, for example, J. Eric Oliver, *Fat Politics: The Real Story behind America's Obesity Epidemic* (Oxford: Oxford University Press, 2006); Gina Kolata, *Rethinking Thin: The New Science of Weight Loss–And the Myths and Realities of Dieting* (New York: Farrar, Strauss & Giroux, 2007); and Paul Campos et al., "The Epidemiology of Overweight and Obesity: Public Health Crisis or Moral Panic?" and "Response: Lifestyle, Not Weight, Should Be the Primary Target," both in *International Journal of Epidemiology* 35 (2006): 55–60, 81–82. I return to a discussion of obesity in the conclusion.

78. Public discourse on obesity, moreover, demonstrates how a neoliberal state can shape citizens' behavior by personalizing responsibility for serious health problems. For example, a 2003 HHS campaign focused on "motivating black men to eat 9 servings of fruits and vegetables a day to reduce their risk for diet-related diseases that disproportionately affect the black community," including certain forms of cancer, high blood pressure, diabetes, and obesity. These leading causes of death, according to then HHS Secretary Tommy Thompson, "are largely preventable through changes in our lifestyle choices." Such a campaign rested on several dubious assumptions: that

eating nine servings of fruits and vegetables can help reduce the incidence of various diseases, an assertion for which medical evidence is inconsistent, at best; that these diseases can be prevented by lifestyle changes, a hypothesis for which compelling evidence is lacking; that diseases can be controlled by disseminating information; that the proper choices are universally available; and that people can and must be taught to make the right choices. "I am a black man who eats more than 9 servings of fruits and vegetables a day, so I know it's doable," said Terry Mason, a physician in Chicago, in an HHS press release. Yet "black men" is not a socioeconomically homogeneous category, and Mason's diet is not "doable" for all or even most black men. If healthy black men eat fresh fruits and vegetables, which are more expensive, less calorie dense, and less accessible than many other foods in poor neighborhoods, lower-income black men cannot but "choose" to be unhealthy. Likewise, if "excess" body fat represents poor health and lack of self-control, people who are genetically "overweight" cannot but fail to be responsible citizens. Regardless of an individual's social location or hereditary disposition, the moral in diet discourse is the same: good health is achievable for responsible people. See www.nih.gov/news/pr/apr2003/nci-24.htm (accessed June 18, 2007).

79. Lorna Weir, *Pregnancy, Risk, and Biopolitics: On the Threshold of the Living Subject* (London: Routledge, 2006), 30.

80. Elisabeth Beck-Gernsheim, "Health and Responsibility: From Social Change to

Technological Change and Vice-Versa," in *The Risk Society and Beyond: Critical Issues for Social Theory*, ed. Barbara Adam, Ulrich Beck, and Joost Van Loon (London: Sage, 2000), 129; W. Van den Daele, "Das zähe Leben des Präventiven Zwanges," quoted in Beck-Gernsheim, "Health and Responsibility," 130.

81. Petersen, "Risk and the Regulated Self," 53.

82. Rose, "The Politics of Life Itself," 218.

83. Fitzpatrick, *The Tyranny of Health*, 70, 118.

84. Petersen and Lupton, *The New Public Health*, 73–74.

85. On republican mothers, see Linda K. Kerber, *Women of the Republic: Intellect and Ideology in Revolutionary America* (Chapel Hill: University of North Carolina Press, 1980).

86. Petersen and Lupton, *The New Public Health*, 73–74.

87. Edward Tenner, *Our Own Devices: The Past and Future of Body Technology* (New York: Knopf, 2003), 31.

Chapter 4

1. Lenore Skenazy, *Free-Range Kids: Giving Our Children the Freedom We Had without Going Nuts with Worry* (San Francisco: Jossey-Bass, 2009). Skenazy also maintains a website, www.freerangekids.com, for parents who "believe in helmets, car seats, and safety belts" but "do NOT believe that every time school-age children go outside they need a security detail" (accessed January 9, 2010).

2. Frank Furedi, *Paranoid Parenting: Why Ignoring the Experts May Be Best for Your Child* (Chicago: Chicago Review Press, 2002), 31 (italics in original).

3. Susan J. Douglas and Meredith W. Michaels, *The Mommy Myth: The Idealization of Motherhood and How It Has Undermined Women* (Boston: Free Press, 2004).

4. Linda Blum, *At the Breast: Breastfeeding and Motherhood in the Contemporary United States* (Boston: Beacon Press, 1999); and Sharon Hays, *The Cultural Contradictions of Motherhood* (New Haven, CT: Yale University Press, 1996).

5. In fact, children's share of domestic spending has shrunk since 1960, and as a percentage of total federal outlays, it is predicted to diminish further over the next ten years. By contrast, spending on the elderly has risen steadily, and the increase over the next decade in the nonchild portions of Medicare, Medicaid, and Social Security alone is predicted to exceed total spending on children. See Julia B. Isaacs et al., *Kids' Share: An Analysis of Federal Expenditures on Children through 2008* (Washington, DC: Brookings Institution, 2009), 4–5.

6. Katha Pollit, "'Fetal Rights': A New Assault on Feminism," in *"Bad" Mothers: The Politics of Blame in Twentieth-Century America*, ed. Molly Ladd-Taylor and Lauri Umansky (New York: New York University Press, 1998), 297.

7. Rima D. Apple, *Perfect Motherhood: Science and Childrearing in America* (New Brunswick, NJ: Rutgers University Press, 2006).

8. Ibid., 1–33.

9. Patricia Bayer Richard, "The Tailor-Made Child: Implications for Women and the State," in *Expecting Trouble: Surrogacy, Fetal Abuse, & New Reproductive Technologies*, ed. Patricia Boling (Boulder, CO: Westview Press, 1995), 9.

10. See Margaret Marsh and Wanda Ronner, *The Empty Cradle: Infertility in America from Colonial Times to the Present* (Baltimore: Johns Hopkins University Press, 1996); William Ray Arney, *Power and the Profession of Obstetrics* (Chicago: University of Chicago Press, 1982), 22–24; Judith Walzer Leavitt, *Brought to Bed: Childbearing in America, 1750–1950* (New York: Oxford University Press, 1986), 20–28; Elizabeth M. Armstrong, *Conceiving Risk, Bearing Responsibility: Fetal Alcohol Syndrome and the Diagnosis of Moral Disorder* (Baltimore: Johns Hopkins University Press, 2003), 23–62; and Richard W. Wertz and Dorothy C. Wertz, *Lying-In: A History of Childbirth in America* (New Haven, CT: Yale University Press, 1977), 120–38.

11. Lealle Ruhl, "Dilemmas of the Will: Uncertainty, Reproduction, and the Rhetoric of Control," *Signs* 27, no. 3 (2002): 644.

12. See Diane Eyer, *Mother–Infant Bonding: A Scientific Fiction* (New Haven, CT: Yale University Press, 1992), 198–99.

13. See www.nichd.nih.gov/health/topics/preconception_care.cfm; familydoctor.org/online/famdocen/home/women/pregnancy/basics/076.html (accessed May 26, 2007).

14. See www.cdc.gov/ncbddd/preconception/QandA_providers.htm (accessed May 26, 2007).

15. See www.cdc.gov/prams/ (accessed August 7, 2008).

16. Kay Johnson et al., "Recommendations to Improve Preconception Health and Health Care—United States: A Report of the CDC/ATSDR Preconception Care Work Group and the Select Panel on Preconception Care," *MMWR Recommendations and Reports* no. 55:RR06, April 21, 2006, 10, 11.

17. See www.acog.org/publications/patient_education/bp056.cfm (accessed May 19, 2009).

18. See Scott D. Grosse and Julianne S. Collins, "Folic Acid Supplementation and Neural Tube Defect Prevention," *Birth Defects Research Part A: Clinical and Molecular Teratology* 79, no. 11 (2007): 737–42; CDC, "Neural Tube Defect Surveillance and Folic Acid Intervention—Texas-Mexico Border, 1993–98," *Morbidity and Mortality Weekly Report* 49, no. 1 (2000): 1–4; and James L. Mills and Caroline Signore, "Neural Tube Defect Rates before and after Food Fortification with Folic Acid," *Birth Defects Research Part A: Clinical and Molecular Teratology* 70, no. 11 (2004): 844–45.

19. Search conducted on amazon.com, May 26, 2007.

20. See www.modernstork.com/category/003691.shtml (accessed May 30, 2007). This was the first website listed in a Google search for "pre-pregnancy."

21. American Society for Reproductive Medicine,

"Frequently Asked Questions about Infertility," available at www.asrm.org/Patients/faqs.html#Q2 (accessed January 20, 2010).

22. Dion Farquhar, *The Other Machine: Discourse and Reproductive Technologies* (New York: Routledge, 1996), 84.

23. As of this writing, *What to Expect When You're Expecting* (1996–2008) had spent 442 weeks on the *New York Times* list of best-selling paperback advice books. Available at www.nytimes.com/2009/05/17/books/bestseller/bestpaperadvice.html (accessed January 20, 2010).

24. Heidi E. Murkoff, Arlene Eisenberg, and Sandee E. Hathaway, *What to Expect When You're Expecting*, 2nd ed. (New York: Workman, 1996), 81.

25. Heidi E. Murkoff, Arlene Eisenberg, and Sandee E. Hathaway, *What to Expect When You're Expecting*, 3rd ed. (New York: Workman, 2002), 84, 74, 69, 178.

26. Search conducted on amazon.com, May 2007.

27. Rayna Rapp, *Testing the Woman, Testing the Fetus: The Social Impact of Amniocentesis in America* (New York: Routledge, 1999). See also Ruth Schwartz Cowan, *Heredity and Hope: The Case for Genetic Screening* (Cambridge, MA: Harvard University Press, 2008), 227–34.

28. Abby Lippman, "The Genetic Construction of Testing: Choice, Consent, or Conformity for Women?" in *Women and Prenatal Testing: Facing the Challenges of Genetic Technology*, ed. Karen H. Rothenberg and Elizabeth J. Thompson (Columbus: Ohio State University Press, 1994), 23.

29. Deborah Lupton, *Risk* (New York: Routledge, 1999), 89–90.

30. Jennifer Gunter, "Intimate Partner Violence," *Obstetrics and Gynecology Clinics of North America* 34 (2007): 367–88; Jay G. Silverman et al., "Intimate Partner Violence Victimization prior to and during Pregnancy among Women Residing in 26 U.S. States: Associations with Maternal and Neonatal Health," *American Journal of Obstetrics and Gynecology* 195 (2006): 140–48; Jacquelyn C. Campbell et al., "Risk Factors for Femicide in Abusive Relationships: Results from a Multisite Case Study," *American Journal of Public Health* 93, no. 7 (2003): 1089–97. Jeanne Flavin argues that because violence is more common against women who are young, unmarried, uneducated, and nonwhite and whose pregnancies are unintended, it is unclear precisely how much violence is the result of pregnancy per se. See Jeanne Flavin, *Our Bodies, Our Crimes: The Policing of Women's Reproduction in America* (New York: New York University Press, 2009), 97.

31. Carol A. Stabile, "Shooting the Mother: Fetal Photography and the Politics of Disappearance," *Camera Obscura* 28 (1992): 178–205.

32. See www.geniusbabies.com/embryonics.html (accessed May 21, 2007).

33. See www.prenatalparenting.com (accessed May 21, 2007). See also Frederick Wirth, *Prenatal Parenting: The Complete Psychological and Spiritual Guide to Loving Your Unborn Child* (New York: HarperCollins, 2001). In fact, "messenger

molecules," which enable "communication" between RNA and DNA, have nothing to do with psychological or emotional communication, and Wirth provides no evidence for either the placental transmission of such molecules or the claim that babies who were not "prenatally parented" are disadvantaged.

34. Deborah Katz, "New Reasons to Watch What You Eat: Nourishment in the Womb May Matter Decades Later," *U.S. News & World Report*, September 22, 2007, available at health.usnews.com/articles/health/2007/09/22/nourishment-in-the-womb-may-matter-decades-later.html (accessed October 22, 2007). The study in question was by Stéphanie A. Bayol, Samantha J. Farrington, and Neil C. Strickland, "A Maternal 'Junk Food' Diet in Pregnancy and Lactation Promotes an Exacerbated Taste for 'Junk Food' and a Greater Propensity for Obesity in Rat Offspring," *British Journal of Nutrition* 98 (2007): 843–51.

35. Daniel DeNoon, "Moms Eat Junk Food, Kids Get Fat," available at www.cbsnews.com/stories/2008/07/01/health/webmd/main4222324.shtml (accessed July 2, 2008).

36. Shari Roan, "Living for Two," *Los Angeles Times*, November 12, 2007.

37. Darshak Sanghavi, "Womb Raider: Do Future Health Problems Begin during Gestation?" available at www.slate.com/id/2201788/ (accessed October 13, 2008).

38. Gideon Koren et al., "Bias against the Null Hypothesis: The Reproductive Hazards of Cocaine," *The Lancet* 1 (1989):

1440–42; Cynthia R. Daniels, "Between Fathers and Fetuses: The Social Construction of Male Reproduction and the Politics of Fetal Harm," *Signs: Journal of Women in Culture and Society* 22, no. 3 (1997): 579–616; Dorothy Roberts, *Killing the Black Body: Race, Reproduction, and the Meaning of Liberty* (New York: Vintage Books, 1997), 154–59.

39. See Flavin, *Our Bodies, Our Crimes*, 95–118.

40. Armstrong, *Conceiving Risk*, 4, 6. The CDC nonetheless warns that "no time during pregnancy is safe to drink alcohol, and harm can occur early, before a woman has realized that she is or might be pregnant. Fetal alcohol syndrome and other alcohol-related birth defects can be prevented if women cease intake of alcohol before conception." See Kay Johnson et al., "Recommendations to Improve Preconception Health and Health Care—United States: A Report of the CDC/ATSDR Preconception Care Work Group and the Select Panel on Preconception Care," *MMWR Recommendations and Reports* no. 55:RR06, April 21, 2006, 5.

41. Rachel Roth, *Making Women Pay: The Hidden Costs of Fetal Rights* (Ithaca, NY: Cornell University Press, 2000), 194.

42. See, for example, Armstrong, *Conceiving Risk*, 3; Family Violence Prevention Fund, available at www.endabuse.org/resources/facts/ReproductiveHealth.pdf (accessed April 13, 2008); and Flavin, *Our Bodies, Our Crimes*, 97–102.

43. R. M. Cantor et al., "Paternal Age and Autism Are Associated in a Family-Based Sample," *Molecular Psychiatry* 12 (2007): 419–23; Alexander

Kolevzon, Raz Gross, and Abraham Reichenberg, "Prenatal and Perinatal Risk Factors for Autism: A Review and Integration of Findings," *Archives of Pediatrics and Adolescent Medicine* 161, no. 4 (2007): 326–33; Lisa A. Croen et al., "Maternal and Paternal Age and Risk of Autism Spectrum Disorders," *Archives of Pediatrics and Adolescent Medicine* 161, no. 4 (2007): 334–40; Abraham Reichenberg et al., "Advancing Paternal Age and Autism," *Archives of General Psychiatry* 63 (2006): 1026–32; Attila Sipos et al., "Paternal Age and Schizophrenia: A Population Based Cohort Study," *British Medical Journal* 329 (2004): 1070–74; Dolores Malaspina et al., "Advancing Paternal Age and the Risk of Schizophrenia," *Archives of General Psychiatry* 58, no. 4 (2001): 361–67. On February 27, 2007, the *New York Times* published a story in its Health section that discussed the association between paternal age and autism and schizophrenia (Roni Rabin, "It Seems the Fertility Clock Ticks for Men, Too"). This research otherwise has received little attention in the mainstream press.

44. Cynthia Daniels, *Exposing Men: The Science and Politics of Male Reproduction* (Oxford: Oxford University Press, 2006), 109–56; and Daniels, "Between Fathers and Fetuses," 596, 601–5, 579 (italics in original); Joan E. Bertin and Laurie R. Beck, "Of Headlines and Hypotheses: The Role of Gender in Popular Press Coverage of Women's Health and Biology," in *Man-Made Medicine: Women's Health, Public Policy, and Reform*, ed. Kary L. Moss (Durham, NC: Duke

University Press, 1996), 44–45. Newspaper accounts of male infertility in the United Kingdom reflect similar gender biases. See Kenneth Gannon, Lesley Glover, and Paul Abel, "Masculinity, Infertility, Stigma and Media Reports," *Social Science & Medicine* 59 (2004): 1169–75.

45. Adria Schwartz, "Taking the Nature out of Mother," in *Representations of Motherhood*, ed. Donna Bassin, Margaret Honey, and Meryle Mahrer Kaplan (New Haven, CT: Yale University Press, 1994), 240–55; Adele E. Clarke, *Disciplining Reproduction: Modernity, American Life Sciences, and the Problems of Sex* (Berkeley: University of California Press, 1998), 248–49.

46. Aviva Jill Romm, *The Natural Pregnancy Book: Herbs, Nutrition, and Other Holistic Choices* (Berkeley, CA: Celestial Arts, 2003), 6, 46, 148.

47. See www.amazon.com/Natural-Child-Parenting-Heart/dp/0865714401/ (accessed May 19, 2009).

48. See www.naturalmom.com/ (accessed June 5, 2007).

49. Peggy O'Mara, Mothering *Magazine's Having a Baby, Naturally*: The Mothering *Magazine Guide to Pregnancy and Childbirth* (New York: Atria, 2003), xviii.

50. Sears and Sears write that mothers and doctors must work together and that mothers should simply make themselves aware of their options before choosing. But their books are essentially treatises on the dangers of medical intervention. For example, in discussing the range of birth options, the authors write that "*positive birth experience* means different things to different women"

(italics in original). Yet they stress "the ideal of a drug-free childbirth" and caution repeatedly that pain medication "is likely to yield a less-than-satisfying birth experience." See William Sears and Martha Sears, *The Birth Book: Everything You Need to Know to Have a Safe and Satisfying Birth* (Boston: Little, Brown, 1994), 11, 51, 82–83, 128.

51. As of this writing, William Sears et al., *The Baby Book: Everything You Need to Know about Your Baby from Birth to Age 2* (Boston: Little, Brown, 2003), ranks 229 in overall sales and is the most popular book in the "Pregnancy and Health" category on Amazon.com. Also in the top fifty best-selling books in "Pregnancy and Health" are William Sears and Martha Sears, *The Discipline Book: How to Have a Better-Behaved Child from Birth to Age Ten* (Boston: Little, Brown, 1995) (no. 22); William Sears and Martha Sears, *The Birth Book: Everything You Need to Know to Have a Satisfying Birth* (Boston: Little, Brown, 1994) (no. 27); Martha Sears and William Sears, *The Breastfeeding Book: Everything You Need to Know about Nursing Your Child from Birth through Weaning* (Boston: Little, Brown, 2000) (no. 31); Martha Sears, William Sears, and Linda Hughey Holt, *The Pregnancy Book: Everything You Need to Know from America's Baby Experts* (Boston: Little, Brown, 1997) (no. 37); and William Sears and Martha Sears, *The Attachment Parenting Book: A Commonsense Guide to Understanding and Nurturing Your Baby* (Boston: Little, Brown, 2001) (no. 50) (accessed amazon. com, May 19, 2009).

52. Sears and Sears, *The Birth Book*, 82–83.

53. Ibid., back cover; available at www.askdrsears.com/about.asp (accessed June 6, 2007).

54. Chris Bobel, *The Paradox of Natural Mothering* (Philadelphia: Temple University Press, 2002), 130 (italics in original).

55. Anthony Giddens, *Modernity and Self-Identity: Self and Society in the Late Modern Age* (Stanford, CA: Stanford University Press, 1991).

56. A natural mother ultimately "redirects the allegiance others pledge to conventional authorities toward a more abstract but nonetheless powerful influence: an ideology of the superiority of nature. . . [which] has become her new religion" (Bobel, *The Paradox of Natural Mothering*, 105–6). For a full analysis of the antinomies of control in natural mothering, see 104–40.

57. Sears and Sears, *The Birth Book*, 82–83.

58. Citing animal and human data, both the American College of Radiology and the ACOG state that the dose of ionizing radiation from radiologic procedures does not raise the risk of congenital malformations, growth restriction, or pregnancy loss. See Anne Drapkin Lyerly et al., "Risks, Values, and Decision-Making Surrounding Pregnancy," *Obstetrics and Gynecology* 109, no. 4 (2007): 982.

59. Sears and Sears, *The Baby Book*, 12.

60. Lyerly et al., "Risks, Values, and Decision Making Surrounding Pregnancy," 981–82.

61. Deborah Lupton, "Risk and the Ontology of Pregnant

Embodiment," in *Risk and Socio-cultural Theory: New Directions and Perspective*, ed. Deborah Lupton (Cambridge: Cambridge University Press, 1999), 82.

62. Elisabeth Beck-Gernsheim, "Life as a Planning Project," in *Risk, Environment, and Modernity: Towards a New Ecology*, ed. Scott Lash, Bronislaw Szerszynski, and Brian Wynne (London: Sage, 1996), 143.

63. Sonja Olin Lauritzen and Lisbeth Sachs, "Normality, Risk and the Future: Implicit Communication of Threat in Health Surveillance," *Sociology of Health and Illness* 23, no. 4 (2001): 504.

64. David Armstrong, "The Rise of Surveillance Medicine," *Sociology of Health and Illness* 17, no. 3 (1995): 396–97.

65. Heidi Murkoff et al., *What to Expect the First Year*, 2nd ed. (New York: Workman, 2003), 310–11.

66. Pamela Paul, *Parenting, Inc.: How We Are Sold on $800 Strollers, Fetal Education, Baby Sign Language, Sleeping Coaches, Toddler Couture, and Diaper Wipe Warmers—and What It Means for Our Children* (New York: Times Books, 2008). Amazon.com offers such titles as *Trillion Dollar Moms: Marketing to a New Generation of Mothers, Marketing to Moms: Getting Your Share of the Trillion-Dollar Market, Marketing to the New Super Consumer: Mom & Kid*, and *The Mom Factor: What Really Drives Where We Shop, Eat, and Play* (search conducted January 10, 2010).

67. Douglas and Michaels, *The Mommy Myth*, 300.

68. See www.toysrus.com/registry/truParentsCheckList.jsp (accessed June 29, 2007).

69. See www.toysrus.com/product/index.jsp?productId=2307234#prod_prodinfo (accessed May 6, 2008).

70. Murkoff et al., *What to Expect the First Year*, 403. I visited a Babies "R" Us store in Austin, Texas, in August 2007.

71. AAP, Task Force on Infant Positioning and Sudden Infant Death Syndrome, "Positioning and Sudden Infant Death Syndrome (SIDS): Update," *Pediatrics* 98, no. 6 (1996): 1216–18.

72. Ibid.

73. AAP, Task Force on Infant Sleep Position and Sudden Infant Death Syndrome, "Changing Concepts of Sudden Infant Death Syndrome: Implications for Infant Sleeping Environment and Sleep Position," *Pediatrics* 105, no. 3 (2000): 650.

74. AAP, Task Force on Sudden Infant Death Syndrome, "The Changing Concept of Sudden Infant Death Syndrome: Diagnostic Coding Shifts, Controversies regarding the Sleeping Environment, and New Variables to Consider in Reducing Risk," *Pediatrics* 116, no. 5 (2005): 1245.

75. Ibid., 1246. The most recent statistics from the CDC indicate 0.54 deaths per 1,000 live births in 2004. See CDC, *National Vital Statistics Reports* 55, no. 14 (May 2, 2007), 25.

76. AAP, Task Force on Sudden Infant Death Syndrome, "The Changing Concept of Sudden Infant Death Syndrome," 1251.

77. See, for example, sids-network.org/risk.htm, www.firstcandle.org/FC-PDF4/Research_Position%20

Statements/triple%20risk%20model%20for%20sids.pdf, and dying.lovetoknow.com/Facts_on_Sudden_Infant_Death_Syndrome (all accessed March 3, 2008). See also www.encyclopedia.com/article-1G2-2830102249/sudden-infant-death-syndrome.html and http://solutions.psu.edu/Parenting_588.htm (accessed January 7, 2010).

78. In responding to a letter raising this possibility, the AAP Task Force noted that motor delays associated with supine sleeping were transient and no longer apparent at one year of age and that other delays were not observed in the first eighteen months. The long-term effects, however, have not been evaluated. See Bradford D. Gessner et al., "Bed Sharing with Unimpaired Parents Is Not an Important Risk for Sudden Infant Death Syndrome," *Pediatrics* 117, no. 3 (2006): 990–96.

79. AAP, Task Force on Sudden Infant Death Syndrome, "The Changing Concept of Sudden Infant Death Syndrome," 1252.

80. AAP, "Identifying Infants and Young Children with Developmental Disorders in the Medical Home: An Algorithm for Developmental Surveillance and Screening," *Pediatrics* 118: (2006): 405–20.

81. Melinda Marshall, "Understanding Autism," *Parenting*, April 2007, available at www.parenting.com/parenting/child/article/0,19840,1597741,00.html (accessed July 14, 2007).

82. Linda M. Blum, "Mother-Blame in the Prozac Nation: Raising Kids with Invisible Disabilities," *Gender & Society*

21, no. 2 (2007): 212. See also Claudia Malacrida, "Alternative Therapies and Attention Deficit Disorder: Discourses of Maternal Responsibility and Risk," *Gender & Society* 16, no. 3 (2002): 366–85; and Jane Taylor McDonnell, "On Being the 'Bad' Mother of an Autistic Child," in *"Bad" Mothers: The Politics of Blame in Twentieth-Century America*, ed. Molly Ladd-Taylor and Lauri Umansky (New York: New York University Press, 1998), 220–29.

83. On concerted cultivation and the accomplishment of natural growth as child-raising strategies, see Annette Lareau, *Unequal Childhoods: Class, Race, and Family Life* (Berkeley: University of California Press, 2003).

84. Lareau, *Unequal Childhoods*, 24–29. In these families, "the cultural logic of child rearing at home is out of sync with the standards of institutions" (3), and this logic leaves working-class and poor children without the skills they need to negotiate with authority later in life.

85. Beck-Gernsheim, "Life as a Planning Project," 139, 143.

86. Lareau, *Unequal Childhoods*, 50.

87. Madeline Levine, *The Price of Privilege: How Parental Pressure and Material Advantage Are Creating a Generation of Disconnected and Unhappy Kids* (New York: HarperCollins, 2006), 29, 10, 31.

88. Jules Law, "The Politics of Breastfeeding," *Signs: Journal of Women in Culture and Society* 25, no. 2 (2000): 444.

89. See Maria Jansson, "Feeding Children and Protecting Women: The Emergence of Breastfeeding as an International Concern," *Women's Studies International Forum* 32 (2009): 240–48, who argues that science is perceived to represent "an indisputable reality that is pre-political and morally good" (242).

90. Dorothy Nelkin, "Foreword: The Social Meanings of Risk," in *Risk, Culture, and Health Inequality: Shifting Perceptions of Danger and Blame*, ed. Barbara Herr Harthorn and Laury Oaks (Westport, CT: Praeger, 2003), viii.

91. See www.llli.org/NB/NBNovDec00p210.html (accessed March 10, 2008).

92. Murkoff et al., *What to Expect When You're Expecting*, 2002, 308–14; ACOG, *Planning Your Pregnancy and Birth*, 3rd ed. (Washington, DC: American College of Obstetricians, 2000), 215. Obstetricians can purchase the latter in bulk for distribution to new patients.

93. Boston Women's Health Book Collective, *Our Bodies, Ourselves: A New Edition for a New Era* (New York: Touchstone, 2005). See also www.ourbodiesourselves.org/book/excerpt.asp?id=31 (accessed May 6, 2009). As Nieca Goldberg, medical director of the New York University Women's Heart Center, told the *New York Times*, breast-feeders "may be healthier women who take better care of themselves" (*New York Times*, April 22, 2009). On lactation and breast cancer, a systematic review concluded "that no consensus about the relationship between breastfeeding and breast cancer is emerging. Expanded consideration of possible confounders for this relationship is required to determine if breastfeeding is protective and how protection might be conferred." See Yang Li and Kathryn H. Jacobsen, "A Systematic Review of the Association between Breastfeeding and Breast Cancer," *Journal of Women's Health* 17, no. 10 (2008): 1635.

94. See www.askdrsears.com/html/2/T020300.asp (accessed March 30, 2008); Sears and Sears, *The Breastfeeding Book*, 7–8.

95. Sears et al., *The Baby Book*, 2003, 124–27. The first edition (1993) advised women about prenatal nipple exams and nipple conditioning (125–26).

96. Breastfeeding.com is advertised as "the leading Web site for breastfeeding information and support" and was the first site retrieved by the Google search engine in a search for "breastfeeding." Its medical advisory board includes physicians Ruth Lawrence, a well-known breastfeeding advocate and author of the standard medical reference book on breastfeeding for physicians; and Audrey Naylor, chair of the U.S. Breastfeeding Committee, an umbrella group of medical and public health organizations committed to protecting, promoting, and supporting breastfeeding. See www.breastfeeding.com/medical.html (accessed March 20, 2008).

97. See www.breastfeeding.com/all_about/all_about_formula.html (accessed March 20, 2008). The stories are reprinted from Naomi Baumslag and Dia L. Michels, *Milk, Money, and Madness: The Culture and Politics of Breastfeeding* (Westport, CT: Bergin & Garvey, 1995).

98. Majia Holmer Nadesan and Patty Sotirin, "The Romance and Science of 'Breast Is Best': Discursive Contradictions and Contexts of Breast-Feeding Choices," *Text and Performance Quarterly* 18, no. 3 (1998): 221.

99. La Leche League International, *The Womanly Art of Breastfeeding*, 7th ed. (New York: Plume, 2004), 339, 375–76. No compelling evidence indicates that either prolactin or breastfeeding leads to better mothering.

100. See Katherine A. Dettwyler, "A Time to Wean: The Hominid Blueprint for the Natural Age of Weaning in Modern Human Populations," 39–74; and "Beauty and the Breast: The Cultural Context of Breastfeeding in the United States," 167–215 both in *Breastfeeding: Biocultural Perspectives*, ed. Patricia Stuart-Macadam and Katherine A. Dettwyler (New York: Aldine de Gruyter, 1995).

101. Nadesan and Sotirin, "The Romance and Science of 'Breast Is Best,'" 219.

102. Pam Carter, *Feminism, Breasts, and Breast-Feeding* (New York: St. Martin's Press, 1995), 69, 66.

103. See www.llli.org/mission.html?m=1,0,2 (accessed August 31, 2008).

104. Bernice L. Hausman, *Mother's Milk: Breastfeeding Controversies in American Culture* (New York: Routledge, 2003), 167.

105. See www.llli.org/FAQ/premresources.html (accessed August 31, 2008).

106. Hausman, *Mother's Milk*, 168, 157.

107. For a discussion of environmental politics and breast milk contamination, see Maia Boswell-Penc, *Tainted Milk: Breastmilk, Feminisms, and the Politics of Environmental Degradation* (Albany: State University of New York Press, 2006).

108. Hausman, *Mother's Milk*, 117.

109. See www.sciencedaily.com/releases/2007/09/070915125155.htm (accessed September 18, 2007). See also www.yessuperbaby.com/superbaby-shirt.html (accessed December 6, 2001), which offers a nursing shirt with straps, rings, and designs that introduce babies and toddlers to textures, colors, shapes, numbers, and the alphabet and "promote tactile and visual stimulation." These shirts originate in England and are available on the Internet.

110. See www.toysrus.com (accessed April 14, 2008). The iPhone also now has several breastfeeding apps.

111. On breastfeeding as a consumer project, see Orit Avishai, "Managing the Lactating Body: The Breast-Feeding Project and Privileged Motherhood," *Qualitative Sociology* 30 (2007): 135–52.

112. Blum, *At the Breast*, 200.

113. See www.breastfeeding.com/all_about/all_about_birth.html (italics in original, accessed March 10, 2008).

114. Sears and Sears, *The Breastfeeding Book*, 25. Women in England describe a similar tendency among maternal and child health educators to avoid talking about formula. One new mother reported being told not to have bottles in the house "'because you will crack. The

baby will be there screaming, and you will crack, and go for that bottle. So don't have it in the house.' They think if they give you information, you will crack." See Ellie J. Lee, "Infant Feeding in Risk Society," *Health, Risk & Society* 9, no. 3 (2007): 295–309.

115. Donna J. Chapman et al., "Breastfeeding Status on U.S. Birth Certificates: Where Do We Go from Here?" *Pediatrics* 122, no. 6 (2008): e1160.

116. For a discussion of breast pumps and "disembodied motherhood," see Blum, *At the Breast*, 55–60.

117. Murkoff et al., *What to Expect When You're Expecting*, 2002, 404; Murkoff et al., *What to Expect the First Year*, 96–98.

118. See www.breastfeeding.com/all_about/all_about_colic_foods.html (accessed March 19, 2008); Sears and Sears, *The Breastfeeding Book*, 399.

119. See www.aap.org/sections/media/Colic.htm (accessed March 20, 2008); Murkoff et al., *What to Expect the First Year*, 187.

120. For a review of this literature, see Katherine Dewey, "Maternal and Fetal Stress Are Associated with Impaired Lactogenesis in Humans," *Journal of Nutrition* 131, no. 11 (2001): 3012S–15S.

121. Sears and Sears, *The Breastfeeding Book*, 60–61.

122. Rima D. Apple, *Mothers and Medicine: A Social History of Infant Feeding, 1890–1950* (Madison: University of Wisconsin Press, 1987), 56.

123. Sears and Sears, *The Breastfeeding Book*, 224–26 (italics in original).

124. See www.askdrsears.com (accessed March 20, 2008).

125. See www.llli.org/NB/NBdepression.html (accessed March 11, 2008).

126. See www.llli.org/NB/NBMayJune04p84.html (accessed March 11, 2008).

127. Because women are trained from a young age to understand themselves *as women* in relation to motherhood, postpartum depression can be tantamount to an identity crisis. As one woman explained her depression, "When you have so much invested in one role like women do in motherhood and you're having negative feelings about it, it goes to the core of questioning your sexuality and your very identity as a woman." See Verta Taylor, *Rock-a-Bye Baby: Feminism, Self-Help, and Postpartum Depression* (New York: Routledge, 1996), 47.

128. See www.breastfeeding.com/all_about/all_about_start.html (accessed March 30, 2008).

129. Priscilla Dunstan, creator of the Dunstan Baby Language Program, was featured on the *Oprah Winfrey Show* in November 2006.

130. Law, "The Politics of Breastfeeding," 200, 415n.

131. Suzanne M. Bianchi, John P. Robinson, and Melissa A. Milkie, *Changing Rhythms of American Family Life* (New York: Russell Sage Foundation, 2006), 66.

132. Douglas and Michaels, *The Mommy Myth*, 299 (italics in original).

133. For a discussion of pure relationships, see chapter 3 and Giddens, *Modernity and Self-Identity*, 87–98, 185–87.

134. Ulrich Beck, *Risk Society: Towards a New Modernity* (London: Sage, 1992), 118 (italics in original).

135. On guilt, shame, and fateful moments, see chapter 3, and Giddens, *Modernity and Self-Identity*, 64–69, 112–14.

136. *New York Times*, June 20, 2006 (accessed June 20, 2006). I discuss the National Breastfeeding Awareness Campaign, which provoked this conversation, in chapter 5.

137. For more on how women reconcile their choices about feeding with maternal identity, see Dana Sullivan and Maureen Connolly, eds., *Unbuttoned: Women Open up about the Pleasures, Pains, and Politics of Breastfeeding* (Boston: Harvard Common Press, 2009); Avishai, "Managing the Lactating Body"; Barbara L.

Behrmann, *The Breastfeeding Café: Mothers Share the Joys, Challenges, and Secrets of Nursing* (Ann Arbor: University of Michigan Press, 2005); Roberta Cricco-Lizza, "Infant-Feeding Beliefs and Experiences of Black Women Enrolled in WIC in the New York Metropolitan Area," *Qualitative Health Research* 14, no. 9 (2004): 1197–1210; and Blum, *At the Breast*. On similar negotiations in Britain, see Ellie Lee and Jennie Bristow, "Rules for Feeding Babies," in *Regulating Autonomy: Sex, Reproduction, and Family*, ed. Shelley Day Sclater et al. (Oxford: Hart Publishing, 2009), 73–91; Ellie J. Lee, "Living with Risk in the Age of 'Intensive Motherhood': Maternal Identity and Infant Feeding," *Health, Risk, and Society* 10, no. 5 (2008): 467–77; and Elizabeth Murphy, "'Breast Is Best': Infant Feeding Decisions and Maternal Deviance," *Sociology of Health and Illness* 21, no. 2 (1999): 187–208.

138. Elizabeth Murphy, "Risk, Responsibility, and Rhetoric in Infant Feeding," *Journal of Contemporary Ethnography* 29, no. 3 (2000): 319. Murphy finds similar narratives among British women who bottle-fed their babies after unsuccessful breastfeeding.

Chapter 5

1. AAP, "Policy Statement Based on Task Force Report: The Promotion of Breastfeeding," *Pediatrics* 69, no. 5 (1982): 655.

2. U.S. Department of Health and Human Services, "Report of the Surgeon General's Workshop on Breastfeeding and Human Lactation," 1984, DHHS Publication no. HRS-D-MC 84–2, 16.

3. U.S. Department of Health and Human Services, *Blueprint for Action on Breastfeeding* (Washington, DC: U.S. Department of Health and Human Services, Office on Women's Health, 2000), 3, 8, 14–17.

4. U.S. Department of Health and Human Services, *Healthy People 2010: Understanding and Improving Health*, 2nd ed. (Washington, DC: U.S. Government Printing Office, November 2000). In linking choice and personal responsibility with health, *Healthy People 2010* (like

its predecessor, *Healthy People 2000*) captures the essence of neoliberal risk culture.

5. U.S. Department of Health and Human Services, *Blueprint for Action on Breastfeeding*, 3.

6. See www.womenshealth. gov/breastfeeding/index. cfm?page=home,and www.cdc. gov/breastfeeding/index.htm (accessed July 20, 2004, and August 30, 2009).

7. Information attributed to Suzanne Haynes was obtained in a phone interview, February 2, 2005.

8. Information about the NBAC was posted on www. adcouncil.org/issues/breast-feeding/, www.adcouncil. org/campaigns/breastfeed-ing/, www.adcouncil.org/research/wga/breastfeed-ing_awareness/?issue3Menu, www.4woman.gov/Breastfeed-ing/bf.cfm?page=Campaign, and www.4woman.gov/Breastfeeding/bf.cfm?page=227 (accessed July 20, 2004). The television ads expired at the end of 2005, the radio spots in April 2006.

9. President Johnston described himself as "embarrassed" that HHS had not informed the academy of the campaign, indeed that he had learned of it first from representatives of the formula industry. According to Amy Spangler, chair of the USBC, "It was never said specifically that the need for keeping the ads under wraps until release was due to anything having to do with infant formula companies, but I think we would have been naïve to assume that this was not one of the reasons why." See Katie Allison Granju, "The Milky Way of Doing Business,"

available at www.hipmama.com/node/view/588 (accessed January 12, 2004). Granju is a well-known breastfeeding advocate, blogger, and author of *Attachment Parenting: Instinctive Care for Your Baby and Young Child* (New York: Simon & Schuster, 1999), to which Dr. William Sears wrote the preface.

10. Precisely how much money the formula industry donates to the AAP is unknown to the public. Three companies—Abbott Laboratories, Mead Johnson Nutritionals, and Nestlé USA, Inc.—are contributors to the AAP's Friends of Children Fund (www.aap. org/donate/fcfhonorroll.htm). The Ross Products unit of Abbott Laboratories, the maker of Similac infant formula, has purchased hundreds of thousands of copies of the academy's breastfeeding guide with the Ross logo printed on them. Ross also donated $500,000 to the academy's operating budget in 2001, but Sanders's staff told the *New York Times* that more current information was not available. See Melody Peterson, "Pediatric Book on Breast-Feeding Stirs Controversy with Its Cover," *New York Times*, September 18, 2002; and Melody Peterson, "Breastfeeding Ads Delayed by a Dispute over Content," *New York Times*, December 4, 2003.

11. Letters by Johnston and Gartner were reprinted on various internet sites (e.g., www. mothering.com/action-alerts/gartner-letter.shtml, and www. promom.org/forum/viewtopic. php?t+2909, accessed January 12, 2004). See also Granju, "The Milky Way of Doing Business";

Peterson, "Breastfeeding Ads" and "Battle over Breastfeeding Ads"; and www.cbsnews.com/stories/2003/12/31/early-show/health/590864.shtml (accessed January 12, 2004).

12. Walker to Thompson, November 21, 2003, posted at www.mothering.com/action-alerts/walker-letter.shtml (accessed March 8, 2004).

13. Yeutter's letter was reproduced at www.abcnews. go.com/sections/2020/investigations/2020-breastfeed-ing-ads-040604.html (accessed June 8, 2004).

14. The USBC press release, "Babies Were Born to Be Breast-fed!" was released to member organizations, including La Leche League, on January 22, 2004. See www.lalecheleague. org/Release/AdCouncil.html (accessed May 4, 2004).

15. See Cesar G. Victora, Jean-Pierre Habicht, and Jennifer Bryce, "Evidence-Based Public Health: Moving beyond Randomized Trials," *American Journal of Public Health* 94, no. 3 (2004): 400–405; Alan R. Andreasen, ed., *Ethics in Social Marketing* (Washington, DC: Georgetown University Press, 2001); Editor in chief, "Our Policy on Policy," *Epidemiology* 124, no. 4 (2001): 371–72; Noel S. Weiss, "Policy Emanating from Epidemiologic Data: What Is the Proper Forum," *Epidemiology* 124, no. 4 (2001): 373–74; Daniel S. Greenbaum, "Epidemiology at the Edge," *Epidemiology* 124, no. 4 (2001): 376–77; Stephen Teret, "Policy and Science: Should Epidemiologists Comment on the Policy Implications of Their Research?" *Epidemiology* 12, no. 4 (2001):

374–75; Jonathan M. Samet and Nora L. Lee, "Bridging the Gap: Perspectives on Translating Epidemiologic Evidence into Policy," *American Journal of Epidemiology* 154, no. 12 (2001): S1–S4; Alfred Sommer, "How Public Health Policy Is Created: Scientific Processes and Political Reality," *American Journal of Epidemiology* 154, no. 12 (2001): S4–S6; Joseph V. Rodricks, "Some Attributes of Risk Influencing Decision-Making by Public Health and Regulatory Officials," *American Journal of Epidemiology* 154, no. 12 (2001): S7–S12; Moyses Szklo, "The Evaluation of Epidemiologic Evidence for Policy-Making," *American Journal of Epidemiology* 154, no. 12 (2001): S13–S17; Genevieve Matanoski, "Conflicts between Two Cultures: Implications for Epidemiologic Researchers in Communicating with Policy-Makers," *American Journal of Epidemiology* 154, no. 12 (2001): S36–S42; William A. Smith, "Ethics and the Social Marketer: A Framework for Practitioners," in *Ethics in Social Marketing*, ed. Alan R. Andreasen (Washington, DC: Georgetown University Press, 2001), 1–16; Michael L. Rothschild, "Ethical Considerations in the Use of Marketing for the Management of Public Health and Social Issues," in *Ethics in Social Marketing*, ed. Alan R. Andreasen (Washington, DC: Georgetown University Press, 2001), 17–38; Alvan R. Feinstein, "Scientific Paradigms and Ethical Problems in Epidemiological Research," *Journal of Clinical Epidemiology* 4 (1991): 119–23; Gary Taubes, "Epidemiology Faces Its Limits,"

Science 269 (July 14, 1995): 164–69; Kim Witte, "The Manipulative Nature of Health Communication Research," *American Behavioral Scientist* 38, no. 2 (1994): 285–93; Tom L. Beauchamp et al., "Ethical Guidelines for Epidemiologists," *Journal of Clinical Epidemiology* 44 (1991): 151S–169S; Leon Gordis, "Ethical and Professional Issues in the Changing Practice of Epidemiology," *Journal of Clinical Epidemiology* 4 (1991): 9–13; Peter M. Sandman, "Emerging Communication Responsibilities of Epidemiologists," *Journal of Clinical Epidemiology* 4 (1991): 41–50; Moyses Szklo, "Issues in Publication and Interpretation in Research Findings," *Journal of Clinical Epidemiology* 4 (1991): 109–13.

16. Sandman, "Emerging Communication Responsibilities," 45.

17. Smith, "Ethics and the Social Marketer," 4.

18. Abigail C. Saguy and Kevin W. Riley, "Weighing Both Sides: Morality, Mortality, and Framing Contests over Obesity," *Journal of Health Politics, Policy and Law* 30, no. 5 (2005): 874; Smith, "Ethics and the Social Marketer," 11.

19. Witte, "The Manipulative Nature," 288, 286.

20. See, for example, American College of Epidemiology, "Ethics Guidelines," January 2000, available at www.acepidemiology.org/policystmts/EthicsGuide.htm, 1–25; Public Health Leadership Society, "Principles of the Ethical Practice of Public Health" (2002), available at www.apha.org/NR/rdonlyres/1CED3CEA-

287E-4185-9CBD-BD405FC60856/0/ethicsbrochure.pdf 2002; CIOMS, "International Guidelines for Ethical Review of Epidemiological Studies" (Geneva: CIOMS, 1991), 1–31; and International Epidemiological Association, "Proposed Guidelines for Epidemiologists" (1990), available at www.akh-wien.ac.at/ROeS/ROeS/ROeS%20Nr.%2031%20Ethik%20for%20Epidemiologists.pdf.

21. Sommer, "How Public Health Policy Is Created," S5.

22. Richard Doll, Marcia Angell, Dimitrios Trichopoulos, and Robert Temple, cited in Taubes, "Epidemiology Faces Its Limits," 168; Joel Best, *More Damned Lies and Statistics: How Numbers Confuse Public Issues* (Berkeley: University of California Press, 2004), 80–81.

23. For a list of studies cited as the "Science behind the Campaign," see www.4women.gov/Breastfeeding/bf.cfm?page=ref (accessed January 14, 2005).

24. Szklo, "The Evaluation of Epidemiologic Evidence," S13.

25. Gordis, "Ethical and Professional Issues," 10.

26. David Sackett, cited in Taubes, "Epidemiology Faces Its Limits," 169.

27. Stephen Arenz and Rüdiger von Kries, "Protective Effect of Breastfeeding against Obesity in Childhood: Can a Meta-Analysis of Observational Studies Help to Validate the Hypothesis?" *Advances in Experimental Medicine and Biology* 569 (2005): 42.

28. James W. Anderson, Bryan M. Johnstone, and Daniel T. Remley, "Breast-feeding and Cognitive Development:

A Meta-Analysis," *American Journal of Clinical Nutrition* 70 (1999): 525–35.

29. A. G. Gordon, "Breast-Feeding, Breast-Milk Feeding, and Intelligence Quotient," *American Journal of Clinical Nutrition* 72 (2000): 1063–64; Anjali Jain, John Concato, and John M. Leventhal, "How Good Is the Evidence Linking Breastfeeding and Intelligence?" *Pediatrics* 109, no. 6 (2002): 1044–53.

30. Kerry Dwan et al., "Systematic Review of the Empirical Evidence of Study Publication Bias and Outcome Reporting Bias," *PloS One* 3, no. 8 (2008): e3081; Petr Skrabanek, "The Epidemiology of Errors," *The Lancet* 342, nos. 8886/8887 (1993): 1502; Moyses Szklo, "Issues in Publication and Interpretation in Research Findings," *Journal of Clinical Epidemiology* 4 (1991): 109–13.

31. Marcia Angell, cited in Taubes, "Epidemiology Faces Its Limits," 169.

32. For example, see Jessica Woo et al., "Breastfeeding Helps Explain Racial and Socioeconomic Status Disparities in Adolescent Adiposity," *Pediatrics* 121, no. 3 (2008): e458–e465; Virginia R. Galton Bachrach, Eleanor Schwarz, and Lela Rose Bachrach, "Breastfeeding and the Risk of Hospitalization for Respiratory Disease in Infancy," *Archives of Pediatric and Adolescent Medicine* 157 (2003): 237–43; Alice H. Cushing et al., "Breastfeeding Reduces Risk of Respiratory Illness in Infants," *American Journal of Epidemiology* 147, no. 9 (1998): 863–70; Paula D. Scariati, Laurence M. Grummer-Strawn, and Sara Beck Fein, "A Longitudinal

Analysis of Infant Morbidity and the Extent of Breastfeeding in the United States," *Pediatrics* 99, no. 6 (1997): e5–e9.

33. See, for example, Elizabeth J. Mayer-Davis et al., "Breast-Feeding and Type 2 Diabetes in the Youth of Three Ethnic Groups," *Diabetes Care* 31 (2008): 470–75; Ute M. Schaefer-Graf et al., "Association of Breast-Feeding and Early Childhood Overweight in Children from Mothers with Gestational Diabetes Mellitus," *Diabetes Care* 29, no. 5 (2006): 1105–7; R. F. Slykerman et al., "Breastfeeding and Intelligence of Preschool Children," *Acta Paediatrica* 94 (2005): 832–37; Xiao Ou Shu et al., "Breastfeeding and Risk of Childhood Acute Leukemia," *Journal of the National Cancer Institute* 91, no. 20 (1999): 1770.

34. See Aimen Chen and Walter J. Rogan, "Breastfeeding and the Risk of Postneonatal Death in the United States," *Pediatrics* 113, no. 5 (2004): e438; Anushua Sinha et al., "Reduced Risk of Neonatal Respiratory Infections among Breastfed Girls but Not Boys," *Pediatrics* 112, no. 4 (2003): e307; Linda C. Duffy et al., "Exclusive Breastfeeding Protects against Bacterial Colonization and Day Care Exposure to Otitis Media," *Pediatrics* 100, no. 4 (1997): e7.

35. For example, see Christina M. Gibson-Davis and Jeanne Brooks-Gunn, "Breastfeeding and Verbal Ability of 3-Year-Olds in a Multicity Sample," *Pediatrics* 118, no. 5 (2006): e1444–51; Laurence M. Grummer-Strawn and Zuguo Mei, "Does Breastfeeding Protect against Pediatric

Overweight? Analysis of Longitudinal Data from the Centers for Disease Control and Prevention Pediatric Nutrition Surveillance System," *Pediatrics* 113, no. 2 (2004): e85; K. E. Bergmann et al., "Early Determinants of Childhood Overweight and Adiposity in a Birth Cohort Study: Role of Breast-Feeding," *International Journal of Obesity* 27 (2003): 169–70; Matthew W. Gillman, "Breast-Feeding and Obesity," *Journal of Pediatrics* 141, no. 6 (2002): 749–50; Erik Lykke Mortensen et al., "The Association between Duration of Breastfeeding and Adult Intelligence," *Journal of the American Medical Association* 287, no. 18 (2002): 2371.

36. Atul Singhal et al., "Breastmilk Feeding and Lipoprotein Profile in Adolescents Born Preterm: Follow-up of a Prospective Randomized Study," *The Lancet* 363 (2004): 1571–78.

37. Elise M. Taveras et al., "Association of Breastfeeding with Maternal Control of Infant Feeding at Age 1 Year," *Pediatrics* 114, no. 5 (2004): 577–83.

38. The names of the first-tier reviewers are confidential, but according to Haynes, members included "a top breastfeeding researcher from the CDC," "a well-known OB-GYN researcher suggested by ACOG (American College of Obstetricians and Gynecologists)," "a well-known pediatrician researcher active in the AAP," "a well-known pediatric educator," "a respected breastfeeding researcher unrelated to any organization," and "a representative from the OWH." They were selected based on their scientific publications in

the area and their membership in the USBC, with "scientific expertise" being the primary criterion. Second-tier reviewers were Duane Alexander, director of the National Institute of Child Health and Human Development; Allen Spiegel, director of the National Institute of Diabetes and Digestive and Kidney Disease; and William Dietz, director of the CDC's Division of Nutrition and Physical Activity. According to Haynes, the second tier served largely as a final check for the first (phone interview, February 2, 2005). On the USBC mission, see www.usbreastfeeding.org/ (accessed July 15, 2008).

39. Beauchamp et al., "Ethical Guidelines for Epidemiologists," 165S.

40. American College of Epidemiology, "Ethics Guidelines," 19.

41. Public Health Leadership Society, "Principles of the Ethical Practice of Public Health," 2002.

42. Steven M. Blair and Michael J. Lamonte, "Commentary: Current Perspectives on Obesity and Health: Black and White, or Shades of Gray," *International Journal of Epidemiology* 35 (2006): 69–72; Paul Campos et al., "The Epidemiology of Overweight and Obesity: Public Health Crisis or Moral Panic?" *International Journal of Epidemiology* 35 (2006): 55–60; J. Eric Oliver, *Fat Politics: The Real Story behind America's Obesity Epidemic* (Oxford: Oxford University Press, 2006); Saguy and Riley, "Weighing Both Sides."

43. According to the 2002 National Immunization Survey, 68 percent of babies were breast fed to any extent at one week; at three, six, and twelve months, the number dropped to 51, 35, and 16 percent, respectively. Sixty-three percent of babies were exclusively breastfed at one week; at one, three, and six months, the number fell to 57, 42, and 13 percent, respectively. Among African Americans, 49 percent were breastfed to any extent at one week; at three, six, and twelve months, the number dropped to 35, 20, and 8 percent, respectively. Forty-six percent of African American babies were exclusively breastfed at one week; at one, three, and six months, the number fell to 39, 29, and 5 percent, respectively. Percentages are rounded to the closest whole number. See Ruowei Li et al., "Breastfeeding Rates in the United States by Characteristics of the Child, Mother, or Family: The 2002 National Immunization Survey," *Pediatrics* 115, no. 1 (2005): e33–34.

44. See Yeutter's letter at www.abcnews. go.com/sections/2020/ investigations/2020-breastfeed-ing-ads-040604.html (accessed June 8, 2004).

45. This account is taken from McKinney+Silver's presentation to the Breastfeeding Task Force of Greater Los Angeles, one of eighteen community-based demonstration projects slated to work in coordination with the OWH and the Ad Council to promote breastfeeding at the local level. See www.breastfeedingtaskforla.org/OW-HGrant/NBAC%20short%20 version.pdf (accessed January 12, 2004).

46. David R. Buchanan and Lawrence Wallack, "This Is the Partnership for a Drug-Free America: Any Questions?" *Journal of Drug Issues* 28, no. 2 (1998): 329–57.

47. Kathleen Woodward, "Statistical Panic," *differences* 11, no. 2 (1999): 185, 187.

48. Whether and under what circumstances fear appeals actually work remains in dispute. See Gerard Hastings, Martine Stead, and John Webb, "Fear Appeals in Social Marketing: Strategic and Ethical Reasons for Concern," *Psychology and Marketing* 21, no. 11 (2004): 961–86; G. Hastings and L. MacFayden, "The Limitations of Fear Messages," *Tobacco Control* 11 (2002): 73–75; Kim Witte and Mike Allen, "A Meta-Analysis of Fear Appeals: Implications for Effective Public Health Campaigns," *Health Education & Behavior* 27, no. 5 (2000): 591–615; Punam Anand Keller, "Converting the Unconverted: The Effect of Inclination and Opportunity to Discount Health-Related Fear Appeals," *Journal of Applied Psychology* 84, no. 3 (1999): 403–15; and Marshall H. Becker, "A Medical Sociologist Looks at Health Promotion," *Journal of Health and Social Behavior* 34 (1993): 106.

49. Jeffrey J. Maciejewski, "Is the Use of Sexual and Fear Appeals Ethical? A Moral Evaluation by Generation Y College Students," *Journal of Current Issues and Research in Advertising* 26, no. 2 (2004): 97–105; Robin L. Snipes et al., "A Model of the Effects of Self-Efficacy on the Perceived Ethicality and Performance of Fear Appeals in Advertising," *Journal of Business Ethics* 19 (1999): 273–85; Suzeanne Benet, Robert E.

Pitts, and Michael LaTour, "The Appropriateness of Fear Appeal Use for Health Care Marketing to the Elderly: Is It Okay to Scare Granny?" *Journal of Business Ethics* 12 (1993): 45–55; Charles R. Duke et al., "A Method for Evaluating the Ethics of Fear Appeals," *Journal of Public Policy and Marketing* 12, no. 1 (1993): 120–29; Witte and Allen, "A Meta-Analysis of Fear Appeals."

50. Nurit Guttman and Charles T. Salmon, "Guilt, Fear, Stigma and Knowledge Gaps: Ethical Issues in Public Health Communication Interventions," *Bioethics* 18, no. 6 (2004): 531–52; Hastings, Stead, and Webb, "Fear Appeals in Social Marketing"; Michael R. Hyman and Richard Tansey, "The Ethics of Psychoactive Ads," *Journal of Business Ethics* 9 (1990): 105–14.

51. Lisa M. Schwartz and Steven Woloshin, "The Case for Letting Information Speak for Itself," *Effective Clinical Practice* 4 (2001): 79 (italics added).

52. Beauchamp et al., "Ethical Guidelines for Epidemiologists," 163S.

53. American College of Epidemiology, "Ethics Guidelines," 21–22.

54. See www.adcouncil.org/about/news_061902 (accessed January 12, 2004).

55. See, for example, Melissa A. Herbst et al., "Relationship of Prenatal Care and Perinatal Morbidity in Low-Birth-Weight Infants," *American Journal of Obstetrics and Gynecology* 189, no. 4 (2003): 930–33; Jennifer Malat, Hyn Joo Oh, and Mary Ann Hamilton, "Poverty Experience, Race, and Child Health," *Public Health Reports* 120 (2005): 442–47; Leiyu Shi and Gregory D. Stevens, "Disparities in Access to Care and Satisfaction among U.S. Children: The Roles of Race/Ethnicity and Poverty Status," *Public Health Reports* 120 (2005): 431–41; Nick Spencer, "Social, Economic, and Political Determinants of Child Health," *Pediatrics* 112, no. 3 (2003): 704–6; David Wood, "Effect of Child and Family Poverty on Child Health in the United States," *Pediatrics* 112, no. 3, suppl. (2003): 707–11.

56. Hyman and Tansey, "The Ethics of Psychoactive Ads."

57. For example, see Dana Sullivan and Maureen Connolly, eds., *Unbuttoned: Women Open up about the Pleasures, Pains, and Politics of Breastfeeding* (Boston: Harvard Common Press, 2009); Katie Allison Granju, *Attachment Parenting: Instinctive Care for Your Baby and Young Child* (New York: Simon & Schuster, 1999); Barbara L. Behrmann, *The Breastfeeding Café: Mothers Share the Joys, Challenges, & Secrets of Nursing* (Ann Arbor: University of Michigan Press, 2005).

58. Sullivan and Connolly, *Unbuttoned*, 111–32, 159–69.

59. Susan Maushart, *The Mask of Motherhood* (New York: Penguin, 1999, 150, 161.

60. Linda Blum, *At the Breast: Ideologies of Breastfeeding and Motherhood in the Contemporary United States* (Boston: Beacon Press, 1999), 178; Pam Carter, *Feminism, Breasts, and Breast-Feeding* (New York: St. Martin's Press, 1995), 106–49.

61. Public Health Leadership Society, "Principles of the Ethical Practice of Public Health."

62. Blum, *At the Breast*, 4. Glenda Wall argues that a similar displacement of mothers occurs in Canadian breastfeeding discourse, in which health benefits for mothers are hardly mentioned. Rather, each mother is cast as the "ecosystem within which the child's optimal food source is produced." See Glenda Wall, "Moral Constructions of Motherhood in Breastfeeding Discourse," *Gender & Society* 15, no. 4 (2001): 601–3.

63. Public health efforts to deter pregnant women from smoking are marked by a similar lack of attention to women's bodies. See Laury Oaks, *Smoking and Pregnancy: The Politics of Fetal Protection* (New Brunswick, NJ: Rutgers University Press, 2001), 80, 103, 200–201.

64. Jules Law, "The Politics of Breastfeeding: Assessing Risk, Dividing Labor," *Signs: Journal of Women in Culture and Society* 25, no. 2 (2000): 421.

65. See Bernice L. Hausman, *Mother's Milk: Breastfeeding Controversies in American Culture* (New York: Routledge, 2003).

66. Petra Büskens, "The Impossibility of 'Natural Parenting' for Modern Mothers: On Social Structure and Formation of Habit," *Journal of the Association for Research on Mothering* 3, no. 1 (2001): 84.

67. Law, "The Politics of Breastfeeding," 423.

68. See www.adcouncil.org/research/wga/breastfeeding_awareness/?issue3Menu (accessed January 12, 2004, and February 7, 2005).

69. Rebecca Kukla, "Ethics and Ideology in Breastfeeding Advocacy Campaigns," *Hypatia* 21, no. 1 (2006): 161–62.

70. In August 2005, to draw attention to National Breastfeeding Awareness Month, Carmona gave interviews to twelve radio stations around the country. The texts were published at www.4woman.gov/breastfeeding/index.cfm?page=Interviews (accessed May 5, 2006).

71. Kukla, "Ethics and Ideology," 175.

72. Ibid., 161, 173 (italics in original).

73. Lucinda Fisher, "Teeth Cut from Breastfeeding Campaign," December 12, 2003, available at www.womensnews.org/article.cfm/dyn/aid/1651/context/archive (accessed April 14, 2004).

74. Brian Ross, "Milk Money," 20/20, ABC News, June 4, 2004.

75. U.S. Department of Health and Human Services, Centers for Disease Control and Prevention, National Center for Chronic Disease Prevention and Health Promotion, Office on Smoking and Health, *The Health Consequences of Smoking: A Report of the Surgeon General* (Washington, DC: U.S. Department of Health and Human Services, 2004). See also CDC, "Health Effects of Cigarette Smoking," available at www.cdc.gov/tobacco/data_statistics/fact_sheets/health_effects/effects_cig_smoking/ (accessed August 12, 2008). On the systematic construction of the scientific case against smoking, see Alan M. Brandt, *The Cigarette Century: The Rise, Fall, and Deadly Persistence of the Product That Defined America* (New York: Basic Books, 2007).

76. Lead has been proven toxic, and one study found longer breastfeeding to be associated with higher lead concentrations in infants "in 3 countries, in 3 different decades, in settings differing in breastfeeding patterns, environmental lead sources, and infant lead levels." See Betsy Lozoff et al., "Higher Infant Blood Levels with Longer Duration of Breastfeeding," *Journal of Pediatrics*, electronic publication (2009): 1–5. The National Children's Study, sponsored by the National Institutes of Health, the CDC, and the Environmental Protection Agency, and slated to begin collecting data in 2010, will provide some longitudinal data. It will track more than 100,000 children across the United States from birth until age twenty-one to examine the effects of environmental influences on health and development. The study defines "environmental" broadly, but it will include "natural and man-made environmental factors" and "biologic and chemical factors." See www.nationalchildrensstudy.gov/about/overview/Pages/default.aspx (accessed December 21, 2008).

77. Philip J. Landrigan et al., "Chemical Contaminants in Breast Milk and Their Impacts on Children's Health: An Overview," *Environmental Health Perspectives* 110, no. 6 (2002): A313–15. See also M. Nathaniel Mead, "Contaminants in Human Milk: Weighing the Risks against the Benefits of Breastfeeding," *Environmental Health Perspectives* 116, no. 10 (2008): A427–34; Marian Condan, "Breast Is Best, but It Could Be Better: What Is in Breast Milk That Should Not Be?" *Pediatric Nursing* 31, no. 4 (2005):

333–38; Larry L. Needham and Richard Y. Wang, "Analytic Considerations for Measuring Environmental Chemicals in Breast Milk," *Environmental Health Perspectives* 110, no. 6 (2002): A317–24; and Gina M. Solomon and Pilar M. Weiss, "Chemical Contaminants in Breast Milk: Time Trends and Regional Variability," *Environmental Health Perspectives* 110, no. 6 (2002): A339–47.

78. Walter J. Rogan, "Pollutants in Breast Milk," *Archives of Pediatric and Adolescent Medicine* 150 (1996): 981.

79. Kathryn Harrison, "Too Close to Home: Dioxin Contamination of Breast Milk and the Political Agenda," *Policy Sciences* 34, no. 1 (2001): 35–62; Maia Boswell-Penc, *Tainted Milk: Breastmilk, Feminisms, and the Politics of Environmental Degradation* (Albany: State University of New York Press, 2006). See also Maryse Arendt, "Communicating Human Biomonitoring Results to Ensure Policy Coherence with Public Health Recommendations: Analyzing Breastmilk Whilst Protecting, Promoting and Supporting Breastfeeding," *Environmental Health* 7, suppl. I (2008): 1–6.

80. Roni Caryn Rabin, "Despite Worries over Toxins, Breast-Feeding Still Best for Infants," *New York Times*, December 20, 2008.

81. See, for example, La Leche League, media release, "Go Green, Breastfeed!" April 2008, available at www.llli.org/Release/GoGreen (accessed December 31, 2008).

82. Scott D. Grosse and Julianne S. Collins, "Folic Acid Supplementation and Neural Tube

Defect Prevention," *Birth Defects Research Part A: Clinical and Molecular Teratology* 79, no. 11 (2007): 737–42; CDC, "Neural Tube Defect Surveillance and Folic Acid Intervention–Texas-Mexico Border, 1993–98," *Morbidity and Mortality Weekly Report* 49, no. 1 (2000): 1–4; James L. Mills and Caroline Signore, "Neural Tube Defect Rates before and after Food Fortification with Folic Acid," *Birth Defects Research Part A: Clinical and Molecular Teratology* 70, no. 11 (2004): 844–45.

83. See Joel B. Mason et al., "A Temporal Association between Folic Acid Fortification and an Increase in Colorectal Cancer Rates May Be Illuminating Important Biological Principles: A Hypothesis," *Cancer Epidemiology Biomarkers & Prevention* 16, no. 7 (2007): 1325–29; J. B. Mason et al., "Folic Acid Fortification and Cancer Risk," *The Lancet* 371 (2008): 1335; and R. Bayston et al., "Authors' Reply," *The Lancet* 371 (2008): 1335–36.

84. Fear appeals have also been employed to persuade women to take folic acid. In a March of Dimes advertisement, a diaper-clad baby crawls next to a manhole in the middle of traffic. "If you think this baby is in danger, it's nothing compared to what can happen as early as the third week of pregnancy, when birth defects of the brain and spinal cord can occur. If you're a woman of childbearing age, take a multivitamin with folic acid every day as part of a healthy diet. Start now, pregnant or not, and help save a baby." See Schwartz and Woloshin, "The Case for Letting Information Speak for Itself," 77.

85. See, for example, Malat, Oh, and Hamilton, "Poverty Experience, Race, and Child Health"; Alan W. Leschied et al., "The Relationship between Maternal Depression and Child Outcomes in a Child Welfare Sample: Implications for Treatment and Policy," *Child and Family Social Work* 10, no. 4 (2005): 281–91; Shi and Stevens, "Disparities in Access to Care and Satisfaction"; Spencer, "Social, Economic, and Political Determinants of Child Health"; Wood, "Effect of Child and Family Poverty"; Steven M. Peterson and Alison Burke Albers, "Effects of Poverty and Maternal Depression on Early Child Development," *Child Development* 72, no. 6 (2001): 1794–1813; Carla Martins and E. A. Gaffan, "Effects of Early Maternal Depression on Patterns of Infant-Mother Attachment: A Meta-Analytic Investigation," *Child Psychology and Psychiatry* 41 (2000): 737–46; Cheryl Tatano Beck, "Maternal Depression and Child Behavior Problems: A Meta-Analysis," *Journal of Advanced Nursing* 29, no. 3 (1999): 623–29; Greg J. Duncan and Jeanne Brooks-Gunn, eds., *Consequences of Growing up Poor* (New York: Russell Sage Foundation, 1997); and National Institute of Child Health and Human Development Early Child Care Research Network: "Affect Dysregulation in the Mother-Child Relationship in the Toddler Years: Antecedents and Consequences," *Development and Psychopathology* 16 (2004): 43–68; "Chronicity of Maternal Depressive Symptoms, Maternal Sensitivity, and Child Functioning at 36 Months,"

Developmental Psychology 35, no. 5 (1999): 1297–1310; and "Familial Factors Associated with the Characteristics of Nonmaternal Care for Infants," *Journal of Marriage and the Family* 59 (1997): 389–408.

86. William Ray Arney, *Power and the Profession of Obstetrics* (Chicago: University of Chicago Press, 1982), 96–97.

87. Joel Best, *Damned Lies and Statistics: Untangling Numbers from the Media, Politicians, and Activists* (Berkeley: University of California Press, 2001), 122; Joel Best, *More Damned Lies and Statistics* (Berkeley: University of California Press, 2004), 88.

88. Cass R. Sunstein, *Laws of Fear: Beyond the Precautionary Principle* (Cambridge: Cambridge University Press, 2005), 45–49.

89. Law, "The Politics of Breastfeeding," 415, 423.

90. In fact, there is some evidence that formula feeding can reduce the risk of asthma (see chapter 2). Kramer was responding to an article in the *Times of London* in which both he and I were quoted as suggesting that many of the benefits associated with breastfeeding had not been demonstrated. Our remarks were taken up on Facebook and in numerous blogs, and Kramer claimed that he had been misquoted. See Helen Rumbelow, "Exposing the Myths of Breastfeeding," and "Benefits of Breastfeeding 'Being Oversold by NHS,'" *Times of London*, July 20, 2009; and Susie Mesure, "Press Twisted My Words, Says Academic in Breast-Milk Row," *The Independent*, August 2, 2009.

91. Judy M. Hopkinson, "Response to 'Is Breast Really Best? Risk and Total Motherhood in the National Breastfeeding Awareness Campaign,'" *Journal of Health Politics, Policy and Law* 32, no. 4 (2007): 641.

92. Daniel J. Taylor et al., "Epidemiology of Insomnia, Depression, and Anxiety," *Sleep* 28, no. 11 (2005): 1457–64. Sleepy drivers also are a public-health problem. The National Highway Transportation Safety Administration estimates that "drowsy driving causes more than 100,000 crashes a year, resulting in 40,000 injuries and 1,550 deaths . . . [and] it is widely recognized that drowsy driving is underreported as a cause of crashes." See National Sleep Foundation, *2008 National Sleep in America Poll: Summary of Findings* (Washington, DC: National Sleep Foundation, 2008).

93. Michael S. Kramer et al., "Promotion of Breastfeeding Intervention Trial," *Journal of the American Medical Association* 285 (2001): 417.

94. On how risk statistics are often misinterpreted by journalists and the public, see Best, *Damned Lies and Statistics*, 46, and *More Damned Lies and Statistics*, 79–83.

95. See www.womenshealth. gov/breastfeeding/index. cfm?page=227 (accessed July 25, 2008).

96. Law points out that parents rarely consider such moves in managing risks to their children ("The Politics of Breastfeeding," 423).

97. Lenore Skenazy points out that each year, around two thousand children die while riding in cars but that only about

fifty are kidnapped and killed by strangers. "This means children are 40 times more likely to die in a car trip to the mall than during a walk home from school." See Lenore Skenazy, *Free-Range Kids: Giving Our Children the Freedom We Had without Going Nuts with Worry* (San Francisco: Jossey-Bass, 2009).

98. International Epidemiological Association, "Proposed Guidelines for Epidemiologists" (1990), available at www. akh-wien.ac.at/ROeS/ROeS/ ROeS%20Nr.%2031%20Ethik% 20for%20Epidemiologists.pdf.

99. American College of Epidemiology, "Ethics Guidelines," 10.

100. Malini D. Persad and Janell L. Mensinger, "Maternal Breastfeeding Attitudes: Association with Breastfeeding Intent and Socio-Demographics among Urban Primiparas," *Journal of Community Health* 33 (2007): 57; Susan M. Ludington-Hoe, Patricia E. McDonald, and Rose-marie Satyshur, "Breastfeeding in African-American Women," *Journal of National Black Nurses Association* 13, no. 1 (2002): 60.

101. See www.omhrc. gov/templates/browse. aspx?lvl=2&lvlID=11 (accessed December 17, 2008). See also Ludington-Hoe, McDonald, and Satyshur, "Breastfeeding in African-American Women," 59–61; Roberta Cricco-Lizza, "Black Non-Hispanic Mothers' Perceptions about the Promotion of Infant-Feeding Methods by Nurses and Physicians," *Journal of Obstetric, Gynecologic and Neonatal Nursing* 35 (2006): 173–80; and Roberta Cricco-Lizza, "The Milk of Human Kindness: Environmental and

Human Interactions in a WIC Clinic That Influence Infant-Feeding Decisions of Black Women," *Qualitative Health Research* 15, no. 4 (2005): 525–38.

102. Research has demonstrated a similar absence of cultural competence in other public health efforts. A study of asthma educational materials in Wisconsin found that those directed at Latino families with asthmatic children were translated into Spanish, often with errors, and that the brochure created for Native American families included a photo of an Indian at a tribal dance. Otherwise, the materials were identical to information targeting white families. See Jane M. Brotanek, Kristen Grimes, and Glenn Flores, "Leave No Asthmatic Child Behind: The Cultural Competency of Asthma Educational Materials," *Ethnicity and Disease* 17 (2007): 744–45.

103. Public Health Leadership Society, "Principles of the Ethical Practice of Public Health."

104. Blum, *At the Breast*, 152.

105. Ludington-Hoe, McDonald, and Satyshur, "Breastfeeding in African-American Women," 58.

106. Blum, *At the Breast*, 167. See also Roberta Cricco-Lizza, "Infant-Feeding Beliefs and Experiences of Black Women Enrolled in WIC in the New York Metropolitan Area," *Qualitative Health Research* 14, no. 9 (2004): 1197–1210; and Jennifer Ludden, "Teaching Black Women to Embrace Breast-Feeding," available at www.npr. org/templates/transcript/transcript.php?storyId=121755349 (accessed January 6, 2010).

107. Mary Douglas, *Risk and Blame: Essays in Cultural Theory* (London: Routledge, 1992), 44.

108. Blum, *At the Breast*, 63.

109. See www.4women. gov/breastfeeding/index. cfm?page=236 (accessed May 8, 2006).

110. Benet, Pitts, and LaTour, "The Appropriateness of Fear Appeal Use"; Duke et al., "A Method for Evaluating the Ethics of Fear Appeals"; Maciejewski, "Is the Use of Sexual and Fear Appeals Ethical?"; Snipes et al., "A Model of the Effects"; Witte and Allen, "A Meta-Analysis of Fear Appeals."

111. Kukla, "Ethics and Ideology," 173.

112. While middle-class women no doubt choose breastfeeding for many reasons, not the least of which is its ostensible risk-reducing qualities, it is also true that guilt associated with working and spending time away from their babies can be at least partially alleviated by buying a breast pump and sustaining the one practice that only they can provide. In this way, breastfeeding makes adherence to the total motherhood ethic more attainable to middle-class working mothers.

113. Rebecca Traister, "Baby, We Were Born to Breast-Feed?" available at www.salon.com/ mwt/broadsheet/2005/12/19/ breastfed/index.html (accessed April 3, 2006), italics added.

114. See www.fns.usda.gov/ wic/Breastfeeding/breastfeedingmainpage.HTM (accessed December 17, 2008). For an example of how the differential allocation of food to breastfeeding and bottle-feeding mothers is implemented within states, see

the Alleghany County Health Department, which encompasses Pittsburgh, at www.achd. net/wic/ (accessed December 17, 2008).

115. Kukla, "Ethics and Ideology," 162.

116. Carter, *Feminism, Breasts, and Breast-Feeding*, 237.

117. Ross, "Milk Money."

118. Chen and Rogan, "Breastfeeding and the Risk of Postneonatal Death," 438, 435.

119. Ross, "Milk Money."

120. Roni Caryn Rabin, "Breast-Feed or Else," *New York Times*, June 13, 2006; "Letters," *New York Times*, June 20, 2006. Near the end of Rabin's lengthy article, the director of medical affairs for the Cato Institute was quoted questioning whether a causal relationship between breastfeeding and better health had been established.

121. Haynes on MSNBC, June 14, 2006, available at www. msnbc.com/id/2113450/ vp/13315821#13315821 (accessed December 9, 2008).

122. See www.salon.com/ mwt/broadsheet/2006/06/14/ breastfeeding_debate/index. html (accessed June 16, 2006).

123. "About Breast-Feeding," *New York Times*, July 2, 2006.

124. Marc Kaufman and Christopher Lee, "HHS Toned Down Breast-Feeding Ads," *Washington Post*, August 31, 2007.

125. Stanley Ip et al., *Breastfeeding and Maternal and Infant Health Outcomes in Developed Countries*, Evidence Report/Technology Assessment no. 153, prepared by Tufts–New England Medical Center, Evidence-Based Practice Center, under contract no. 290-02-0022, AHRQ publication no.

07-E007 (Rockville, MD: Agency for Healthcare Research and Quality, April 2007), 6.

126. abcnews.com, September 1, 2007 (accessed September 3, 2007).

127. *Los Angeles Times*, September 30, 2007 (accessed October 2, 2007).

128. *Boston Globe*, September 10, 2007 (accessed September 10, 2007).

129. *Ms.*, September 5, 2007 (accessed September 11, 2007).

130. Rebecca Goldin, director of research at STATS, a nonprofit research organization associated with George Mason University, writes that the formula industry's opposition "doesn't make the government corrupt for pulling the [insulin] ad—it misrepresented the science, and would have prompted a pointless guilt trip among an untold number of women who can't or don't want to nurse." See www.stats.org/stories/2007/diabetes_and_nursing_oct22_07.htm (accessed October 26, 2007).

131. "National Breastfeeding Awareness Campaign Results," available at www.womenshealth. gov/breastfeeding/campaign_ results.pdf (accessed July 23, 2008).

132. Margaret M. McDowell, Chia-Yih Wang, and Jocelyn Kennedy-Stephenson, "Breastfeeding in the United States: Findings from the National Health and Nutrition Examination Surveys, 1999–2006," NCHS data briefs no. 5 (Hyattsville, MD: National Center for Health Statistics, 2008).

133. See www.cdc.gov/nccd-php/dnpa/obesity/childhood/ index.htm (accessed December 29, 2008).

134. Michael Baker and Kevin S. Milligan, "Maternal Employment, Breastfeeding, and Health: Evidence from Maternity Leave Mandates," *Journal of Health Economics* 27, no. 4 (2008): 871–87. In their call for the Canadian government to extend maternity leave policies, Jody Heyman and Michael Kramer, the latter of whom was the primary author of the PROBIT study, do not cite this study. See Jody Heyman and Michael S. Kramer, "Public Policy and Breastfeeding: A Straightforward and Significant Solution," *Canadian Journal of Public Health* 100 (2009), 381–83.

135. Sunstein, *Laws of Fear*, 98–101.

136. Sheldon Ungar and Dennis Bray, "Silencing Science: Partisanship and the Career of a Publication Disputing the Dangers of Secondhand Smoke," *Public Understanding of Science* 14, no. 1 (2005): 8, 9.

137. AAP, "The Changing Concept of Sudden Infant Death Syndrome: Diagnostic Coding Shifts, Controversies regarding the Sleep Environment, and New Variables to Consider in Reducing Risk," *Pediatrics* 116, no. 5 (2005): 1252.

138. USBC press release, "Mixed Credibility of the Revised AAP SIDS Prevention Recommendations,"

October 17, 2005, available at www.usbreastfeeding.org/News-and-Events/USBC-SIDS-PR-10-17-2005.pdf (accessed December 22, 2008).

139. Claudia Kalb, "Big Binky Brouhaha," *Newsweek*, October 31, 2005.

140. Bradford D. Gessner et al., "Bed Sharing with Unimpaired Parents Is Not an Important Risk for Sudden Infant Death Syndrome," *Pediatrics* 117, no. 3 (2006): 992.

141. Nikolas Rose, "The Politics of Life Itself," *Theory, Culture & Society* 18, no. 6 (2001): 17.

142. George M. Gray and David P. Ropeik, "Dealing with the Dangers of Fear: The Role of Risk Communication," *Health Affairs* 21, no. 6 (2002): 112.

143. Ibid.

144. Steven Woloshin, Lisa M. Schwartz, and H. Gilbert Welch, "The Risk of Death by Age, Sex, and Smoking Status in the United States: Putting Health Risks in Context," *Journal of the National Cancer Institute* 100, no. 12 (2008): 846.

145. Phillip Cole, "The Moral Bases for Public Health Interventions," *Epidemiology* 6, no. 1 (1995): 81.

146. Hastings and MacFadyen, "The Limitations of Fear Messages," 74.

147. Elizabeth Murphy, "Risk, Maternal Ideologies, and

Infant Feeding," in *A Sociology of Food and Nutrition*, ed. John Germov and Lauren Williams (Oxford: Oxford University Press, 2004), 208.

148. Walker to Thompson, November 21, 2003, posted at www.mothering.com/action-alerts/walker-letter.shtml (accessed March 8, 2004), italics added. Copious evidence, on the Internet and in various media, demonstrates that many mothers feel tremendous guilt for not breastfeeding. See, for example, "Letters," *New York Times*, June 20, 2006. On white working-class women, see Blum, *At the Breast*, 114–23.

149. Laura Stanley, "The Breastfeeding Police," *Parenting*, n.d., available at www.parenting.com/article/Baby/Feeding/The-Breastfeeding-Police (accessed March 29, 2007).

150. Laura Cook-Crotty, "My Turn: In Defense of Formula-Fed Babies," *Newsweek*, June 14, 2007, available at www.newsweek.com/id/33605 (accessed June 17, 2007), and Comments, available at www.health.talk.newsweek.com/default.asp?item=625386 (accessed June 17, 2007).

151. Charles E. Rosenberg, "Banishing Risk: Or the More Things Change, the More They Remain the Same," *Perspectives in Biology and Medicine* 39, no. 1 (1995): 36.

Chapter 6

1. For an analysis of how antismoking activists waged a battle against secondhand tobacco smoke despite the absence of compelling evidence that it posed health risks, see Ronald Bayer and James

Colgrove, "Science, Politics, and Ideology in the Campaign against Environmental Tobacco Smoke," *American Journal of Public Health* 92, no. 6 (2002): 949–54. For a discussion of how public health campaigns

create social divisions and moral stigma, see also James A. Morone, "Enemies of the People: The Moral Dimension to Public Health," *Journal of Health Politics, Policy and Law* 22, no. 4 (1997): 993–1020.

2. Stephen T. Ziliak and Deirdre N. McCloskey, *The Cult of Statistical Significance: How the Standard Error Costs Us Jobs, Justice, and Lives* (Ann Arbor: University of Michigan Press, 2008), 4, 9, 6. The authors acknowledge but bracket the problem of causality and instead focus on effect size and its practical implications (xvii, 5).

3. Ziliak and McCloskey, *The Cult of Statistical Significance*, xv–xvi.

4. Kramer and Young, quoted in Andreas von Bubnoff, "Numbers Can Lie," *Los Angeles Times*, September 17, 2007.

5. See, for example, Paul Campos et al., "The Epidemiology of Overweight and Obesity: Public Health Crisis or Moral Panic?" *International Journal of Epidemiology* 35 (2006): 55–60; and Gina Kolata, *Rethinking Thin: The New Science of Weight Loss—and the Myths and Realities of Dieting* (New York: Farrar, Strauss & Giroux, 2007).

6. J. Eric Oliver, *Fat Politics: The Real Story behind America's Obesity Epidemic* (Oxford: Oxford University Press, 2006), 23.

7. Oliver, *Fat Politics*, 8–9, 25–26, 2, italics in original.

8. Oliver, *Fat Politics*, 165.

9. Ibid., 12. On the construction of the "obesity epidemic," see also Julie Guthman and Melanie DuPuis, "Embodying Neoliberalism: Economy, Culture, and the Politics of Fat," *Environment and Planning D: Society and Space* 24 (2006): 427–48. Scholars, too, can engage in this kind of hyperbole. The lead author of a recent study projecting that every American would be obese by 2048 said the dubious prediction was intended "to send a message" to citizens and public health officials and that this political goal was not in conflict with basic standards of scientific inquiry, which preclude misleading statistical extrapolation. Not unlike the NBAC's claim that formula feeding is dangerous, this study's rhetorical excesses suggest that distortion is morally justifiable when the science is presumed to be irrefutable. See Youfa Wang et al., "Will All Americans Become Overweight or Obese? Estimating the Progression and Cost of the US Obesity Epidemic," *Obesity* 16, no. 10 (2008): 2323–30; and Carl Bialik, "Obesity Study Looks Thin: Results Warn That Everyone in the U.S. Will Be Overweight by the Year 2048," *Wall Street Journal*, August 15, 2008.

10. See Jacqueline H. Wolf, "Low Breastfeeding Rates and Public Health in the United States," *American Journal of Public Health* 93, no. 12 (2003): 2000–2010. Wolf argues that "today's medical community recognizes what their predecessors knew a century ago—that the American propensity to shun human milk is a public health problem and should be exposed as such" (2006). She characterizes the U.S. Department of Health and Human Services' *Blueprint for Action on Breastfeeding*, published in 2000, as "reminiscent of the early-20th-century public health campaigns' insistence that having been breastfed was the single-most powerful predictor of an infant's ability to survive childhood" (2006).

11. See the remarks of Suzanne Haynes, HHS Office of Women's Health senior science adviser, in an Ad Council press release at the beginning of the NBAC, available at www.adcouncil.org/about/news_061902 (accessed January 12, 2004).

12. Matthew W. Gillman et al., "Breastfeeding and Overweight in Adolescence," *Epidemiology* 17, no. 1 (2006): 112.

13. Jerome Kagan argues that the belief in infant determinism, or the notion that experiences in the first few years of life have a lasting impact on adult mental health, is similarly entrenched yet lacking in empirical support. Psychologists tend to interpret the research finding little significance for the early years as anomalous, not as a challenge to the fundamental principle of infant determinism, despite a large body of evidence indicating that the first two years of life do not, in themselves, have much predictive power. See Jerome Kagan, *Three Seductive Ideas* (Cambridge, MA: Harvard University Press, 1998), 105–12.

14. This account is drawn from www.cdc.gov/ulcer/history.htm (accessed April 4, 2009).

15. Kolata, *Rethinking Thin*, passim.

16. Cass R. Sunstein, *Laws of Fear: Beyond the Precautionary Principle* (Cambridge: Cambridge University Press, 2005), 13.

17. Daniel Engber, "The Paranoid Style in American Science," April 15–17, 2008, available at www.slate.com/id/2189178/pagenum/all/ (accessed April 17, 2008).

18. Brian Berry, *Why Social Justice Matters* (Cambridge:

Polity Press, 2005), 129. Indeed, Americans promote personal responsibility even when it costs them money. Under the terms of the 1996 Personal Responsibility and Work Opportunity Reconciliation Act, for example, mothers must have a job, participate in job training, or be actively searching for a job in order to receive benefits. In fact, it costs more for American taxpayers to provide these mothers with child care subsidies than it would to send them welfare checks so they could stay home with their children. See Sharon Hays, *Flat Broke with Children: Women in the Age of Welfare Reform* (New York: Oxford University Press, 2003), 71–72.

19. Susan Yadlon notes that the actual effects of putatively healthy behavior can be less important than the sense of agency they give to women concerned about breast cancer. See Susan Yadlon, "Skinny Women and Good Mothers: The Rhetoric of Risk, Control, and Culpability in the Production of Knowledge about Breast Cancer," *Feminist Studies* 23, no. 3 (1997): 664.

20. Ziliak and McCloskey, *The Cult of Statistical Significance*, 13.

21. Gina Kolata, "Grant System Leads Cancer Researchers to Play It Safe," *New York Times*, June 28, 2009.

22. Judy M. Hopkinson, "Response to 'Is Breast Really Best? Risk and Total Motherhood in the National Breastfeeding Awareness Campaign,'" *Journal*

of Health Politics, Policy and Law 32, no. 4 (2007): 638.

23. Institute of Medicine (IOM) and National Research Council, *Local Government Actions to Prevent Childhood Obesity* (Washington, DC: National Academies Press, 2009), 8, 61. An Associated Press article described the recommendation as "encourage breastfeeding, which prevents obesity later in childhood." See Lauran Neergaard, "Report: Tips on Creating Fat-Fighting Communities," Associated Press, September 1, 2009.

24. Michael S. Kramer, "Randomized Trials and Public Health Interventions: Time to End the Scientific Double Standard," *Clinical Perinatology* 30 (2003): 358–59.

25. Oliver, *Fat Politics*, 2.

26. Kagan again makes a similar argument about the first two years of a baby's life. "It is a bit dishonest," he writes, "to suggest to poor parents that playing with and talking to their infant will protect the child from future academic failure and guarantee life success." All sorts of social influences, including schools, peers, and especially class status, are at least as important, and it is considerably more expensive for the government to address social problems in these areas than it is to advise mothers, in particular, to talk to and interact consistently with their babies. "Although a change in maternal behavior in this direction will have benevolent effects, those effects will be slim compared with the effect of changing

current social policies." See Kagan, *Three Seductive Ideas*, 91.

27. Bernice L. Hausman, "Motherhood and Inequality: A Commentary on Hanna Rosin's 'The Case against Breastfeeding,'" *Journal of Human Lactation* 25, no. 3 (2009): 266, 267.

28. On "ideal workers," see Joan Williams, *Unbending Gender: Why Family and Work Conflict and What to Do about It* (Oxford: Oxford University Press, 2000).

29. Linda Blum, *At the Breast: Ideologies of Breastfeeding and Motherhood in the Contemporary United States* (Boston: Beacon Press, 1999); and Pam Carter, *Feminism, Breasts, and Breast-Feeding* (New York: St. Martin's Press, 1995).

30. Margaret M. McDowell, Chia-Yih Wang, and Jocelyn Kennedy-Stephenson. "Breastfeeding in the United States: Findings from the National Health and Nutrition Examination Surveys, 1999–2006," NCHS data briefs no. 5 (Hyattsville, MD: National Center for Health Statistics, 2008); Laurence M. Grummer-Strawn et al., "Infant Feeding and Feeding Transitions during the First Year of Life," *Pediatrics* 122 (2008): S36–S42.

31. For a discussion of how restructuring market work and benefits would advantage families, see Joan Williams, *Unbending Gender*, esp. 72–100.

32. See www.nlm.nih.gov/medlineplus/news/fullstory_88117.html (accessed September 2, 2009).

Bibliography

Adam, Barbara, Ulrich Beck, and Joost Van Loon, eds. *The Risk Society and Beyond: Critical Issues for Social Theory*. London: Sage, 2000.

Adami, Hans-Olov, and Dimitrios Trichopoulos. "Epidemiology, Medicine and Public Health." *International Journal of Epidemiology* 28 (1999): S1005–8.

Ahluwalia, Indu B., Brian Morrow, Jason Hsia, and Laurence M. Grummer-Strawn. "Who Is Breast-Feeding? Recent Trends from the Pregnancy Risk Assessment and Monitoring System." *Journal of Pediatrics* 142 (2003): 486–93.

Ainsworth, Mary D. Salter, Mary C. Blehar, Everett Waters, and Sally Wall. *Patterns of Attachment: A Psychological Study of the Strange Situation*. Hillsdale, NJ: Erlbaum, 1978.

Alcalay, Rina. "The Impact of Mass Communication Campaigns in the Health Field." *Social Science & Medicine* 17, no. 2 (1983): 87–94.

Alper, Brian S., Jason A. Hand, Susan G. Elliott, Scott Kinkade, Michael J. Hauan, Daniel K. Onion, and Bernard M. Sklar. "How Much Effort Is Needed to Keep up with the Literature Relevant for Primary Care?" *Journal of the American Medical Association* 92, no. 4 (2004): 429–37.

Al-Qaoud, N., and P. Prakash. "Can Breastfeeding and Its Duration Determine the Overweight Status of Kuwaiti Children at the Age of 3–6 Years?" *European Journal of Clinical Medicine* 63 (2009): 1041–43.

Altheide, David L. *Creating Fear: News and the Construction of Crisis*. New York: Aldine de Gruyter, 2002.

American Academy of Family Physicians. "AAFP Policy Statement on Breastfeeding" (2001). Available at www.aafp.org/x6633.xml.

American Academy of Pediatrics (AAP). "Identifying Infants and Young Children with Developmental Disorders in the Medical Home: An Algorithm for Developmental Surveillance and Screening." *Pediatrics* 118 (2006): 405–20.

———. "Policy Statement Based on Task Force Report: The Promotion of Breastfeeding." *Pediatrics* 69, no. 5 (1982): 654–61.

American Academy of Pediatrics (AAP) and American Academy of Family Physicians, Subcommittee on Management of Acute Otitis Media. "Diagnosis and Management of Acute Otitis Media." *Pediatrics* 113, no. 5 (2004): 1451–65.

American Academy of Pediatrics (AAP), Committee on Injury, Violence, and Poison Prevention. "Policy Statement—Role of the Pediatrician in Youth Violence Prevention." *Pediatrics* 124, no. 1 (2009): 393–402.

American Academy of Pediatrics (AAP), Committee on Nutrition. "Prevention of Pediatric Overweight and Obesity." *Pediatrics* 112, no. 2 (2003): 424–30.

American Academy of Pediatrics (AAP), Section on Breastfeeding. "Policy Statement: Breastfeeding and the Use of Human Milk." *Pediatrics* 115, no. 2 (2005): 496–506.

American Academy of Pediatrics (AAP), Task Force on Infant Sleep Position and Sudden Infant Death Syndrome [SIDS]. "The Changing Concept of Sudden Infant Death Syndrome: Diagnostic Coding Shifts, Controversies regarding the Sleeping Environment, and New Variables to Consider in Reducing Risk." *Pediatrics* 116, no. 5 (2005): 1245–55.

———. "Changing Concepts of Sudden Infant Death Syndrome: Implications for Infant Sleeping Environment and Sleep Position." *Pediatrics* 105, no. 3 (2000): 650–56.

———. "Positioning and SIDS." *Pediatrics* 89, no. 6 (1992): 1120–26.

———. "Positioning and Sudden Infant Death Syndrome (SIDS): Update." *Pediatrics* 98, no. 6 (1996): 1216–18.

American Academy of Pediatrics (AAP), Work Group on Breastfeeding. "Policy Statement: Breastfeeding and the Use of Human Milk." *Pediatrics* 100, no. 6 (1997): 1035–39.

American Association of Health Plans and Office on Women's Health, U.S. Department of Health and Human Services. "Advancing Women's Health: Health Plans' Innovative Programs in Breastfeeding Promotion." 2001. Available at http://www.ahip.org/content/default.aspx?bc=38|65|369|412|424, 1–90.

American College of Epidemiology. "Ethics Guidelines." January 2000. Available at www.acepidemiology.org/policystmts/EthicsGuide.htm, 1–25.

American College of Obstetricians and Gynecologists (ACOG). "Breastfeeding: Maternal and Infant Aspects." *International Journal of Gynecology and Obstetrics* 74 (2001): 217–32.

———. *Planning Your Pregnancy and Birth.* 3rd ed. Washington, DC: American College of Obstetricians, 2000.

American Dietetic Association. "Breaking the Barriers to Breastfeeding." *Journal of the American Dietetic Association* 101, no. 10 (2001): 1213–20.

———. "Position of the American Dietetic Association: Promoting and Supporting Breastfeeding." *Journal of the American Dietetic Association* 109, no. 11 (2009): 1926–42.

Anderson, James W., Bryan M. Johnstone, and Daniel T. Remley. "Breast-Feeding and Cognitive Development: A Meta-Analysis." *American Journal of Clinical Nutrition* 70 (1999): 525–35.

Andreasen, Alan R., ed. *Ethics in Social Marketing.* Washington, DC: Georgetown University Press, 2001.

Andregg, David. *Worried All the Time: Rediscovering the Joy in Parenthood in an Age of Anxiety.* New York: Free Press, 2003.

Angell, Marcia, and Jerome P. Kassirer. "Clinical Research—What Should the Public Believe?" *New England Journal of Medicine* 331, no. 3 (1994): 189–90.

Angelsen, N. K., T. Vik, G. Jacobsen, and L. S. Bakketeig. "Breastfeeding and Cognitive Development at Age 1 and 5 Years." *Archives of Disease in Childhood* 85 (2001): 183–88.

Aniansson, G., B. Alm, B. Andersson, A. Håkansson, P. Larsson, O. Nylén, H. Peterson, R. Rignér, M. Svanborg, H. Sabharwal, and C. Svanborg. "A Prospective Cohort Study on Breast-Feeding and Otitis Media in Swedish Infants." *Pediatric Infectious Disease Journal* 13 (1994): 183–88.

Apple, Rima D. "Constructing Mothers: Scientific Motherhood in the Nineteenth and Twentieth Centuries." *Social History of Medicine* 8, no. 2 (1995): 161–78.

———. *Mothers and Medicine: A Social History of Infant Feeding, 1890–1950.* Madison: University of Wisconsin Press, 1987.

———. *Perfect Motherhood: Science and Childrearing in America.* New Brunswick, NJ: Rutgers University Press, 2006.

Apple, Rima D., and Janet Golden, eds. *Mothers and Motherhood: Readings in American History.* Columbus: Ohio State University Press, 1997.

Arditti, Joyce A. "Women, Divorce, and Economic Risk." *Family and Conciliation Courts Review* 35, no. 1 (1997): 79–89.

Arendt, Maryse. "Communicating Human Biomonitoring Results to Ensure Policy Coherence with Public Health Recommendations: Analyzing Breastmilk Whilst Protecting, Promoting and Supporting Breastfeeding." *Environmental Health* 7, suppl. I (2008): 1–6.

Arenz, S., R. Rückerl, B. Koletzko, and R. von Kries. "Breast-Feeding and Childhood Obesity—A Systematic Review." *International Journal of Obesity* 28 (2004): 1247–56.

Arenz, Stephan, and Rüdiger von Kries. "Protective Effect of Breastfeeding against

Obesity in Childhood: Can a Meta-Analysis of Observational Studies Help to Validate the Hypothesis?" *Advances in Experimental Medicine and Biology* 569 (2005): 40–48.

Armstrong, David. "The Invention of Infant Mortality." *Sociology of Health and Illness* 8, no. 3 (1986): 211–32.

———. "The Rise of Surveillance Medicine." *Sociology of Health and Illness* 17, no. 3 (1995): 393–404.

Armstrong, Elizabeth M. *Conceiving Risk, Bearing Responsibility: Fetal Alcohol Syndrome and the Diagnosis of Moral Disorder.* Baltimore: Johns Hopkins University Press, 2003.

Armstrong, Julie, John J. Reilly, and the Child Health Information Team. "Breastfeeding and Lowering the Risk of Childhood Obesity." *The Lancet* 359 (2002): 2003–4.

Arney, William Ray. *Power and the Profession of Obstetrics.* Chicago: University of Chicago Press, 1980.

Atkinson, Mark, and Edwin A. M. Gale. "Infant Diets and Type 1 Diabetes: Too Early, Too Late, or Just Too Complicated?" *Journal of the American Medical Association* 290, no. 13 (2003): 1771–72.

Avishai, Orit. "Managing the Lactating Body: The Breast-Feeding Project and Privileged Motherhood." *Qualitative Sociology* 30 (2007): 135–52.

Bachrach, Virginia R., Per Nafsted, Wendy Odd, Malcolm R. Sears, and D. Robin Taylor. "Long-Term Follow-up

of Asthma." *New England Journal of Medicine* 350, no. 3 (2004): 304.

Bachrach, Virginia R. Galton, Eleanor Schwarz, and Lela Rose Bachrach. "Breastfeeding and the Risk of Hospitalization for Respiratory Disease in Infancy." *Archives of Pediatric and Adolescent Medicine* 157 (2003): 237–43.

Baker, Michael, and Kevin S. Milligan. "Maternal Employment, Breastfeeding, and Health: Evidence from Maternity Leave Mandates." *Journal of Health Economics* 27, no. 4 (2008): 871–87.

Baker, Robin. *Fragile Science: The Reality behind the Headlines.* London: Macmillan, 2001.

Ball, Thomas M., Catharine J. Holberg, Michael B. Aldous, Fernando D. Martinez, and Anne L. Wright. "Influence of Attendance at Day Care on the Common Cold from Birth through 13 Years of Age." *Archives of Pediatric and Adolescent Medicine* 156 (2002): 121–26.

Ball, Thomas M., and Anne L. Wright. "Health Care Costs of Formula-Feeding in the First Year of Life." *Pediatrics* 103, no. 4 (1999): 870–76.

Barone, Joseph, et al. "Breastfeeding during Infancy May Protect against Bed-Wetting during Childhood." *Pediatrics* 118, no. 1 (2006): 254–59.

Barr, Donald A. *Health Disparities in the United States: Social Class, Race, Ethnicity, and Health.* Baltimore: Johns Hopkins University Press, 2008.

Bartels, M., C. E. M. van Beijsterveldt, and D. I. Boomsma. "Breastfeeding, Maternal Education and Cognitive Function: A Prospective Study in Twins." *Behavior Genetics* 39 (2009): 616–22.

Bartlett, Allison. "Breastfeeding as Headwork: Corporeal Feminism and Meanings for Breastfeeding." *Women's Studies International Forum* 25, no. 3 (2002): 373–82.

———. *Breastwork.* Sydney: University of New South Wales Press, 2005.

Bassin, Donna, Margaret Honey, and Meryle Mahrer Kaplan, eds. *Representations of Motherhood.* New Haven, CT: Yale University Press, 1994.

Battersby, Sue. "Breastfeeding and Bullying: Who's Putting the Pressure On?" *The Practicing Midwife* 3, no. 8 (2000): 36–38.

Baumslag, Naomi, and Dia L. Michels. *Milk, Money, and Madness: The Culture and Politics of Breastfeeding.* Westport, CT: Bergin & Garvey, 1995.

Bayer, Ronald, and James Colgrove. "Science, Politics, and Ideology in the Campaign against Environmental Tobacco Smoke." *American Journal of Public Health* 92, no. 6 (2002): 949–54.

Bayol, Stéphanie A., Samantha J. Farrington, and Neil C. Strickland. "A Maternal 'Junk Food' Diet in Pregnancy and Lactation Promotes an Exacerbated Taste for 'Junk Food' and a Greater Propensity for Obesity in Rat Offspring." *British Journal of Nutrition* 98 (2007): 843–51.

Bayston, R. A., Andrew Russell, N. J. Wald, and A. V. Hoffbrand. "Authors' Reply." *The Lancet* 371 (2008): 1335–36.

Beauchamp, Tom L., Ralph R. Cook, William E. Fayerweather, Gerhard K. Raabe, William E. Thar, Sally R. Cowles, and Gary H. Spivey. "Ethical Guidelines for Epidemiologists." *Journal of Clinical Epidemiology* 44 (1991): 151S–169S.

Beaudry, Micheline, Renee Dufour, and Sylvie Marcoux. "Relation between Infant Feeding and Infections during the First Six Months of Life." *Journal of Pediatrics* 126, no. 2 (1995): 191–97.

Beck, Cheryl Tatano. "Maternal Depression and Child Behavior Problems: A Meta-Analysis." *Journal of Advanced Nursing* 29, no. 3 (1999): 623–29.

Beck, Ulrich. "From Industrial Society to Risk Society: Questions of Survival, Social Structure and Ecological Environment." *Theory, Culture & Society* 9 (1992): 97–123.

———. "Politics of Risk Society." In *The Politics of Risk Society*, ed. Jane Franklin, 9–22. Cambridge: Polity Press, 1998.

———. "Risk Society Revisited: Theory, Politics and Research Programmes." In *The Risk Society and Beyond: Critical Issues for Social Theory*, ed. Barbara Adam, Ulrich Beck, and Joost Van Loon, 211–29. London: Sage, 2000.

———. *Risk Society: Towards a New Modernity*. London: Sage, 1992.

Beck, Ulrich, and Elisabeth Beck-Gernsheim. *The Normal Chaos of Love*. Cambridge: Polity Press, 1995.

Beck, Ulrich, Anthony Giddens, and Scott Lash. *Reflexive Modernization: Politics, Tradition and Aesthetics in the Modern Social Order*. Stanford, CA: Stanford University Press, 1994.

Becker, Marshall H. "A Medical Sociologist Looks at Health Promotion." *Journal of Health and Social Behavior* 34 (1993): 106.

Beck-Gernsheim, Elisabeth. "Health and Responsibility: From Social Change to Technological Change and Vice-Versa." In *The Risk Society and Beyond: Critical Issues for Social Theory*, ed. Barbara Adam, Ulrich Beck, and Joost Van Loon, 122–35. London: Sage, 2000.

———. "Life as a Planning Project." In *Risk, Environment, and Modernity: Towards a New Ecology*, ed. Scott Lash, Bronislaw Szerszynski, and Brian Wynne, 139–53. London: Sage, 1996.

Behrmann, Barbara L. *The Breastfeeding Café: Mothers Share the Joys, Challenges, & Secrets of Nursing*. Ann Arbor: University of Michigan Press, 2005.

Belsky, Jay. Emanuel Miller Lecture: "Developmental Risks (Still) Associated with Early Child Care." *Journal of Child Psychology and Psychiatry* 42, no. 7 (2001): 845–59.

———. "Quantity Counts: Amount of Child Care and Children's Socioemotional Development." *Journal of Developmental and Behavioral Pediatrics* 23, no. 3 (2002): 167–71.

Benet, Suzeanne, Robert E. Pitts, and Michael LaTour. "The Appropriateness of Fear Appeal Use for Health Care Marketing to the Elderly: Is It Okay to Scare Granny?" *Journal of Business Ethics* 12 (1993): 45–55.

Benjamin, Jessica. "The Omnipotent Mother: A Psychoanalytic Study of Fantasy." In *Representations of Motherhood*, ed. Donna Bassin, Margaret Honey, and Meryle Mahrer Kaplan, 129–46. New Haven, CT: Yale University Press, 1994.

Berger, Peter. "Towards a Religion of Health Activism." In *Health, Lifestyle and Environment: Countering the Panic*, ed. Social Affairs Unit / Manhattan Institute, 25–30. London: SAU/MI, 1991.

Bergman, Abraham B. "Colds with a Silver Lining." *Archive of Pediatric and Adolescent Medicine* 156 (2002): 104.

———. "Wrong Turns in Sudden Infant Death Syndrome Research." *Pediatrics* 99, no. 1 (1997): 119–21.

Bergmann, K. E., R. L. Bergmann, R. Von Kries, O Böhm, R. Richter, J. W. Dudenhausen, and U. Wahn. "Early Determinants of Childhood Overweight and Adiposity in a Birth Cohort Study: Role of Breastfeeding." *International Journal of Obesity* 27 (2003): 162–72.

Berry, Brian. *Why Social Justice Matters*. Cambridge: Polity Press, 2005.

Berry, Mary Frances. *The Politics of Parenthood: Child Care, Women's Rights, and the Myth* of the Good Mother. New York: Viking Press, 1993.

Bertin, Joan E., and Laurie R. Beck. "Of Headlines and Hypotheses: The Role of Gender in Popular Press Coverage of Women's Health and Biology." In Man-Made Medicine: Women's Health, Public Policy, and Reform, ed. Kary L. Moss, 37–56. Durham, NC: Duke University Press, 1996.

Best, Joel. Damned Lies and Statistics: Untangling Numbers from the Media, Politicians, and Activists. Berkeley: University of California Press, 2001.

———. More Damned Lies and Statistics: How Numbers Confuse Public Issues. Berkeley: University of California Press, 2004.

———. "Social Progress and Social Problems: Toward a Sociology of Doom." Sociological Quarterly 42, no. 1 (2001): 1–12.

———. Threatened Children: Rhetoric and Concern about Child-Victims. Chicago: University of Chicago Press, 1990.

Bettelheim, Bruno. The Empty Fortress: Infantile Autism and the Birth of the Self. New York: Free Press, 1967.

Bialik, Carl. "Obesity Study Looks Thin: Results Warn That Everyone in the U.S. Will Be Overweight by the Year 2048." Wall Street Journal, August 15, 2008.

Bianchi, Suzanne M. "Maternal Employment and Time with Children: Dramatic Change or Surprising Continuity?" Demography 37, no. 4 (2000): 401–14.

Bianchi, Suzanne M., John P. Robinson, and Melissa A. Milkie. Changing Rhythms of American Family Life. New York: Russell Sage Foundation, 2006.

Birken, Catherine S., and Patricia C. Parkin. "In Which Journals Will Pediatricians Find the Best Evidence for Clinical Practice?" Pediatrics 103, no. 5 (1999): 941–47.

Blades, Joan, and Kristin Rowe-Finkbeiner. The Motherhood Manifesto: What America's Moms Want—And What to do about It. New York: Nation Books, 2006.

Blair, Steven M., and Michael J. Lamonte. "Commentary: Current Perspectives on Obesity and Health: Black and White, or Shades of Gray." International Journal of Epidemiology 35 (2006): 69–72.

Blum, Linda M. At the Breast: Ideologies of Breastfeeding and Motherhood in the Contemporary United States. Boston: Beacon Press, 1999.

———. "Mother-Blame in the Prozac Nation: Raising Kids with Invisible Disabilities." Gender & Society 21, no. 2 (2007): 202–26.

Bobel, Chris. The Paradox of Natural Mothering. Philadelphia: Temple University Press, 2002.

Boling, Patricia, ed. Expecting Trouble: Surrogacy, Fetal Abuse, & New Reproductive Technologies. Boulder, CO: Westview Press, 1995.

Borge, Anne I. H., Michael Ruttner, Sylvana Côté, and Richard E. Tremblay. "Early Childcare and Physical Aggression: Differentiating Social Selection and Social Causation." Journal of Child Psychology and Psychiatry 45, no. 2 (2004): 367–76.

Bornstein, Marc H., ed. Handbook of Parenting: Becoming a Parent. Vol. 3. Mahweh, NJ: Erlbaum, 2002.

Borradaile, Kelley E., Gary D. Foster, Henry May, Allison Karapyn, Sandy Sherman, Karen Grundy, Joan Nachmani, Stephanie Vander Veur, and Robert F. Boruch. "Associations between the Youth/Adolescent Questionnaire, the Youth/Adolescent Activity Questionnaire, and Body Mass Index z Score in Low-Income Inner-City Fourth through Sixth Grade Children." American Journal of Clinical Nutrition 87 (2008): 1650–55.

Boston Women's Health Collective. Our Bodies, Ourselves: A Book by and for Women. 1st and 2nd eds. New York: Simon & Schuster, 1973, 1976.

———. Our Bodies, Ourselves: A New Edition for a New Era. New York: Touchstone, 2005.

Boswell-Penc, Maia. Tainted Milk: Breastmilk, Feminisms, and the Politics of Environmental Degradation. Albany: State University of New York Press, 2006.

Bourke, Joanna. Fear: A Cultural History. Emeryville, CA: Shoemaker and Hoard, 2006.

Brandt, Alan M. "Antagonism and Accommodation: Interpreting the Relationship between Public Health and Medicine in the United States during the 20th Century." American Journal of Public Health 90, no. 5 (2000): 707–15.

————. *The Cigarette Century: The Rise, Fall, and Deadly Persistence of the Product That Defined America.* New York: Basic Books, 2007.

Brooks-Gunn, Jeanne, Allison Sidle Fuligni, and Lisa J. Berlin, eds. *Early Child Development in the 21st Century: Profiles of Current Research Initiatives.* New York: Teachers College Press, 2003.

Brosco, Jeffrey P. "Weight Charts and Well-Child Care: How the Pediatrician Became the Expert in Child Health." *Archives of Pediatric and Adolescent Medicine* 155 (2001): 1385–89.

Brotanek, Jane M., Kristen Grimes, and Glenn Flores. "Leave No Asthmatic Child Behind: The Cultural Competency of Asthma Educational Materials." *Ethnicity and Disease* 17 (2007): 742–48.

Brown, Linda P., Angel H. Bair, and Paula P. Meier. "Does Federal Funding for Breastfeeding Research Target Our National Health Objectives?" *Pediatrics* 111, no. 4 (2003): 360–64.

Browning, Robert. "Who Are the Health Activists?" In *Health, Lifestyle and Environment: Countering the Panic,* by Social Affairs Unit / Manhattan Institute, 31–38. London: SAU/MI, 1991.

Bruer, John T. *The Myth of the First Three Years: A New Understanding of Early Brain Development and Lifelong Learning.* New York: Free Press, 1999.

Buchanan, David R. *An Ethic for Health Promotion: Rethinking the Sources of Human Well-Being.* New York: Oxford University Press, 2000.

Buchanan, David R., Susan Shaw, Amy Ford, and Merrill Singer. "Empirical Science Meets Moral Panic: An Analysis of the Politics of Needle Exchange." *Journal of Public Health Policy* 24, nos. 3/4 (2003): 427–44.

Buchanan, David R., and Lawrence Wallack. "This Is the Partnership for a Drug-Free America: Any Questions?" *Journal of Drug Issues* 28, no. 2 (1998): 329–57.

Bunton, Robin, Sarah Nettleton, and Roger Burrows, eds. *The Sociology of Health Promotion.* London: Routledge, 1995.

Burchell, Graham, Colin Gordon, and Peter Miller, eds. *The Foucault Effect: Studies in Governmentality.* Chicago: University of Chicago Press, 1991.

Burgess, Adam. *Cellular Phones, Public Fears, and a Culture of Precaution.* Cambridge: Cambridge University Press, 2004.

Burke, David T., Andrew L. Judelson, Jeffrey C. Schneider, Melissa C. DeVito, and Danielle Latta. "Reading Habits of Practicing Physiatrists." *American Journal of Physical Medicine & Rehabilitation* 81, no. 10 (2002): 779–87.

Burke, Valerie, Lawrie J. Beilin, Karen Simmer, Wendy H. Oddy, Kevin V. Blake, Dorota Doherty, Garth E. Kendall, John P. Newnham, Louis I. Landau, and Fiona J. Stanley. "Breastfeeding and Overweight: Longitudinal Analysis in an Australian Birth Cohort." *Journal of Pediatrics* 147 (2005): 56–61.

Bury, Michael. *Health and Illness in a Changing Society.* London: Routledge, 1997.

Büskens, Petra. "The Impossibility of 'Natural Parenting' for Modern Mothers: On Social Structure and Formation of Habit." *Journal of the Association for Research on Mothering* 3, no. 1 (2001): 75–86.

Butte, Nancy F. "Impact of Infant Feeding Practices on Childhood Obesity." *Journal of Nutrition* 139, no. 2 (2009): 412S–16S.

————. "The Role of Breastfeeding in Obesity." *Pediatric Clinics of North America* 48, no. 1 (2001): 189–98.

Butte, Nancy F., William W. Wong, Judy M. Hopkinson, E. O'Brian Smith, and Kenneth J. Ellis. "Infant Feeding Mode Affects Early Growth and Body Composition." *Pediatrics* 106, no. 6 (2000): 1355–66.

Buyken, Anette E., Nadina Karaolis-Danckert, Thomas Remer, Katja Bolzenius, Beate Landsberg, and Anja Kroke. "Effects of Breastfeeding on Trajectories of Body Fat and BMI throughout Childhood." *Obesity* 16, no. 2 (2008): 389–95.

Byam-Cook, Clare. *What to Expect When You're Breastfeeding . . . and What If You Can't.* London: Vermillion, 2001.

Byers, Tim, Barbara Lyle, and Workshop Participants. "Summary Statement." *American Journal of Clinical Nutrition* 69 (1999): 1365S–67S.

Cadwell, Karin, ed. *Reclaiming Breastfeeding for the United States: Protection, Promotion, and Support.* Boston: Jones and Bartlett, 2002.

Callahan, Daniel, and Bruce Jennings. "Ethics and Public Health: Forging a Strong Relationship." *American Journal of Public Health* 92, no. 2 (2002): 169–76.

Campbell, Jacquelyn C., Daniel Webster, Jane Koziol-McLain, Carolyn Block, Doris Campbell, Mary Ann Curry, Faye Gary, Nancy Glass, Judith Mc-Farlane, Carolyn Sachs, Phyllis Sharps, Yvonne Ulrich, Susan A. Wilt, Jennifer Manganello, Xiao Xu, Janet Schollenberger, Victoria Frye, and Kathryn Laughon. "Risk Factors for Femicide in Abusive Relationships: Results from a Multisite Case Study." *American Journal of Public Health* 93, no. 7 (2003): 1089–97.

Campos, Paul, Abigail Saguy, Paul Ernsberger, Eric Oliver, and Glen Gaesser. "The Epidemiology of Overweight and Obesity: Public Health Crisis or Moral Panic?" *International Journal of Epidemiology* 35 (2006): 55–60.

———. "Response: Lifestyle, Not Weight, Should Be the Primary Target." *International Journal of Epidemiology* 35 (2006): 81–82.

Cantor, R. M., J. L. Yoon, J. Furr, and C. M. Lajonchere. "Paternal Age and Autism Are Associated in a Family-Based Sample." *Molecular Psychiatry* 12 (2007): 419–23.

Carey, Benedict. "Poor Behavior Is Linked to Time in Day Care." *New York Times,* March 26, 2007.

Carter, Pam. *Feminism, Breasts, and Breast-Feeding.* New York: St. Martin's Press, 1995.

Carter, Simon. "Boundaries of Danger and Uncertainty: An Analysis of the Technological Culture of Risk Assessment." In *Medicine, Health and Risk: Sociological Approaches,* ed. Jonathan Gabe, 133–50. Oxford: Blackwell, 1995.

Cartwright, Rosalind. "Sleeping Together: A Pilot Study of the Effects of Shared Sleeping on Adherence to CPAP Treatment of Obstructive Sleep Apnea." *Journal of Clinical Sleep Medicine* 4, no. 2 (2008): 123–27.

Caspi, Avshalom, Benjamin Williams, Julia Kim-Cohen, Ian W. Craig, Barry J. Milne, Richie Poulton, Leonard C. Schalkwyk, Alan Taylor, Helen Werts, and Terrie E. Moffitt. "Moderation of Breastfeeding Effects on the IQ by Genetic Variation in Fatty Acid Metabolism." *Proceedings of the National Academy of Sciences* 104, no. 47 (2007): 18860–65.

Cassidy, Tina. *Birth: The Surprising History of How We Are Born.* New York: Grove Press, 2006.

Castel, Robert. "From Dangerousness to Risk." In *The Foucault Effect: Studies in Governmentality,* ed. Graham Burchell, Colin Gordon, and Peter Miller, 281–98. Chicago: University of Chicago Press, 1991.

CBS News. "The Benefits of Breastfeeding." *The Early Show,* September 4, 2004.

(CDC) Centers for Disease Control and Prevention. "Health Effects of Cigarette Smoking." Available at www.cdc.gov/tobacco/data_statistics/fact_sheets/health_effects/effects_cig_smoking/ (accessed August 12, 2008).

———. "Neural Tube Defect Surveillance and Folic Acid Intervention—Texas-Mexico Border, 1993–98." *Morbidity and Mortality Weekly Report* 49, no. 1 (2000): 1–4.

———. "Recommendations to Improve Preconception Health and Health Care—United States." *Morbidity and Mortality Weekly Report* 55:RR06, April 21, 2006, 1–23.

Chamberlain, James M., Jill G. Joseph, Kantilal M. Patel, and Murray M. Pollack. "Differences in Severity-Adjusted Pediatric Hospitalization Rates Are Associated with Race/Ethnicity." *Pediatrics* 119, no. 6 (2007): e1319–24.

Chantry, Caroline J., Cynthia R. Howard, and Peggy Auinger. "Full Breastfeeding Duration and Associated Decrease in Respiratory Tract Infection in U.S. Children." *Pediatrics* 117, no. 2 (2006): 425–32.

Chapman, Donna J., Anne Merewood, Robert Ackatia Armah, and Rafael Pérez-Escamilla. "Breastfeeding Status on U.S. Birth Certificates: Where Do We Go from Here?" *Pediatrics* 122, no. 6 (2008): e1159–63.

Chatterji, Pinka, Karen Bonuck, Simi Dhawan, and Nandini Deb. "WIC Participation and the Initiation and Duration of Breastfeeding." Institute for Research on Poverty, discussion paper no. 1246–02, 2002.

Chen, Aimen, and Walter J. Rogan. "Breastfeeding and the Risk of Postneonatal Death in the United States." Pediatrics 113, no. 5 (2004): e435–39.

Chetley, Andrew. The Politics of Baby Foods: Successful Challenges to an International Marketing Strategy. New York: St. Martin's Press, 1986.

Childress, James F., Ruth R. Faden, Ruth D. Gaare, Lawrence O. Gostin, Jeffrey Kahn, Richard J. Bonnie, Nancy E. Kass, Anna C. Mastroianni, Jonathan D. Moreno, and Phillip Nieburg. "Public Health Ethics: Mapping the Terrain." Journal of Law, Medicine & Ethics 30 (2002): 170–78.

Chodorow, Nancy. The Reproduction of Mothering: Psychoanalysis and the Sociology of Gender. Berkeley: University of California Press, 1979.

Chodorow, Nancy, and Susan Contratto. "The Fantasy of the Perfect Mother." In Rethinking the Family: Some Feminist Questions, ed. Barrie Thorne and Marilyn Yalom, 54–75. New York: Longman, 1982.

Council for International Organizations of Medical Sciences (CIOMS). "International Guidelines for Ethical Review of Epidemiological Studies." Geneva: CIOMS, 1991.

Clark, Roseanne, Janet Shibley Hyde, Marily J. Essex, and Marjorie H. Klein. "Length of Maternity Leave and Quality of Mother-Infant Interactions." Child Development 68, no. 2 (1997): 364–83.

Clarke, Adele E. Disciplining Reproduction: Modernity, American Life Sciences, and the Problems of Sex. Berkeley: University of California Press, 1998.

Clarke-Stewart, Alison. "Infant Day Care: Maligned or Malignant?" American Psychologist 44, no. 2 (1989): 266–73.

Clarke-Stewart, Alison, and Virginia D. Allhusen. What We Know about Childcare. Cambridge, MA: Harvard University Press, 2005.

Clifford, Tammy J. "Breast Feeding and Obesity." British Medical Journal 327 (2003): 879–80.

Coker, Tumaini, Lawrence P. Casalino, G. Caleb Alexander, and John Lantos. "Should Our Well-Child Care System Be Redesigned? A National Survey of Pediatricians." Pediatrics 118, no. 5 (2006): 1852–57.

Cole, Philip. "The Moral Bases for Public Health Interventions." Epidemiology 6, no. 1 (1995): 78–83.

Collman, James P. Naturally Dangerous: Surprising Facts about Food, Health, and the Environment. Sausalito, CA: University Science Books, 2001.

Condan, Marian. "Breast Is Best, but It Could Be Better: What Is in Breast Milk That Should Not Be?" Pediatric Nursing 31, no. 4 (2005): 333–38.

Connolly, Maureen, and Dana Sullivan. Unbuttoned: Women Open up about the Pleasures, Pains, and Politics of Breastfeeding. Boston: Harvard Common Press, 2009.

Cook-Crotty, Laura. "Comments." Available at www.health.talk.newsweek.com/default.asp?item=625386 (accessed June 17, 2007).

———. "My Turn: In Defense of Formula-Fed Babies." Newsweek, June 14, 2007. Available at www.newsweek.com/id/33605 (accessed June 17, 2007).

Cooklin, Amanda R., Susan M. Donath, and Lisa H. Amir. "Maternal Employment and Breastfeeding: Results from the Longitudinal Study of Australian Children." Acta Paediatrica 97 (2008): 620–23.

Cope, Mark Bradley, and David B. Allison. "Critical Review of the World Health Organization's (WHO) 2007 Report on 'Evidence of the Long-Term Effects of Breastfeeding: Systematic Reviews and Meta-Analysis' with Respect to Obesity." Obesity Reviews 9, no. 6 (2008): 594–605.

Correll, Shelley J., Stephen Benard, and In Paik. "Getting a Job: Is There a Motherhood Penalty?" American Journal of Sociology 112, no. 5 (2007): 1297–1338.

Cost, Quality & Child Outcomes Study Team. Cost, Quality, and Child Outcomes in Child Care Centers, Public Report. 2nd ed. Denver: Economics Department, University of Colorado at Denver, 1995.

Coveney, John. "The Government of the Table: Nutrition Expertise and the Social Organization of Family Food Habits." In *A Sociology of Food and Nutrition*, ed. John Germov and Lauren Williams, 220–38. Oxford: Oxford University Press, 2004.

Cowan, Ruth Schwartz. *Heredity and Hope: The Case for Genetic Screening*. Cambridge, MA: Harvard University Press, 2008.

Crandall, Lee A. "Should Epidemiologists and Other Health Scientists Become Advocates for Social Policies?" *Professional Ethics* 11, no. 3 (2003): 83–94.

Cricco-Lizza, Roberta. "Black Non-Hispanic Mothers' Perceptions about the Promotion of Infant-Feeding Methods by Nurses and Physicians." *Journal of Obstetric, Gynocologic and Neonatal Nursing* 35 (2006): 173–80.

———. "Ethnography and the Generation of Trust in Breastfeeding Disparities Research." *Applied Nursing Research* 20 (2007): 200.

———. "Infant-Feeding Beliefs and Experiences of Black Women Enrolled in WIC in the New York Metropolitan Area." *Qualitative Health Research* 14, no. 9 (2004): 1197–1210.

———. "The Milk of Human Kindness: Environmental and Human Interactions in a WIC Clinic That Influence Infant-Feeding Decisions of Black Women." *Qualitative Health Research* 15, no. 4 (2005): 525–38.

Crittenden, Ann. *The Price of Motherhood: Why the Most Important Job in the World Is Still the Least Valued*. New York: Owl Books, 2001.

Croen, Lisa A., Daniel V. Najjar, Bruce Fireman, and Judith K. Grether. "Maternal and Paternal Age and Risk of Autism Spectrum Disorders." *Archives of Pediatrics and Adolescent Medicine* 161, no. 4 (2007): 334–40.

Cronon, William. "Introduction: In Search of Nature." In *Uncommon Ground: Toward Reinventing Nature*, ed. William Cronon, 23–56. New York: Norton, 1995.

———, ed. *Uncommon Ground: Toward Reinventing Nature*. New York: Norton, 1995.

Crotty, Pat, and John Germov. "Food and Class." In *A Sociology of Food and Nutrition*, ed. John Germov and Lauren Williams, 241–62. Oxford: Oxford University Press, 2004.

Cushing, Alice H., Jonathan M. Samet, William E. Lambert, Betty J. Skipper, William C. Hunt, Stephen A. Young, and Leroy C. McLaren. "Breastfeeding Reduces Risk of Respiratory Illness in Infants." *American Journal of Epidemiology* 147, no. 9 (1998): 863–70.

Daly, Kathleen A., and G. Scott Giebink. "Clinical Epidemiology of Otitis Media." *Pediatric Infectious Disease Journal* 19, no. 5 (2000): S31–36.

Daniels, Cynthia R. "Between Fathers and Fetuses: The Social Construction of Male Reproduction and the Politics of Fetal Harm." *Signs: Journal of Women in Culture and Society* 22, no. 3 (1997): 579–616.

———. *Exposing Men: The Science and Politics of Male Reproduction*. Oxford: Oxford University Press, 2006.

Davies, A. Michael, E. Maurice Backett, Angele Petros-Barvazian, Jack Dowie, Robyn M. Dawes, Kenneth S. Warren, and Michael V. Hayes. "Comment: The Risk Approach." *Social Science & Medicine* 33, no. 1 (1991): 64–70.

Davis, Jaimie, Marc J. Weigensberg, Gabriel Q. Shaibi, Noe C. Crespo, Louise A. Kelly, Christianne J. Lane, and Michael I. Goran. "Influence of Breastfeeding on Obesity and Type 2 Diabetes Risk Factors in Latino Youth with a Family History of Type 2 Diabetes." *Diabetes Care* 30, no. 4 (2007): 784–89.

Davison, Charlie, and George Davey Smith. "The Baby and the Bath Water: Examining Socio-Cultural and Free-Market Critiques of Health Promotion." In *The Sociology of Health Promotion*, ed. Robin Bunton, Sarah Nettleton, and Roger Burrows, 91–99. London: Routledge, 1995.

Davison, Charlie, Stephen Frankel, and George Davey Smith. "The Limits of Lifestyle: Re-Assessing 'Fatalism' in the Popular Culture of Illness Prevention." *Social Science & Medicine* 34, no. 6 (1992): 675–85.

Dean, Cornelia. "New Complications in Reporting Science." *Nieman Reports* 56, no. 3 (2002): 25–26.

Dean, Mitchell. *Governmentality: Power and Rule in Modern Society*. Thousand Oaks, CA: Sage, 1999.

Denney, David. *Risk and Society*. London: Sage, 2005.

DeNoon, Daniel. "Moms Eat Junk Food, Kids Get Fat." Available at www.cbsnews.com/stories/2008/07/01/health/webmd/main4222324.shtml (accessed July 2, 2008).

Der, Geoff, G. David Batty, and Ian J. Deary. "Effect of Breastfeeding on Intelligence in Children: Prospective Study, Sibling Pairs Analysis, and Meta-Analysis." *British Medical Journal* 333 (2006): 945–48.

de Silva, A., P. W. Jones, and S. A. Spencer. "Does Human Milk Reduce Infection Rates in Preterm Infants? A Systematic Review." *Archives of Disease in Childhood, Fetal Neonatal Edition* 89 (2004): F509–F513.

Des Jarlais, Don C., Cynthia Lyles, Nicole Crepaz, and the TREND Group. "Improving the Reporting Quality of Nonrandomized Evaluations of Behavioral and Public Health Interventions: The TREND Statement." *American Journal of Public Health* 94, no. 3 (2004): 361–66.

Dettwyler, Katherine A. "Beauty and the Breast: The Cultural Context of Breastfeeding in the United States." In *Breastfeeding: Biocultural Perspectives*, ed. Patricia Stuart-Macadam and Katherine A. Dettwyler, 167–215. New York: Aldine de Gruyter, 1995.

———. "Formula Is Bad for Babies." *Chicago Parent* (January 2004).

———. "A Time to Wean: The Hominid Blueprint for the Natural Age of Weaning in Modern Human Populations." In *Breastfeeding: Biocultural Perspectives*, ed. Patricia Stuart-Macadam and Katherine A. Dettwyler, 39–74. New York: Aldine de Gruyter, 1995.

Devries, Raymond, Cecilia Benoit, Edwin R. Van Teijlingen, and Sirpa Wrede. *Birth by Design: Pregnancy, Maternity Care, and Midwifery in North America and Europe*. New York: Routledge, 2001.

Dewey, Katherine. "Maternal and Fetal Stress Are Associated with Impaired Lactogenesis." *Journal of Nutrition* 131, no. 11 (2001): 3012S–15S.

Dewey, Kathryn G., M. Jane Heinig, and Laurie A. Nommsen-Rivers. "Differences in Morbidity between Breast-Fed and Formula-Fed Infants." *Journal of Pediatrics* 126, no. 5 (1995): 696–702.

Dietz, William H. "Breastfeeding May Help Prevent Childhood Overweight." *Journal of the American Medical Association* 285, no. 19 (2001): 2506–7.

DiGirolamo, A. M., L. M. Grummer-Strawn, and S. B. Fein. "Do Perceived Attitudes of Physicians and Hospital Staff Affect Breastfeeding Decisions?" *Birth* 30, no. 2 (2003): 94–100.

Doll, Sir Richard. "Weak Associations in Epidemiology." *Radiological Protection Bulletin* 192 (1997): 10–15.

Dolnick, Edward. *Madness on the Couch: Blaming the Victim in the Heyday of Psychoanalysis*. New York: Simon & Schuster, 1998.

Douglas, Mary. *Risk and Blame: Essays in Cultural Theory*. London: Routledge, 1992.

Douglas, Mary, and Aaron Wildavsky. *Risk and Culture: An Essay on the Selection of Technical and Environmental Dangers*. Berkeley: University of California Press, 1982.

Douglas, Susan J., and Meredith W. Michaels. *The Mommy Myth: The Idealization of Motherhood and How It Has Undermined Women*. Boston: Free Press, 2004.

Doyle, Lex W., Anne L. Rickards, Elaine A. Kelly, Geoffrey W. Ford, and Catherine Callanan. "Breastfeeding and Intelligence." *The Lancet* 339 (1992): 744–45.

Drane, Denise L., and Jeri A. Logemann. "A Critical Evaluation of the Evidence on the Association between Type of Infant Feeding and Cognitive Development." *Paediatric and Perinatal Epidemiology* 14 (2000): 349–56.

Duden, Barbara. *Disembodying Women: Perspectives on Pregnancy and the Unborn*. Cambridge, MA: Harvard University Press, 1993.

Duffy, Linda C., Howard Faden, Raymond Wasielewski, Judy Wolf, Debra Krystofik, and Tonawanda/Williamsville Pediatrics. "Exclusive Breastfeeding Protects against Bacterial Colonization and Day Care Exposure to Otitis Media." *Pediatrics* 100, no. 4 (1997): e7–e15.

Duke, Charles R., Gregory M. Pickett, Les Carlson, and Stephen J. Grove. "A Method for Evaluating the Ethics of Fear Appeals." *Journal of Public Policy and Marketing* 12, no. 1 (1993): 120–29.

Duncan, Burris, John Ey, Catherine J. Holberg, Anne L. Wright, Fernando D. Martinez, and Lynn M. Taussig. "Exclusive Breast-Feeding for at Least 4 Months Protects against Otitis Media." *Pediatrics* 91, no. 5 (1993): 867–72.

Duncan, Greg J., and Jeanne Brooks-Gunn, eds. *Consequences of Growing up Poor.* New York: Russell Sage Foundation, 1997.

Duncan, Joanne M., and Malcolm R. Sears. "Breastfeeding and Allergies: Time for a Change in Paradigm?" *Current Opinion in Allergy and Clinical Immunology* 8, no. 5 (2008): 398–405.

Dwan, Kerry, Douglas G. Altman, Juan A. Arnaiz, Jill Bloom, An-Wen Chan, Eugenia Cronin, Evelyne Decullier, Philippa J. Easterbrook, Erik Von Elm, Carrol Gamble, Davina Ghersi, John P. A. Ioannidis, John Sims, and Paula R. Williamson. "Systematic Review of the Empirical Evidence of Study Publication Bias and Outcome Reporting Bias." *PloS One* 3, no. 8 (2008): e3081.

Dykes, Fiona. "'Supply' and 'Demand': Breastfeeding as Labour." *Social Sciences & Medicine* 60 (2005): 2283–93.

Earle, Sarah. "Is Breast Best? Breastfeeding, Motherhood and Identity." In *Gender, Identity & Reproduction: Social Perspectives,* ed. Sarah Earle and Gayle Letherby, 135–50. New York: Palgrave Macmillan, 2003.

Earle, Sarah, and Gayle Letherby, eds. *Gender, Identity & Reproduction: Social Perspectives.* New York: Palgrave Macmillan, 2003.

Easterbrook, Gregg. *The Progress Paradox: How Life Gets Better While People Feel Worse.* New York: Random House, 2003.

Editor in Chief. "Our Policy on Policy." *Epidemiology* 124, no. 4 (2001): 371–72.

Ehrenreich, Barbara, and Deirdre English. *For Her Own Good: Two Centuries of the Experts' Advice to Women.* New York: Anchor Books, 2005.

Eisenberg, Arlene, Heidi E. Murkoff, and Sandee E. Hathaway. *What to Expect When You're Expecting.* 2nd and 3rd eds. New York: Workman, 1996, 2002.

———. *What to Expect the First Year.* 2nd ed. New York: Workman, 1996.

Elliott, Kristen G., Chris L. Kjolhede, Effie Gournis, and Kathleen M. Rasmussen. "Duration of Breastfeeding Associated with Obesity during Adolescence." *Obesity Research* 5, no. 6 (1997): 538–41.

Elliott, Leslie, John Henderson, Kate Northstone, Grace Y. Chiu, David Dunson, and Stephanie J. London. "Prospective Study of

Breast-Feeding in Relation to Wheeze, Atopy, and Bronchial Hyperresponsiveness in the Avon Longitudinal Study of Parents and Children (ALSPAC)." *Journal of Allergy and Clinical Immunology* 122, no. 1 (2008): 49–54.

Engber, Daniel. "The Paranoid Style in American Science." April 15–17, 2008. Available at www.slate.com/id/2189178 (accessed April 17, 2008).

Engel, Kirsten G., Michael Heisler, Dylan M. Smith, Claire H. Robinson, Jane H. Forman, and Peter A. Ubel. "Patient Comprehension of Emergency Department Care and Instructions: Are Patients Aware of When They Do Not Understand?" *Annals of Emergency Medicine* 53, no. 4 (2008): 454–61.

Ericson, Richard V., and Kevin D. Haggerty. *Policing the Risk Society.* Toronto: University of Toronto Press, 1997.

Evenhouse, Eirik, and Siobhan Reilly. "Improved Estimates of the Benefits of Breastfeeding Using Sibling Comparisons to Reduce Selection Bias." *Health Sciences Research* 40, no. 6, part I (2005): 1781–1802.

Eyer, Diane. *Motherguilt: How Our Culture Blames Mothers for What's Wrong with Society.* New York: Times Books, 1996.

———. *Mother–Infant Bonding: A Scientific Fiction.* New Haven, CT: Yale University Press, 1992.

Faden, Ruth R. "Ethical Issues in Government Sponsored Public Health Campaigns." *Health Education Quarterly* 14, no. 1 (1987): 27–37.

Farquhar, Dion. *The Other Machine: Discourse and Reproductive Technologies.* New York: Routledge, 1996.

Feinstein, Alvan R. "Meta-Analysis: Statistical Alchemy for the 21st Century." *Journal of Clinical Epidemiology* 48, no. 1 (1995): 71–79.

———. "Scientific Paradigms and Ethical Problems in Epidemiological Research." *Journal of Clinical Epidemiology* 4 (1991): 119–23.

Feldman-Winter, Lori B., Richard J. Schanler, Karen G. O'Connor, and Ruth A. Lawrence. "Pediatricians and the Promotion and Support of Breastfeeding." *Archives of Pediatric and Adolescent Medicine* 162, no. 12 (2008): 1142–49.

Fisher, Jonathan, and Angela Lyons. "The Ability of Women to Pay Debt after Divorce." Paper presented at "Women Working to Make a Difference," International Women's Policy Research Conference, Washington, DC, June 2003.

Fisher, Lucinda. "Teeth Cut from Breastfeeding Campaign." December 12, 2003. Available at www.womensenews.org/article.cfm/dyn/aid/1651/context/archive (accessed April 14, 2004).

Fitzpatrick, Michael. *The Tyranny of Health: Doctors and the Regulation of Lifestyle.* New York: Routledge, 2001.

Flacking, Renée, Uwe Ewald, and Bengt Starrin. "'I Wanted to Do a Good Job': Experiences of 'Becoming a Mother' and Breastfeeding in Mothers of Very Preterm Infants after Discharge from a Neonatal Unit." *Social Science & Medicine* 64 (2007): 2405–16.

Flavin, Jeanne. *Our Bodies, Our Crimes: The Policing of Women's Reproduction in America.* New York: New York University Press, 2009.

Flynn, James, Paul Slovic, and Howard Kunreuther, eds. *Risk, Media, and Stigma: Understanding Public Challenges to Modern Science and Technology.* London: Earthscan, 2001.

Forste, Renata, Jessica Weiss, and Emily Lippincott. "The Decision to Breastfeed in the United States: Does Race Matter?" *Pediatrics* 108, no. 1 (2001): 291–96.

Foucault, Michel. "Governmentality." In *The Foucault Effect: Studies in Governmentality,* ed. Graham Burchell, Colin Gordon, and Peter Miller, 87–104. Chicago: University of Chicago Press, 1991.

Francis, Charles M., Edythe L. P. Anthony, Jennifer A. Brunton, and Thomas H. Kunz. "Lactation in Male Fruit Bats." *Nature* 367 (1994): 1691–92.

Francis, Solveig, Selma James, Phoebe Jones Schellenberg, and Nina Lopez-Jones. *The Milk of Human Kindness: Defending Breastfeeding from the Global Market and the AIDS Industry.* London: Crossroads, 2002.

Franklin, Jane, ed. *The Politics of Risk Society.* Cambridge: Polity Press, 1998.

Franklin, Jon. "The Extraordinary Adventure That Is Science Writing." *Nieman Reports* 56, no. 3 (2002): 8–10.

Fredriksson, Niina Jaakkola, and Jouni J. K. Jaakkola. "Breastfeeding and Childhood Asthma: A Six-Year Population-Based Cohort Study." *BMC Pediatrics* 7, no. 39 (2007): 1–7.

Friedman, Sharon M., Sharon Dunwoody, and Carol L. Rogers, eds. *Communicating Uncertainty: Media Coverage of New and Controversial Science.* Mahweh, NJ: Erlbaum, 1999.

Furedi, Frank. *Paranoid Parenting: Why Ignoring the Experts May Be Best for Your Child.* Chicago: Chicago Review Press, 2002.

———. *Therapy Culture: Cultivating Vulnerability in an Uncertain Age.* London: Routledge, 2004.

Furstenberg, Frank Jr. "Family Change and the Welfare of Children: What Do We Know and What Can We Do about It?" In *Gender and Family Change in Industrialized Countries,* ed. Karen Oppenheim Mason and An-Magrit Jensen, 245–57. Oxford: Clarendon Press, 1995.

Gabe, Jonathan, ed. *Medicine, Health and Risk: Sociological Approaches.* Oxford: Blackwell, 1995.

Gahagan, Sheila. "Breast Feeding and the Risk of Allergy and Asthma." *British Medical Journal* 355 (2007): 782–83.

Gale, Catharine, Lynne D. Mariott, Christopher N. Martyn, Jennifer Limond, Hazel M. Inskip, Keith M. Godfrey,

Catherine M. Law, Cyrus Cooper, Carolyn West, and Siân M. Robinson, for the Southampton Women's Survey Study Group. "Breast-feeding, the Use of Docosahexaenoic Acid-Fortified Formulas in Infancy and Neuropsychological Function in Childhood." *Archives of Disease in Childhood*, electronic publication (2009): 1–6.

Gannon, Kenneth, Lesley Glover, and Paul Abel. "Masculinity, Infertility, Stigma and Media Reports." *Social Science & Medicine* 59 (2004): 1169–75.

Gardner, Kristen E. *Early Detection: Women, Cancer, and Awareness Campaigns in the Twentieth-Century United States.* Chapel Hill: University of North Carolina Press, 2006.

Geist-Martin, Patricia, Eileen Berlin Ray, and Barbara F. Sharf. *Communicating Health: Personal, Cultural, and Political Complexities.* Belmont, CA: Wadsworth / Thomson Learning, 2003.

Germov, John, and Lauren Williams, eds. *A Sociology of Food and Nutrition.* Oxford: Oxford University Press, 2004.

Gessner, Bradford D., Thomas J. Porter, Arthur I. Eidelman, Lawrence M. Garnter, Melissa Bartick, Rafael Pelayo, Judith Owens, Jodi Mindell, Stephen Sheldon, John Kattwinkel, Fern R. Hauck, Rachel Y. Moon, Michael Malloy, and Marian Willinger. "Bed Sharing with Unimpaired Parents Is Not an Important Risk for Sudden Infant Death Syndrome." *Pediatrics* 117, no. 3 (2006): 990–96.

Gibbs, W. Wyat. "Obesity: An Overblown Epidemic?" Available at www.sciam.com/.cfm?articleID=000E5065-2345-128A-9E1583414B7.

Gibson-Davis, Christina M., and Jeanne Brooks-Gunn. "Breastfeeding and Verbal Ability of 3-Year-Olds in a Multicity Sample." *Pediatrics* 118, no. 5 (2006): e1444–51.

Giddens, Anthony. *Modernity and Self-Identity: Self and Society in the Late Modern Age.* Stanford, CA: Stanford University Press, 1991.

Gieryn, Thomas F. *Cultural Boundaries of Science: Credibility on the Line.* Chicago: University of Chicago Press, 1999.

Gigliotti, Eileen. "When Women Decide *Not* to Breastfeed." *MCN, the American Journal of Maternal/Child Nursing* 20 (1995): 315–21.

Gillman, Matthew W. "Breast-Feeding and Obesity." *Journal of Pediatrics* 141, no. 6 (2002): 749–50.

Gillman, Matthew W., Carlos A. Camargo Jr., A. Lindsay Frazier, and Graham A. Colditz. "Risk of Overweight among Adolescents Who Were Breastfed as Infants." *Journal of the American Medical Association* 285, no. 19 (2001): 2461–67.

Gillman, Matthew W., and Christos S. Mantzoros. "Breast-Feeding, Adipokines, and Childhood Obesity." *Epidemiology* 18, no. 6 (2007): 730–32.

Gillman, Matthew W., Sheryl L. Rifas-Shiman, Catherine S. Berkey, A. Lindsay Frazier, Helaine R. H. Rockett,

Carlos A. Camargo Jr., Alison E. Field, and Graham A. Colditz. "Breast-Feeding and Overweight in Adolescence." *Epidemiology* 17, no. 1 (2006): 112–14.

Ginsburg, Faye, and Anna Lowenhaupt Tsing, eds. *Uncertain Terms: Negotiating Gender in American Culture.* Boston: Beacon Press, 1990.

Gitlin, Todd. *Media Unlimited: How the Torrent of Images and Sounds Overwhelms Our Lives.* New York: Henry Holt, 2002.

Gladwell, Malcolm. "Big and Bad: How the S.U.V. Ran over Automotive Safety." *New Yorker*, January 12, 2004, 28–33.

Glassner, Barry. *The Culture of Fear.* New York: Basic Books, 1999.

Glenn, Evelyn Nakano, Grace Chang, and Linda Rennie Forcey, eds. *Mothering: Ideology, Experience, and Agency.* New York: Routledge, 1994.

Glick, Daniel. "Rooting for Intelligence." *Newsweek*, March 1, 1997.

Godfrey, Jodi R., and David Meyers. "Toward Optimal Health: Maternal Benefits of Breastfeeding." *Journal of Women's Health* 18, no. 9 (2009): 1–4.

Golden, Janet. *A Social History of Wet Nursing in America: From Breast to Bottle.* Cambridge: Cambridge University Press, 1996.

Goodman, Elizabeth, Beth R. Hinden, and Seema Khandelwal. "Accuracy of Teen and Parental Reports of Obesity and Body Mass Index." *Pediatrics* 106, no. 1 (2000): 52–58.

Goodman, Lenn E., and Madeleine J. Goodman. "Prevention—How Misuse of a Concept Undercuts Its Worth." *Hastings Center Report* (1986): 26–38.

Gordis, Leon. "Ethical and Professional Issues in the Changing Practice of Epidemiology." *Journal of Clinical Epidemiology* 4 (1991): 9–13.

Gordon, A. G. "Breast-Feeding, Breast-Milk Feeding, and Intelligence Quotient." *American Journal of Clinical Nutrition* 72 (2000): 1063–64.

Gordon, Colin. "Governmental Rationality: An Introduction." In *The Foucault Effect: Studies in Governmentality*, ed. Graham Burchell, Colin Gordon, and Peter Miller, 1–51. Chicago: University of Chicago Press, 1991.

Gori, Gio Batta. "Epidemiology and Public Health: Is a New Paradigm Needed or a New Ethic?" *Journal of Clinical Epidemiology* 51, no. 8 (1998): 637–41.

———. "Science, Imaginable Risks, and Public Policy: Anatomy of a Mirage." *Regulatory Toxicology and Pharmacology* 23 (1996): 304–11.

Goutman, Thomas M. *Medical Monitoring: How Bad Science Makes Bad Law.* Washington, DC: National Legal Center for the Public Interest, 2001.

Graham, John D. *Risk versus Risk: Tradeoffs in Protecting Health and the Environment.* Cambridge, MA: Harvard University Press, 1995.

Granju, Katie Allison. *Attachment Parenting: Instinctive Care for Your Baby and Young Child.* New York: Simon & Schuster, 1999.

———. "The Milky Way of Doing Business." Available at www.hipmama.com/node/view/588 (accessed January 12, 2004).

Gray, George M., and David P. Ropeik. "Dealing with the Dangers of Fear: The Role of Risk Communication." *Health Affairs* 21, no. 6 (2002): 106–16.

Greenbaum, Daniel S. "Epidemiology at the Edge." *Epidemiology* 124, no. 4 (2001): 376–77.

Greenspan, Stanley I., and Jacqueline Salmon. *The Four-Thirds Solution: Solving the Childcare Crisis in America Today.* Cambridge, MA: Perseus, 2001.

Greer, Frank R. "Breastfeeding and Cardiovascular Disease: Where's the Beef?" *Pediatrics* 115, no. 6 (2005): 1765.

Greer, Frank R., Scott H. Sicherer, A. Wesley Burks, and the Committee on Nutrition and Section on Allergy and Immunology. "Effects of Early Nutritional Interventions on the Development of Atopic Disease in Infants and Children: The Role of Maternal Dietary Restriction, Breastfeeding, Timing of Introduction of Complementary Foods, and Hydrolyzed Formulas." *Pediatrics* 121, no. 1 (2008): 183–91.

Gregory, Robin, James Flynn, and Paul Slovic. "Technological Stigma." In *Risk, Media, and Stigma: Understanding Public Challenges to Modern Science and Technology*, ed. James Flynn,

Paul Slovic, and Howard Kunreuther, 3–8. London: Earthscan, 2001.

Gresky, Dana M., Laura L. Ten Eyck, Charles G. Lord, and Rusty B. McIntyre. "Effects of Salient Multiple Identities on Women's Performance under Mathematics Stereotype Threat." *Sex Roles* 53, nos. 9/10 (2005): 703–16.

Grosse, Scott D., and Julianne S. Collins. "Folic Acid Supplementation and Neural Tube Defect Prevention." *Birth Defects Research Part A: Clinical and Molecular Teratology* 79, no. 11 (2007): 737–42.

Grummer-Strawn, Laurence M., and Zuguo Mei. "Does Breastfeeding Protect against Pediatric Overweight? Analysis of Longitudinal Data from the Centers for Disease Control and Prevention Pediatric Nutrition Surveillance System." *Pediatrics* 113, no. 2 (2004): e81–e86.

Grummer-Strawn, Laurence M., Kelley S. Scanlon, and Sara B. Fine. "Infant Feeding and Feeding Transitions during the First Year of Life." *Pediatrics* 122 (2008): S36–S42.

Guilbert, Theresa W., Debra A. Stern, Wayne J. Morgan, Fernando D. Martinez, and Anne L. Wright. "Effect of Breastfeeding on Lung Function in Childhood and Modulation by Maternal Asthma and Atopy." *American Journal of Respiratory and Critical Care Medicine* 176 (2007): 843–48.

Gunter, Jennifer. "Intimate Partner Violence." *Obstetrics and Gynecology Clinics of North America* 34 (2007): 367–88.

Guthman, Julie. "Fast Food/ Organic Food: Reflexive Tastes and the Making of 'Yuppie Chow.'" *Social and Cultural Geography* 4, no. 1 (2003): 45–58.

Guthman, Julie, and Melanie DuPuis. "Embodying Neoliberalism: Economy, Culture, and the Politics of Fat." *Environment and Planning D: Society and Space* 24 (2006): 427–48.

Guttman, Nurit, and William Harris Ressler. "On Being Responsible: Ethical Issues in Appeals to Personal Responsibility in Health Campaigns." *Journal of Health Communication* 6 (2001): 117–36.

Guttman, Nurit, and Charles T. Salmon. "Guilt, Fear, Stigma and Knowledge Gaps: Ethical Issues in Public Health Communication Interventions." *Bioethics* 18, no. 6 (2004): 531–52.

Guttman, Nurit, and Deena R. Zimmerman. "Low-Income Mothers' Views on Breastfeeding." *Social Science & Medicine* 50 (2000): 1457–73.

Gwyn, Richard. *Communicating Health and Illness.* London: Sage, 2002.

Hacking, Ian. *The Taming of Chance.* Cambridge: Cambridge University Press, 1990.

Haisma, H., W. A. Coward, E. Albernaz, G. H. Visser, J. C. K. Wells, A. Wright, and C. G. Victora. "Breast Milk and Energy Intake in Exclusively, Predominantly, and Partially Breast-Fed Infants." *European Journal of Clinical Nutrition* 57 (2003): 1633–42.

Handwerker, Lisa. "Medical Risk: Implicating Poor Pregnant Women." *Social Science and Medicine* 38, no. 5 (1994): 665–75.

Hanigsberg, Julia E., and Sara Ruddick, eds. *Mother Troubles: Rethinking Contemporary Maternal Dilemmas.* Boston: Beacon Press, 1999.

Haraway, Donna. "Situated Knowledges: The Science Question in Feminism and the Privilege of Partial Perspective." *Feminist Studies* 14, no. 3 (1988): 575–99.

Harder, Thomas, Renate Bergmann, Gerd Kallischnigg, and Andreas Plagemann. "Duration of Breastfeeding and Risk of Overweight: A Meta-Analysis." *American Journal of Epidemiology* 162 (2005): 397–403.

Harris, Judith Rich. *The Nurture Assumption: Why Children Turn out the Way They Do.* New York: Free Press, 1998.

Harrison, Kathryn. "Too Close to Home: Dioxin Contamination of Breast Milk and the Political Agenda." *Policy Sciences* 34, no. 1 (2001): 35–62.

Harthorn, Barbara Herr, and Laury Oaks, eds. *Risk, Culture, and Health Inequality: Shifting Perceptions of Danger and Blame.* Westport, CT: Praeger, 2003.

Hastings, G., and L. MacFadyen. "The Limitations of Fear Messages." *Tobacco Control* 11 (2002): 73–75.

Hastings, Gerard, Martine Stead, and John Webb. "Fear Appeals in Social Marketing: Strategic and Ethical Reasons for Concern." *Psychology and Marketing* 21, no. 11 (2004): 961–86.

Hausman, Bernice L. "Motherhood and Inequality: A Commentary on Hanna Rosin's 'The Case against Breastfeeding.'" *Journal of Human Lactation* 25, no. 3 (2009): 266–68.

———. *Mother's Milk: Breastfeeding Controversies in American Culture.* New York: Routledge, 2003.

———. "Risky Business: Framing Childbirth in Hospital Settings." *Journal of Medical Humanities* 26, no. 1 (2005): 23–38.

Hayes, Michael V. "On the Epistemology of Risk: Language, Logic, and Social Science." *Social Science & Medicine* 35, no. 4 (1992): 401–7.

———. The Risk Approach: Unassailable Logic?" *Social Science & Medicine* 33, no. 1 (1991): 55–61.

Hays, Sharon. *The Cultural Contradictions of Motherhood.* New Haven, CT: Yale University Press, 1996.

———. *Flat Broke with Children: Women in the Age of Welfare Reform.* New York: Oxford University Press, 2003.

Hazinski, Thomas A., Howard T. Chatterton, Marcia Angell, and Jerome P. Kassirer. "Which Results Should the Public Believe?" *New England Journal of Medicine* 332, no. 14 (1995): 963–64.

Hediger, Mary L., Mary D. Overpeck, Robert J. Kuczmarski, and W. June Ruan. "Association between Infant Breastfeeding and Overweight in Young Children." *Journal of the American Medical Association* 285, no. 19 (2001): 2453–60.

Heery, Lee B., Catharine J. Holberg, Burris Duncan, and John Ey. "Exclusive Breast-Feeding for at Least 4 Months Protects against Otitis Media." *Pediatrics* 93, no. 3 (1994): 537–38.

Heinig, M. Jane. "The Burden of Proof: A Commentary on 'Is Breast Really Best: Risk and Total Motherhood in the National Breastfeeding Awareness Campaign.'" *Journal of Human Lactation* 23, no. 4 (2007): 374–76.

Heinig, M. Jane, and Kathryn G. Dewey. "Health Advantages of Breastfeeding for Infants: A Critical Review." *Nutrition Research Reviews* 9 (1996): 89–110.

———. "Health Effects of Breast Feeding for Mothers: A Critical Review." *Nutrition Research Reviews* 10 (1997): 35–56.

Herbst, Melissa A., Brian M. Mercer, Dorothy Beazley, Norman Meyer, and Teresa Carr. "Relationship of Prenatal Care and Perinatal Morbidity in Low-Birth-Weight Infants." *American Journal of Obstetrics and Gynecology* 189, no. 4 (2003): 930–33.

Heyman, Jody, and Michael S. Kramer. "Public Policy and Breastfeeding: A Straightforward and Significant Solution." *Canadian Journal of Public Health* 100 (2009): 381–83.

Hilgartner, Stephen. *Science on Stage: Expert Advice as Public Drama.* Stanford, CA: Stanford University Press, 2000.

Hirshleifer, David. "The Blind Leading the Blind: Social Influence, Fads, and Informational Cascades." In *The New Economics of Human Behavior*, ed. Mariano Tommasi and Kathryn Ierulli, 188–215. Cambridge: Cambridge University Press, 1995.

Hochschild, Arlie Russell. *The Commercialization of Intimate Life: Notes from Home and Work.* Berkeley: University of California Press, 2003.

———. *The Second Shift.* New York: Penguin, 2003.

Hoffmeister, H., and M. Szklo. "'Epidemiologic Practices in Assessing Small Effects': Conclusions from a Conference Held in Berlin/Potsdam, Germany, 10–13 October 1995." *International Archives of Occupational and Environmental Health* 70 (1997): 67–70.

Holberg, Catharine J., Anne L. Wright, Fernando D. Martinez, C. George Ray, Lynn M. Taussig, Michael D. Lebowitz, and Group Health Medical Associates. "Risk Factors for Respiratory Syncytial Virus–Associated Lower Respiratory Illnesses in the First Year of Life." *American Journal of Epidemiology* 133, no. 11 (1991): 1135–51.

Hopkinson, Judy M. "Response to 'Is Breast Really Best? Risk and Total Motherhood in the National Breastfeeding Awareness Campaign.'" *Journal of Health Politics, Policy and Law* 32, no. 4 (2007): 649–54.

Horwood, L. John, and David M. Fergusson. "Breastfeeding and Later Cognitive and Academic Outcomes." *Pediatrics* 101, no. 1 (1998): e9–e15.

Hotz, Robert Lee. "The Difficulty of Finding Impartial Sources in Science." *Nieman Reports* 56, no. 3 (2002): 6–7.

Howie, Peter W., J. Stewart Forsyth, Simon A. Ogston, Ann Clark, and Charles du V. Florey. "Protective Effect of Breast Feeding Against Infection." *British Medical Journal* 300 (1990): 11–16.

Huang, Ze, Victoria Cabanela, and Timothy Howell. "Stress, Bottlefeeding, and Diabetes." *The Lancet* 350 (1997): 889.

Huus, Karina, Jonas F. Ludvigsson, Karin Enskar, and Johnny Ludvigsson. "Exclusive Breastfeeding of Swedish Children and Its Possible Influence on Development of Obesity: A Prospective Cohort Study." *BMC Pediatrics* 8, no. 42 (2008): 106.

Hyman, Michael R., and Richard Tansey. "The Ethics of Psychoactive Ads." *Journal of Business Ethics* 9 (1990): 105–14.

Infante-Rivard, Claire, Devendra Amre, Denyse Gautrin, and Jean-Luc Malo. "Family Size, Day-Care Attendance, and Breastfeeding in Relation to the Incidence of Childhood Asthma." *American Journal of Epidemiology* 153 (2001): 653–58.

Institute of Medicine (IOM) and National Research Council. *Local Government Actions to Prevent Childhood Obesity.* Washington, DC: National Academies Press, 2009.

International Epidemiological Association. "Proposed Ethics Guidelines for Epidemiologists" (1990). Available at www.akh-wien.ac.at/ROeS/ROeS/ROeS%20 Nr.%2031%20Ethik%20 for%20Epidemiologists.pdf.

International Journal of Epidemiology (special issue on obesity) 35, no. 1 (2006).

Ioannidis, John P. A. "Contradicted and Initially Stronger Effects in Highly Cited Clinical Research." *Journal of the American Medical Association* 294, no. 2 (2005): 218–28.

Ip, Stanley, M. Chung, G. Raman, P. Chew, N. Magula, D. DeVine, T. Trikalinos, and J. Lau. *Breastfeeding and Maternal and Infant Health Outcomes in Developed Countries.* Evidence Report / Technology Assessment no. 153. Prepared by Tufts–New England Medical Center, Evidence-Based Practice Center, under contract no. 290-02-0022. AHRQ Publication no. 07-E007. Rockville, MD: Agency for Healthcare Research and Quality, April 2007.

Isaacs, Elizabeth B., David G. Gadian, Stuart Sabatini, Wui K. Chong, Brian T. Quinn, Bruce R. Fischl, and Alan Lucas. "The Effect of Early Human Diet on Caudate Volumes and IQ." *Pediatric Research* 63 (2008): 308–14.

Isaacs, Julia B., Tracy Vericker, Jennifer Macomber, and Adam Kent. *Kids' Share: An Analysis of Federal Expenditures on Children through 2008.* Washington, DC: Brookings Institution, 2009.

Jackson, Leila W., Nora L. Lee, and Jonathan M. Samet. "Frequency of Policy Recommendations in Epidemiologic Publications." *American Journal of Public Health* 89, no. 8 (1999): 1206–11.

Jackson, Peter. "The Development of a Scientific Fact: The Case of Passive Smoking." In *The Sociology of Health Promotion*, ed. Robin Bunton, Sarah Nettleton, and Roger Burrows, 104–15. London: Routledge, 1995.

Jackson, Stevi, and Sue Scott. "Risk Anxiety and the Social Construction of Childhood." In *Risk and Sociocultural Theory: New Directions and Perspective*, ed. Deborah Lupton, 86–107. Cambridge: Cambridge University Press, 1999.

Jacobs, Jerry A., and Kathleen Gerson. *The Time Divide: Work, Family, and Gender Inequality.* Cambridge, MA: Harvard University Press, 2004.

Jacobson, Sandra W., and Joseph L. Jacobson. "Breastfeeding and Intelligence." *The Lancet* 339 (1992): 926–27.

———. Editorial: "Breast Feeding and Intelligence in Children." *British Medical Journal* 333 (2006): 929–30.

Jacobson, Sandra W., Lisa M. Chiodo, and Joseph L. Jacobson. "Breastfeeding Effects on Intelligence Quotient in 4- and 11-Year-Old Children." *Pediatrics* 103, no. 5 (1999): e71–e76.

Jain, Anjali, John Concato, and John M. Leventhal. "How Good Is the Evidence Linking Breastfeeding and Intelligence?" *Pediatrics* 109, no. 6 (2002): 1044–53.

Jansson, Maria. "Feeding Children and Protecting Women: The Emergence of Breastfeeding as an International Concern." *Women's Studies International Forum* 32 (2009): 240–48.

Jasanoff, Sheila, Gerald E. Markle, James C. Petersen, and Trevor Pinch, eds. *Handbook of Science and Technology Studies.* Thousand Oaks, CA: Sage, 1995.

Jelliffe, Derrick B., and E. F. Patrice Jelliffe, eds. *Programmes to Promote Breastfeeding.* Oxford: Oxford University Press, 1988.

Job, R. F. Soames. "Effective and Ineffective Use of Fear in Health Promotion Campaigns." *American Journal of Public Health* 78, no. 2 (1988): 163–67.

Johnson, Kay, Samuel F. Posner, Janis Bierman, José F. Cordero, Hani K. Atrash, Christopher S. Parker, Sheree Boulet, and Michele G. Curtis. "Recommendations to Improve Preconception Health and Health Care—United States: A Report of the CDC/ATSDR Preconception Care Work Group and the Select Panel on Preconception Care." *MMWR Recommendations and Reports* no. 55:RR06, April 21, 2006, 1–23.

Johnson, Timothy. "Shattuck Lecture—Medicine and the Media." *New England Journal of Medicine* 339, no. 2 (1998): 87–92.

Joint Commission. *What Did the Doctor Say? Improving Health Literacy to Protect Patient Safety.* Oakbrook Terrace, IL: Joint Commission, 2007.

Julvez, Jordi, Núria Ribas-Fitó, Maria Forns, Raquel Garcia-Esteban, Maries Torrent, and Jordi Sunyer. "Attention Behaviour and Hyperactivity at Age 4 and Duration of Breast-Feeding." *Acta Paediatrica* 96 (2007): 842–47.

Kagan, Jerome. *Three Seductive Ideas*. Cambridge, MA: Harvard University Press, 1998.

Kalb, Claudia. "Big Binky Brouhaha." *Newsweek*, October 31, 2005.

Kaplan, E. Ann. "Look Who's Talking, Indeed: Fetal Images in Recent North American Visual Culture." In *Mothering: Ideology, Experience, and Agency*, ed. Evelyn Nakano Glenn, Grace Chang, and Linda Rennie Forcey, 121–38. New York: Routledge, 1994.

———. "Sex, Work, and Motherhood: Maternal Subjectivity in Recent Visual Culture." In *Representations of Motherhood*, ed. Donna Bassin, Margaret Honey, and Meryle Mahrer Kaplan, 256–71. New Haven, CT: Yale University Press, 1994.

Karbo, Karen. "Goodbye, Moon." *New York Times*, December 4, 2005.

Kasperson, Roger E. "The Social Amplification of Risk: Progress in Developing an Integrative Framework." In *Social Theories of Risk*, ed. Sheldon Krimsky and Dominic Golding, 153–78. Westport, CT: Praeger, 1992.

Kasperson, Roger E., Nayna Jhaveri, and Jeanne X. Kasperson. "Stigma and the Social Amplification of Risk: Toward a Framework of Analysis." In *Risk, Media, and*

Stigma: Understanding Public Challenges to Modern Science and Technology, ed. James Flynn, Paul Slovic, and Howard Kunreuther, 9–27. London: Earthscan, 2001.

Kass, Nancy E. "An Ethics Framework for Public Health." *American Journal of Public Health* 91, no. 11 (2001): 1776–82.

Katz, Deborah. "New Reasons to Watch What You Eat: Nourishment in the Womb May Matter Decades Later." *U.S. News & World Report*, September 22, 2007. Available at health.usnews.com/articles/health/2007/09/22/nourishment-in-the-womb-may-matter-decades-later.html (accessed October 22, 2007).

Kaufman, Marc, and Christopher Lee. "HHS Toned down Breast-Feeding Ads." *Washington Post*, August 31, 2007.

Kelleher, Christa M. "The Physical Challenges of Early Breastfeeding." *Social Science & Medicine* 63 (2006): 2727–38.

Kelleher, Shannon L., and B. Lönnderdal. "Immunological Activities Associated with Milk." In *Advances in Nutritional Research*, ed. B. Woodward and H. Draper, 39–65. New York: Plenum Press, 2001.

Keller, Punam Anand. "Converting the Unconverted: The Effect of Inclination and Opportunity to Discount Health-Related Fear Appeals." *Journal of Applied Psychology* 84, no. 3 (1999): 403–15.

Kempner, Joanna, Clifford S. Perlis, and Jon F. Merz. "Forbidden Knowledge." *Science* 307 (2005): 854.

Kerber, Linda K. *Women of the Republic: Intellect and Ideology in Revolutionary America*. Chapel Hill: University of North Carolina Press, 1980.

Kersh, Rogan, and James Morone. "How the Personal Becomes Political: Prohibitions, Public Health, and Obesity." *Studies in American Political Development* 16 (2002): 162–75.

Kirkwood, William G., and Dan Brown. "Public Communication about the Causes of Disease: The Rhetoric of Responsibility." *Journal of Communication* 45, no. 1 (1995): 55–76.

Klein, M. Inés, Eduardo Bergel, Luz Gibbons, Silvina Coviello, Gabriela Bauer, Alicia Benitez, M. Elina Serra, M. Florencia Delgado, Guillermina A. Melendi, Susana Rodriguez, Steven R. Kleeberger, and Fernando P. Polack. "Differential Gender Response to Respiratory Infections and to the Protective Effect of Breast Milk in Preterm Infants." *Pediatrics* 121 (2008): 1510–16.

Klement, Eyal, Regev V. Cohen, Jonathan Boxman, Aviva Joseph, and Shimon Reif. "Breastfeeding and Risk of Inflammatory Bowel Disease: A Systematic Review with Meta-Analysis." *American Journal of Clinical Nutrition* 80, no. 5 (2004): 1342–52.

Knobler, Michael Davidson, and Ezra Susser. "Advancing Paternal Age and Autism." *Archives of General Psychiatry* 63, no. 9 (2006): 1026–32.

Kolata, Gina. "Grant System Leads Cancer Researchers to Play It Safe." *New York Times*, June 28, 2009.

———. *Rethinking Thin: The New Science of Weight Loss— And the Myths and Realities of Dieting*. New York: Farrar, Strauss & Giroux, 2007.

———. "10 Million Women Who Lack Cervices Still Get Pap Tests." *New York Times*, June 23, 2004.

Kolevzon, Alexander, Raz Gross, and Abraham Reichenberg. "Prenatal and Perinatal Risk Factors for Autism: A Review and Integration of Findings." *Archives of Pediatrics and Adolescent Medicine* 161, no. 4 (2007): 326–33.

Koren, Gideon, and Naomi Klein. "Bias against Negative Studies in Newspaper Reports of Medical Research." *Journal of the American Medical Association* 266, no. 13 (1991): 1824–26.

Koren, Gideon, Heather Shear, Karen Graham, and Tom Einarson. "Bias against the Null Hypothesis: The Reproductive Hazards of Cocaine." *The Lancet* 1 (1989): 1440–42.

Kraemer, Helena C., Ellen Frank, and David J. Kupfer. "Moderators of Treatment Outcomes: Clinical, Research, and Policy Importance." *Journal of the American Medical Association* 296, no. 10 (2006): 1286–89.

Kramer, Michael S. "Does Breast Feeding Help Protect against Atopic Disease? Biology, Methodology, and a Golden Jubilee of Controversy." *Journal of Pediatrics* 112 (1988): 181–90.

———. "Randomized Trials and Public Health Interventions: Time to End the Scientific Double Standard." *Clinical Perinatology* 30 (2003): 351–61.

———. "Testing Hypotheses: Reply." *British Medical Journal* 335 (2007): 1061.

Kramer, Michael S., Frances Aboud, Elena Mironova, Irina Vanilovich, Robert W. Platt, Lidia Matush, Sergei Igumnov, Eric Fombonne, Natalia Bogdanovich, Thierry Ducruet, Jean-Paul Collet, Beverley Chalmers, Ellen Hodnett, Sergei Davidovsky, Oleg Skugarevsky, Oleg Trofimovich, Ludmila Kozlova, and Stanley Shapiro. "Breastfeeding and Child Cognitive Development: New Evidence from a Large Randomized Trial." *Archives of General Psychiatry* 65, no. 5 (2008): 578–84.

Kramer, Michael S., B. Chalmers, E. D. Hodnet, et al. for the PROBIT Study Group. "Promotion of Breastfeeding Intervention Trial (PROBIT): A Randomized Trial in the Republic of Belarus." *Journal of the American Medical Association* 285 (2001): 413–20.

Kramer, Michael S., Eric Fombonne, Sergei Igumnov, Irina Vanilovich, Lidia Matush, Elena Mironova, Natalia Bogdanovich, Richard E. Tremblay, Beverley Chalmers, Xun-Zhang, and Robert W. Platt. "Effects of Prolonged and Exclusive Breastfeeding on Child Behavior and Maternal Adjustment: Evidence from a Large, Randomized Trial."

Pediatrics 121, no. 3 (2008): 435–40.

Kramer, Michael S., Lidia Matush, Irina Vanilovich, Robert W. Platt, Natalia Bogdanovich, Zinaida Sevkovskaya, Irina Dzikovich, Gyorgy Shishko, Jean-Paul Collet, Richard M. Martin, George Davey Smith, Matthew W. Gillman, Beverley Chalmers, Ellen Hodnett, and Stanley Shapiro. "Effects of Prolonged and Exclusive Breastfeeding on Child Height, Weight, Adiposity, and Blood Pressure at Age 6.5 Y: Evidence from a Large Randomized Trial." *American Journal of Clinical Nutrition* 86 (2007): 1717–21.

Kramer, Michael S., Lidia Matush, Irina Vanilovich, Robert Platt, Natalia Bogdanovich, Zinaida Sevkovskaya, Irina Dzikovich, Gyorgy Shishko, and Bruce Mazer. "Effect of Prolonged and Exclusive Breast Feeding on Risk of Allergy and Asthma: Cluster Randomized Trial." *British Medical Journal* 335 (2007): 385–90.

Kramer, M. S., I. Vanilovich, L. Matush, N. Bogdanovich, X. Zhang, G. Shishko, M. Muller-Bolla, and R. W. Platt. "The Effect of Prolonged and Exclusive Breast-Feeding on Dental Caries in Early School-Age Children." *Caries Research* 41 (2007): 484–88.

Krieger, Nancy. "Questioning Epidemiology: Objectivity, Advocacy, and Socially Responsible Science." *American Journal of Public Health* 89, no. 8 (1999): 1151–53.

Krimsky, Sheldon, and Dominic Golding, eds. *Social Theories of Risk*. Westport, CT: Praeger, 1992.

Krugman, Scott, Paul Law, David Fergusson, and L. John Horwood. "Breastfeeding and IQ." *Pediatrics* 103 (1999): 193–94.

Kua, Eunice, Micheal Reder, and Martha J. Grossel. "Science in the News: A Study of Reporting Genomics." *Public Understanding of Science* 13 (2004): 309–22.

Kuhn, Thomas. *The Structure of Scientific Revolutions*. 3rd ed. Chicago: University of Chicago Press, 1996.

Kukla, Rebecca. "Ethics and Ideology in Breastfeeding Advocacy Campaigns." *Hypatia* 21, no. 1 (2006): 157–80.

Kull, Inger, Catarina Almqvist, Gunnar Lilja, Göran Pershagen, and Magnus Wickman. "Breast-Feeding Reduces the Risk of Asthma during the First 4 Years of Life." *Journal of Allergy and Clinical Immunology* 114 (2004): 755–60.

Kunreuther, Howard, and Paul Slovic. "Coping with Stigma: Challenges and Opportunities." In *Risk, Media, and Stigma: Understanding Public Challenges to Modern Science and Technology*, ed. James Flynn, Paul Slovic, and Howard Kunreuther, 331–52. London: Earthscan, 2001.

Kunz, Thomas H., and David J. Hosken. "Male Lactation: Why, Why Not and Is It Care?" *Trends in Ecology and Evolution* 24, no. 2 (2009): 80–85.

Kuran, Timur, and Cass R. Sunstein. "Availability Cascades and Risk Regulation." *Stanford Law Review* 51, no. 4 (1999): 683–768.

Kutner, Mark, Elaine Greenberg, Ying Jin, and Christine Paulsen. *The Health Literacy of America's Adults: Results from the 2003 National Assessment of Adult Literacy* (NCES-483). Washington, DC: National Center for Education Statistics, U.S. Department of Education, 2006.

Kwok, Man Ki, C. Mary Schooling, Tai Hing Lam, and Gabriel M. Leung. "Does Breastfeeding Protect against Childhood Overweight? Hong Kong's 'Children of 1997' Birth Cohort." *International Journal of Epidemiology*, electronic publication (2009): 1–9.

La Leche League International. *The Womanly Art of Breastfeeding*. 2nd ed. Franklin Park, IL: La Leche League International, 1963.

———. *The Womanly Art of Breastfeeding*. 7th ed. New York: Plume, 2004.

Ladd-Taylor, Molly, and Lauri Umansky, eds. *"Bad" Mothers: The Politics of Blame in Twentieth-Century America*. New York: New York University Press, 1998.

Ladomenou, Fani, Anthony Kafatos, and Emmanouil Galanakis. "Risk Factors Related to Intention to Breastfeed, Early Weaning and Suboptimal Duration of Breastfeeding." *Acta Paediatrica* 96 (2007): 1441–44.

LaKind, Judy S., Cheston M. Berlin Jr., and Donald R. Mattison. "The Heart of the Matter on Breastmilk and Environmental Chemicals: Essential Points for Healthcare Providers and New Parents." *Breastfeeding Medicine* 3, no. 4 (2008): 251–59.

LaKind, Judy S., Cheston M. Berlin Jr., Andreas Sjödin, Wayman Turner, Richard Y. Wang, Larry L. Needham, Ian M. Paul, Jennifer L. Stokes, Daniel Q. Naiman, and Donald G. Patterson Jr. "Do Human Milk Concentrations of Persistent Organic Chemicals Really Decline during Lactation? Chemical Concentrations during Lactation and Milk/Serum Partitioning." *Environmental Health Perspectives* 117, no. 10 (2009): 1625–31.

Landrigan, Philip J., Babasaheb Sonawane, Donald Mattison, Michael McAlly, and Anjali Garg. "Chemical Contaminants in Breast Milk and Their Impacts on Children's Health: An Overview." *Environmental Health Perspectives* 110, no. 6 (2002): A313–15.

Lane, Karen. "The Medical Model of the Body as a Site of Risk: A Case Study of Childbirth." In *Medicine, Health and Risk: Sociological Approaches*, ed. Jonathan Gabe, 53–72. Oxford: Blackwell, 1995.

Lareau, Annette. *Unequal Childhoods: Class, Race, and Family Life*. Berkeley: University of California Press, 2003.

Lash, Scott. "Risk Culture." In *The Risk Society and Beyond: Critical Issues for Social Theory*, ed. Barbara Adam, Ulrich Beck, and Joost Van Loon, 47–62. London: Sage, 2000.

Lash, Scott, Bronislaw Szerszynski, and Brian Wynne, eds. *Risk, Environment, and Modernity: Towards a New Ecology*. London: Sage, 1996.

Lauritzen, Sonja Olin, and Lisbeth Sachs. "Normality, Risk and the Future: Implicit Communication of Threat in Health Surveillance." *Sociology of Health and Illness* 23, no. 4 (2001): 497–516.

Law, Jules. "The Politics of Breastfeeding: Assessing Risk, Dividing Labor." *Signs: Journal of Women in Culture and Society* 25, no. 2 (2000): 407–50.

Lawrence, Ruth A. "Breastfeeding in Belarus." *Journal of the American Medical Association* 285, no. 4 (2001): 463–64.

———. "Major Difficulties in Promoting Breastfeeding: US Perspectives." In *Programmes to Support Breastfeeding*, ed. Derrick B. Jelliffe and E. F. Jelliffe, 267–71. Oxford: Oxford University Press, 1988.

Leavitt, Judith Walzer. *Brought to Bed: Childbearing in America, 1750–1950*. New York: Oxford University Press, 1986.

Lebow, Morton A. "The Pill and the Press: Reporting Risk." *Obstetrics and Gynecology* 99, no. 3 (1999): 453–56.

Lee, Ellie J. "Infant Feeding in Risk Society." *Health, Risk & Society* 9, no. 3 (2007): 295–309.

———. "Living with Risk in the Age of 'Intensive Motherhood': Maternal Identity and Infant Feeding." *Health, Risk, and Society* 10, no. 5 (2008): 467–77.

Lee, Ellie, and Jennie Bristow. "Rules for Feeding Babies." In *Regulating Autonomy: Sex, Reproduction, and Family*, ed. Shelley Day Sclater, Shelley Day, Fatemah Ebtehaj, Emily Jackson, and Martin Richards, 73–91. Oxford: Hart Publishing, 2009.

Lemke, Thomas. "Disposition and Determinism—Genetic Diagnostics in Risk Society." *Sociological Review* 52, no. 4 (2004): 550–66.

León-Cava, Natalia. *Quantifying the Benefits of Breastfeeding: A Summary of the Evidence*. Washington, DC: Pan American Health Organization, 2002.

Leschied, Alan W., Debbie Chiodo, Paul C. Whitehead, and Dermot Hurley. "The Relationship between Maternal Depression and Child Outcomes in a Child Welfare Sample: Implications for Treatment and Policy." *Child and Family Social Work* 10, no. 4 (2005): 281–91.

Levi, Ragnar. *Medical Journalism: Exposing Fact, Fiction, Fraud*. Ames: Iowa State University Press, 2001.

Levine, Madeline. *The Price of Privilege: How Parental Pressure and Material Advantage Are Creating a Generation of Disconnected and Unhappy Kids*. New York: HarperCollins, 2006.

Levitas, Ruth. "Discourses of Risk and Utopia." In *The Risk Society and Beyond: Critical Issues for Social Theory*, ed. Barbara Adam, Ulrich Beck, and Joost Van Loon, 198–210. London: Sage, 2000.

Lewin, Ellen. "Negotiating Lesbian Motherhood: The Dialectics of Resistance and Accommodation." In *Mothering: Ideology, Experience, and Agency*, ed. Evelyn Nakano Glenn, Grace Chang, and Linda Rennie Forcey, 333–54. New York: Routledge, 1994.

Lewin, Tamar. "Study Links Working Mothers to Slow Learning." *New York Times*, July 17, 2002.

Li, L., T. J. Parsons, and C. Power. "Breast Feeding and Obesity in Childhood: Cross-Sectional Study." *British Medical Journal* 327 (2003): 904–5.

Li, Ruowei, Natalie Darling, Emmanuel Maurice, Lawrence Barker, and Laurence M. Grummer-Strawn. "Breastfeeding Rates in the United States by Characteristics of the Child, Mother, or Family: The 2002 National Immunization Survey." *Pediatrics* 115, no. 1 (2005): e31–e37.

Li, Ruowei, Cynthia Ogden, Carol Ballew, Cathleen Gillespie, and Laurence Grummer-Strawn. "Prevalence of Exclusive Breastfeeding among US Infants: The Third National Health and Nutrition Examination Survey (Phase II, 1991–1994)." *American Journal of Public Health* 92, no. 7 (2002): 1107–10.

Li, Yang, and Kathryn Jacobsen. "A Systematic Review of the Association between Breastfeeding and Breast Cancer." *Journal of Women's Health* 17, no. 10 (2008): 1635–45.

Liberati, Alessandro. "'Meta-Analysis: Statistical Alchemy for the 21st Century': Discussion. A Plea for a More Balanced View of Meta-Analysis and Systematic Overviews of the Effect of Health Care Interventions." *Journal of Clinical Epidemiology* 48, no. 1 (1995): 81–86.

Libster, Romina, Jimena Bugna Hortoneda, Federico R. Laham, Javier M. Cassellas, Victor Israel, Norberto R. Polack, Maria Florenica Delgado, Maria Inés Klein, and Fernando P. Polack. "Breastfeeding Prevents Severe Disease in Full Term Infants with Acute Respiratory Infection." *Pediatric Infectious Disease Journal* 28, no. 2 (2009): 131–34.

Lima, Rosângela da Costa, Cesar G. Victora, Ana Maria B. Menezes, and Fernando C. Barros. "Do Risk Factors for Childhood Infections and Malnutrition Protect against Asthma? A Study of Brazilian Male Adolescents." *American Journal of Public Health* 93, no. 11 (2003): 1858–64.

Lipkus, Isaac M., Monica Biradavolu, Kathryn Fenn, Punam Keller, and Barbara K. Rimer. "Informing Women about Their Breast Cancer Risks: Truth and Consequences." *Health Communication* 13, no. 2 (2001): 205–26.

Lippman, Abby. "The Genetic Construction of Prenatal Testing: Choice, Consent, or Conformity for Women?" In *Women and Prenatal Testing: Facing the Challenges of Genetic Technology*, ed. Karen H. Rothenberg and Elizabeth J. Thompson, 9–34. Columbus: Ohio State University Press, 1994.

Little, Miles. "Assignments of Meaning in Epidemiology." *Social Science and Medicine* 47, no. 9 (1998): 1135–45.

Lloyd, Elisabeth. *The Case of the Female Orgasm.* Cambridge, MA: Harvard University Press, 2005.

Loke, Yoon K., and Sheena Derry. "Does Anybody Read 'Evidence-Based' Articles?" *BMC Medical Research Methodology* 3 (2003): 14–18.

Lovaglia, Michael, Jeffrey W. Lucas, Jeffrey A. Houser, Shane Thye, and Barry Markovsky. "Status Processes and Mental Ability Test Scores." *American Journal of Sociology* 104 (1998): 195–228.

Lowenberg, June S. "Health Promotion and the 'Ideology of Choice.'" *Public Health Nursing* 12, no. 5 (1995): 319–23.

Lozoff, Betsy, Elias Jiminez, Abraham W. Wolf, Mary Lu Anginelli, Jigna Zatakia, Sandra W. Jacobson, Niko Kaciroti, Katy M. Clark, Min Tao, Marcela Castillo, Tomas Walter, and Paulino Pino. "Higher Infant Blood Levels with Longer Duration of Breastfeeding." *Journal of Pediatrics*, electronic publication (2009): 1–5.

Lu, M. C., L. Lange, W. Slusser, J. Hamilton, and N. Halfon. "Provider Encouragement of Breast-Feeding: Evidence from a National Survey." *Obstetrics and Gynecology* 97, no. 2 (2001): 290–95.

Lucas, A., R. Morley, T. J. Cole, G. Lister, and C. Leeson-Payne. "Breast Milk and Subsequent Intelligence Quotient in Children Born Preterm." *The Lancet* 339 (1992): 261–64.

Ludden, Jennifer. "Teaching Black Women to Embrace Breast-Feeding." Available at www.npr.org/templates/transcript/transcript.php?storyId=121755349 (accessed January 6, 2010).

Ludington-Hoe, Susan M., Patricia E. McDonald, and Rosemarie Satyshur. "Breastfeeding in African-American Women." *Journal of National Black Nurses Association* 13, no. 1 (2002): 56–64.

Luhmann, Niklas. *Risk: A Sociological Theory.* New York: Aldine de Gruyter, 1993.

Lupton, Deborah. *The Imperative of Health: Public Health and the Regulated Body.* London: Sage, 1995.

———. *Risk.* New York: Routledge, 1999.

———. "Risk and the Ontology of Pregnant Embodiment." In *Risk and Sociocultural Theory: New Directions and Perspective*, ed. Deborah Lupton, 59–85. Cambridge: Cambridge University Press, 1999.

———, ed. *Risk and Sociocultural Theory: New Directions and Perspectives.* Cambridge: Cambridge University Press, 1999.

Lyerly, Anne Drapkin, Lisa M. Mitchell, Elizabeth M. Armstrong, Lisa H. Harris, Rebecca Kukla, Miriam Kupperman, and Margaret Olivia Little. "Risks, Values, and Decision-Making Surrounding Pregnancy." *Obstetrics and Gynecology* 109, no. 4 (2007): 979–84.

Maciejewski, Jeffrey J. "Is the Use of Sexual and Fear Appeals Ethical? A Moral Evaluation by Generation Y College Students." *Journal of Current Issues and Research in Advertising* 26, no. 2 (2004): 97–105.

Maddux, James E. "Social Science, Social Policy, and Scientific Research." *American Psychologist* 48 (1993): 689–91.

Maguire, John. "The Tears inside a Stone: Reflections on the Ecology of Fear." In *Risk, Environment and Modernity: Towards a New Ecology,* ed. Scott Lash, Bronislaw Szerszynski, and Brian Wynne, 169–88. London: Sage, 1996.

Maher, Vanessa, ed. *The Anthropology of Breast-Feeding: Natural Law or Social Construct?* Oxford: Berg, 1992.

———. "Breast-Feeding in Cross-Cultural Perspective." In *The Anthropology of Breast-Feeding: Natural Law or Social Construct?* ed. Vanessa Maher, 1–36. Oxford: Berg, 1992.

———. "Breast-Feeding and Maternal Depletion: Natural Law or Cultural Arrangements?" In *The Anthropology of Breast-Feeding: Natural Law or Social Construct?* ed. Vanessa Maher, 151–80. Oxford: Berg, 1992.

Mahnke, C. Becket. "The Growth and Development of a Specialty: The History of Pediatrics." *Clinical Pediatrics* 39 (2000): 705–14.

Mahony, Rhona. *Kidding Ourselves: Breadwinning, Babies, and Bargaining Power.* New York: Basic Books, 1995.

Mahowald, Mary Briody. *Women and Children in Health Care: An Unequal Majority.* Oxford: Oxford University Press, 1993.

Mai, Xiao-Mei, Allan B. Becker, Elizabeth A. C. Sellers, Joel J. Liem, and Anita L. Kozyrskyj. "The Relationship of Breast-Feeding, Overweight, and Asthma in Preadolescents." *Journal of Allergy and Clinical Immunology* 120 (2007): 551–56.

Malacrida, Claudia. "Alternative Therapies and Attention Deficit Disorder: Discourses of Maternal Responsibility and Risk." *Gender & Society* 16, no. 3 (2002): 366–85.

Malaspina, Delores, Susan Harlap, Shmuel Fennig, Dov Heiman, Daniella Nahon, Dina Feldman, and Ezra S. Susser. "Advancing Paternal Age and the Risk of Schizophrenia." *Archives of General Psychiatry* 58, no. 4 (2001): 361–67.

Malat, Jennifer, Hyn Joo Oh, and Mary Ann Hamilton. "Poverty Experience, Race, and Child Health." *Public Health Reports* 120 (2005): 442–47.

Mandhane, Piush J., Justina M. Greene, and Malcolm R. Sears. "Interactions between Breast-Feeding, Specific Parental Atopy, and Sex on Development of Asthma and Atopy." *Journal of Allergy and Clinical Immunology* 119, no. 6 (2007): 1359–66.

Mann, Jonathan M. "Medicine and Public Health, Ethics and Human Rights." *Hastings Center Report* 27, no. 3 (1997): 6–13.

Mark, Anne P. *The Complete Idiot's Guide to Breastfeeding.*

Indianapolis: Macmillan, 2001.

Marmot, Michael. *The Status Syndrome: How Social Standing Affects Our Health and Longevity.* New York: Henry Holt, 2004.

Marsh, Margaret S., and Wanda Ronner. *The Empty Cradle: Infertility in America from Colonial Times to the Present.* Baltimore: Johns Hopkins University Press, 1996.

Marshall, Joyce L., Mary Godfrey, and Mary J. Renfrew. "Being a 'Good Mother': Managing Breastfeeding and Merging Identities." *Social Science & Medicine* 65 (2007): 2147–59.

Marshall, Melinda. "Understanding Autism." *Parenting,* April 2007. Available at www.parenting.com/ parenting/child/article/0,19840,1597741,00. html (accessed July 14, 2007).

Martin, Richard Michael, Sarah Goodhall, David J. Gunnell, and George Davey Smith. "Breastfeeding in Infancy and Social Mobility: 60 Year Follow-up of the Boyd Orr Cohort." *Archives of Disease in Childhood* 92, no. 4 (2007): 317–21.

Martins, Carla, and E. A. Gaffan. "Effects of Early Maternal Depression on Patterns of Infant-Mother Attachment: A Meta-Analytic Investigation." *Child Psychology and Psychiatry* 41 (2000): 737–46.

Mason, J. B., B. F. Cole, J. A. Baron, Y-I Kim, and A. D. Smith. "Folic Acid Fortification and Cancer Risk." *The Lancet* 371 (2008): 1335.

Mason, Jason B., Aaron Dickstein, Paul F. Jacques, Paul Haggarty, Jacob Selhub, Gerard Dallal, and Irwin Rosenberg. "A Temporal Association between Folic Acid Fortification and an Increase in Colorectal Cancer Rates May Be Illuminating Important Biological Principles: A Hypothesis." *Cancer Epidemiology Biomarkers & Prevention* 16, no. 7 (2007): 1325–29.

Mason, Karen Oppenheim, and An-Magrit Jensen, eds. *Gender and Family Change in Industrialized Countries.* Oxford: Clarendon Press, 1995.

Massumi, Brian, ed. *The Politics of Everyday Fear.* Minneapolis: University of Minnesota Press, 1993.

Matanoski, Genevieve. "Conflicts between Two Cultures: Implications for Epidemiologic Researchers in Communicating with Policy-Makers." *American Journal of Epidemiology* 154, no. 12 (2001): S36–S42.

Matheson, Melanie Claire, Bircan Erbas, Aindralal Belasuriya, Mark Andrew Jenkins, Cathryn Leisa Wharton, Mimi Lai-Kuan Tang, Michael John Abramson, Eugene Hayden Walters, John Llewelyn Hopper, and Shyamali Chandrika Dharmage. "Breast-Feeding and Atopic Disease: A Cohort Study from Childhood to Middle Age." *Journal of Allergy and Clinical Immunology* 120 (2007): 1051–57.

Maurer, Donna, and Jeffrey Sobal, eds. *Eating Agendas: Food and Nutrition as Social Problems.* New York: Aldine de Gruyter, 1995.

Maushart, Susan. *The Mask of Motherhood.* New York: Penguin, 1999.

May, Elaine Tyler. "Nonmothers as Bad Mothers: Infertility and the 'Maternal Instinct.'" In *"Bad" Mothers: The Politics of Blame in Twentieth-Century America*, ed. Molly Ladd-Taylor and Lauri Umansky, 198–219. New York: New York University Press, 1998.

Mayer-Davis, Elizabeth J., Dana Dabelea, Archana Pande Lamichhane, Ralph B. D'Agostino Jr., Angela D. Liese, Joan Thomas, Robert E. McKeown, and Richard F. Hamman. "Breast-Feeding and Type 2 Diabetes in the Youth of Three Ethnic Groups." *Diabetes Care* 31 (2008): 470–75.

McDonnell, Jane Taylor. "On Being the 'Bad' Mother of an Autistic Child." In *"Bad" Mothers: The Politics of Blame in Twentieth-Century America*, ed. Molly Ladd-Taylor and Lauri Umansky, 220–29. New York: New York University Press, 1998.

McDowell, Margaret M., Chia-Yih Wang, and Jocelyn Kennedy-Stephenson. "Breastfeeding in the United States: Findings from the National Health and Nutrition Examination Surveys, 1999–2006." NCHS data briefs no. 5. Hyattsville, MD: National Center for Health Statistics, 2008.

McGrath, John J. "The Surprisingly Rich Contours of Schizophrenia Epidemiology." *Archives of General Psychiatry* 64 (2007): 14–16.

McKinlay, John B., and Lisa D. Marceau. "To Boldly Go. . . ." *American Journal of Public Health* 90, no. 1 (2000): 25–33.

McMichael, A. J. "Prisoners of the Proximate: Loosening the Constraints on Epidemiology in an Age of Change." *American Journal of Epidemiology* 149, no. 10 (1999): 887–97.

Mead, M. Nathaniel. "Contaminants in Human Milk: Weighing the Risks against the Benefits of Breastfeeding." *Environmental Health Perspectives* 116, no. 10 (2008): A427–34.

Mesure, Susie. "Press Twisted My Words, Says Academic in Breast-Milk Row." *The Independent*, August 2, 2009.

Michel, Sonya. *Children's Interest, Mothers' Rights: The Shaping of America's Child Care Policy.* New Haven, CT: Yale University Press, 1999.

Michels, Dia, ed. *Breastfeeding Annual International 2001.* Washington, DC: Platypus Media LLC, 2001.

Michels, K. B., W. C. Willett, B. I. Graubard, R. L. Vaidya, M. M. Cantwell, L. B. Sansbury, and M. R. Forman. "A Longitudinal Study of Infant Feeding and Obesity throughout the Life Course." *International Journal of Obesity* 31 (2007): 1078–95.

Mihrshahi, S., R. Ampon, C. Almqvist, A. S. Kemp, D. Hector, and G. B. Marks. "The Association between Infant Feeding Practices and Subsequent Atopy among Children with a Family History of Asthma." *Clinical and Experimental Allergy* 37 (2007): 671–79.

Miller, Jon D. "Public Under-standing of, and Attitudes toward, Scientific Research: What We Know and What We Need to Know." *Public Understanding of Science* 13 (2004): 273–94.

Millman, Sara. "Breastfeeding and Infant Mortality: Un-tangling the Complex Web of Causality." *Sociological Quarterly* 26, no. 1 (1985): 65–79.

Milloy, Steven J. *Junk Science Judo: Self-Defense against Health Scares and Scams*. Washington, DC: Cato Institute, 2001.

Mills, James L., and Caroline Signore. "Neural Tube De-fect Rates before and after Food Fortification with Folic Acid." *Birth Defects Research Part A: Clinical and Molecular Teratology* 70, no. 11 (2004): 844–45.

Monterrosa, Eva C., Edward A. Frongillo, Edgar M. Vásquez-Garibay, Enrique Romero Velarde, Linda M. Casey, and Noreen D. Wil-lows. "Predominant Breast-Feeding from Birth to Six Months Is Associated with Fewer Gastrointestinal Infections and Increased Risk for Iron Deficiency among Infants." *Journal of Nutrition* 138 (2008): 1499–1504.

Montgomery, Scott L. *The Scientific Voice*. New York: Guilford Press, 1996.

Montgomery, Scott M., Anna Ehlin, and Amanda Sacker. "Breast Feeding and Resil-ience against Psychosocial Stress." *Archives of Disease in Childhood* 91 (2006): 990–94.

Morgen, Sandra. *Into Our Own Hands: The Women's Health Movement in the United States, 1969–1990*. New Brunswick, NJ: Rutgers University Press, 2002.

Morone, James A. "Enemies of the People: The Moral Di-mension to Public Health." *Journal of Health Politics, Policy and Law* 22, no. 4 (1997): 993–1020.

Morris, Richard J. "Are Breast-feeding and Diet Strategies Overrated for the Preven-tion of Atopy?" *American Journal of Clinical Nutrition* 101 (2008): 113.

Mortensen, Erik Lykke. "Neuro-Developmental Effects of Breastfeeding." *Acta Paediat-rica* 96 (2007): 796–97.

Mortensen, Erik Lykke, Kim Fleischer Michaelsen, Steph-anie A. Sanders, and June Machover Reinisch. "The As-sociation between Duration of Breastfeeding and Adult Intelligence." *Journal of the American Medical Association* 287, no. 18 (2002): 2365–72.

Moss, Kary L., ed. *Man-Made Medicine: Women's Health, Public Policy, and Reform*. Durham, NC: Duke Univer-sity Press, 1996.

Moynihan, Ray, Lisa Bero, Den-nis Ross-Degnan, David Henry, Kirby Lee, Judy Watkins, Connie Mah, and Stephen B. Soumerai. "Cov-erage by the News Media of the Benefits and Risks of Medications." *New England Journal of Medicine* 342, no. 22 (2000): 1645–50.

Muller, Mike. *The Baby Killer: A War on Want Investigation into the Promotion and Sale of Powdered Baby Milks in the Third World*. London: War on Want, 1974.

Murkoff, Heidi E., Arlene Eisen-berg, Sandee E. Hathaway, and Sharon Mazel. *What to Expect the First Year*. 2nd ed. New York: Workman, 2003.

Murkoff, Heidi E., Arlene Eisen-berg, and Sandee E. Hatha-way. *What to Expect When You're Expecting*. 2nd to 4th eds. New York: Workman, 1996–2008.

Murphy, Elizabeth. "'Breast Is Best': Infant Feeding Deci-sions and Maternal Deviance." *Sociology of Health and Illness* 21, no. 2 (1999): 187–208.

———. "Risk, Maternal Ideolo-gies, and Infant Feeding." In *A Sociology of Food and Nu-trition*, ed. John Germov and Lauren Williams, 200–219. Oxford: Oxford University Press, 2004.

———. "Risk, Responsibility, and Rhetoric in Infant Feed-ing." *Journal of Contempo-rary Ethnography* 29, no. 3 (2000): 291–325.

Murray, David, Joel Schwarz, and S. Robert Lichter. *It Ain't Necessarily So: How Media Make and Unmake the Scientific Picture of Reality*. New York: Penguin, 2002.

Mythen, Gabe, and Sandra Walklate, eds. *Beyond the Risk Society: Critical Reflec-tions on Risk and Human Security*. New York: Open University Press, 2006.

Nadesan, Majia Holmer, and Patty Sotirin. "The Romance and Science of 'Breast Is Best': Discursive Contradic-tions and Contexts of Breast-Feeding Choices." *Text and Performance Quarterly* 18, no. 3 (1998): 217–32.

Nafsted, Per, J. J. K. Jaakkola, J. A. Hagen, G. Botten, and J. Kongerud. "Breastfeeding, Maternal Smoking and Lower Respiratory Tract Infections." *European Respiratory Journal* 9 (1996): 2623–29.

Nagel, G., G. Büchele, G. Weinmayr, B. Björkstén, Y.-Z. Chen, H. Wang, W. Nystad, Y. Saraclar, L. Bråbäck, J. Batlles-Garrido, G. Garcia-Hernandez, S. K. Weiland, and the ISAAC Phase II Study Group. "Effect of Breastfeeding on Asthma, Lung Function and Bronchial Hyperreactivity in ISAAC Phase II." *European Respiratory Journal* 33, no. 5 (2009): 993–1002.

National Institute of Child Health and Human Development Early Child Care Research Network. "Affect Dysregulation in the Mother-Child Relationship in the Toddler Years: Antecedents and Consequences." *Development and Psychopathology* 16 (2004): 43–68.

———. "Chronicity of Maternal Depressive Symptoms, Maternal Sensitivity, and Child Functioning at 36 Months." *Developmental Psychology* 35, no. 5 (1999): 1297–1310.

———. "Familial Factors Associated with the Characteristics of Nonmaternal Care for Infants." *Journal of Marriage and the Family* 59 (1997): 389–408.

———. "Poverty and Patterns of Child Care." In *Consequences of Growing up Poor*, ed. Greg J. Duncan and Jeanne Brooks-Gunn, 100–31. New York: Russell Sage Foundation, 1997.

National Institutes of Health. "Breastfeeding Has Minor Effect in Reducing Risk of Childhood Overweight." NIH News Release, May 15, 2001.

National Science Foundation. *Science and Engineering Indicators 2008.* Arlington, VA: NSB 08-01; NSB 08-01A, June 2008. Available at www.nsf.gov/statistics/seind08 (accessed April 23, 2008).

National Sleep Foundation. *2008 National Sleep in America Poll: Summary of Findings.* Washington, DC: National Sleep Foundation, 2008.

Needham, Larry L., and Richard Y. Wang. "Analytic Considerations for Measuring Environmental Chemicals in Breast Milk." *Environmental Health Perspectives* 110, no. 6 (2002): A317–24.

Neergaard, Lauran. "Report: Tips on Creating Fat-Fighting Communities." Associated Press, September 1, 2009.

Nelkin, Dorothy. "Foreword: The Social Meanings of Risk." In *Risk, Culture, and Health Inequality: Shifting Perceptions of Danger and Blame*, ed. Barbara Herr Harthorn and Laury Oaks, vii–xiii. Westport, CT: Praeger, 2003.

———. *Selling Science: How the Press Covers Science and Technology.* New York: Freeman, 1995.

Nelson, Melissa C., Penny Gordon-Larsen, and Linda S. Adair. "Are Adolescents Who Were Breast-fed Less Likely to Be Overweight: Analysis of Sibling Pairs to Reduce Confounding." *Epidemiology* 16, no. 2 (2005): 247–53.

Nickerson, Krista. "Environmental Contaminants in Breast Milk." *Journal of Midwifery and Women's Health* 51, no. 1 (2006): 26–34.

Nicolson, Paula. *Post-Natal Depression: Psychology, Science, and the Transition to Motherhood.* New York: Routledge, 1998.

Nielsen-Bohlman, Lynn, Allison M. Panzer, and David A. Kindig, eds. *Health Literacy: A Prescription to End Confusion.* Washington, DC: National Academies Press, 2004.

Norris, Jill M., and Fraser W. Scott. "A Meta-Analysis of Infant Diet and Insulin-Dependent Diabetes Mellitus: Do Biases Play a Role?" *Epidemiology* 7 (1996): 87–92.

Norris, Stephen P., Linda M. Phillips, and Connie A. Korpan. "University Students' Interpretation of Media Reports of Science and Its Relationship to Background Knowledge, Interest, and Reading Difficulty." *Public Understanding of Science* 12, no. 2 (2003): 123–45.

Novas, Carlos, and Nikolas Rose. "Genetic Risk and the Birth of the Somatic Individual." *Economy and Society* 29, no. 4 (2000): 458–513.

Oakley, Ann. *Social Support and Motherhood: The Natural History of a Research Project.* Oxford: Blackwell, 1992.

Oaks, Laury. *Smoking and Pregnancy: The Politics of Fetal Protection.* New Brunswick, NJ: Rutgers University Press, 2001.

Oddy, Wendy H. "Breastfeeding and Childhood Asthma." *Thorax* 64, no. 7 (2009): 558–59.

Oddy, W. H., P. G. Holt, P. D. Sly, A. W. Read, L. I. Landeau, F. J. Stanley, G. E. Kendall, and P. R. Burton. "Association between Breast Feeding and Asthma in 6 Year Old Children: Findings of a Prospective Birth Cohort Study." *British Medical Journal* 319 (1999): 815–19.

Oddy, Wendy H., Garth E. Kendall, Eve Blair, Nicholas H. de Klerk, Fiona J. Stanley, Louis I. Landau, S. Silburn, and Stephen Zubrick. "Breastfeeding and Cognitive Development in Childhood: A Prospective Birth Cohort Study." *Paediatric and Perinatal Epidemiology* 17 (2003): 81–90.

Oddy, Wendy H., Garth E. Kendall, Jianghong Li, Peter Jacoby, Monique Robinson, Nicholas H. de Klerk, Sven R. Silburn, Stephen R. Zubrick, Louis I. Landau, and Fiona J. Stanley. "The Long-Term Effects of Breastfeeding on Child and Adolescent Mental Health: A Pregnancy Cohort Study Followed for 14 Years" (2009), electronic publication, 1–7.

Oddy, Wendy H., Jill L. Sheriff, Nicholas H. de Klerk, Garth E. Kendall, Peter D. Sly, Lawrence J. Beilin, Kevin B. Blake, Louis I. Landau, and Fiona J. Stanley. "The Relation of Breastfeeding and Body Mass Index to Asthma and Atopy in Children: A Prospective Cohort Study to Age 6 Years." *American Journal of Public Health* 94, no. 9 (2004): 1531–37.

Oddy, W. H., P. D. Sly, N. H. de Klerk, L. I. Landeau, G. E. Kendall, P. G. Holt, and F. J. Stanley. "Breast Feeding and Respiratory Morbidity in Infancy: A Birth Cohort Study." *Archives of Disease in Childhood* 88 (2003): 224–28.

Ogbuano, I. U., W. Karmaus, S. H. Arshad, R. J. Kurukulaaratchy, and S. Ewart. "Effect of Breastfeeding Duration on Lung Function at Age 10 Years: A Prospective Birth Cohort Study." *Thorax* 64 (2009): 62–66.

O'Keefe, Daniel J. "Guilt and Social Influence." In *Communication Yearbook*, vol. 23, ed. Michael E. Roloff, 67–101. Thousand Oaks, CA: Sage, 2000.

Oken, Emily, Marie Louise Østerdal, Matthew W. Gillma, Vibeke K. Knudsen, Thorhallur I. Halldorsson, Marin Strøm, David C. Bellinger, Minja Hadders-Algra, Kim Fleischer Michaelsen, and Sjurdur F. Olsen. "Associations of Maternal Fish Intake during Pregnancy and Breastfeeding Duration with Attainment of Developmental Milestones in Early Childhood: A Study from the Danish National Birth Cohort." *American Journal of Clinical Nutrition* 88 (2009): 789–96.

Oliver, J. Eric. *Fat Politics: The Real Story behind America's Obesity Epidemic.* Oxford: Oxford University Press, 2006.

Olsen, J. "What Characterizes a Useful Concept of Causation in Epidemiology." *Journal of Epidemiology and Community Health* 57 (2003): 86–88.

O'Mara, Peggy. *Mothering Magazine's Having a Baby, Naturally: The Mothering Magazine Guide to Pregnancy and Childbirth.* New York: Atria, 2003.

Owen, Christopher G., Richard M. Martin, Peter H. Whincup, George Davey-Smith, Matthew W. Gillman, and Derek G. Cook. "The Effect of Breastfeeding on Mean Body Mass Index throughout Life: A Quantitative Review of Published and Unpublished Observational Evidence." *American Journal of Clinical Nutrition* 82 (2005): 1298–1307.

Owen, Mary Jean, Constance D. Baldwin, Paul R. Swank, Amarjit K. Pannu, Dale L. Johnson, and Virgil M. Howle. "Relation of Infant Feeding Practices, Cigarette Exposure, and Group Child Care to the Onset and Duration of Otitis Media with Effusion in the First Two Years of Life." *Journal of Pediatrics* 123 (1993): 702–11.

Palmer, Gabrielle. *The Politics of Breastfeeding.* London: Pandora, 1988.

Palmlund, Ingar. "Social Drama and Risk Evaluation." In *Social Theories of Risk*, ed. Sheldon Krimsky and Dominic Golding, 197–212. Westport, CT: Praeger, 1992.

Paltrow, Lynn M. "Punishment and Prejudice: Judging Drug-Using Pregnant Women." In *Mother*

Troubles: Rethinking Contemporary Maternal Dilemmas, ed. Julia E. Hanigsberg and Sara Ruddick, 59–80. Boston: Beacon Press, 1999.

Paradise, Jack L., Howard E. Rockette, D. Kathleen Colborn, Beverly S. Bernard, Clyde G. Smith, Marcia Kurs-Lasky, and Janine E. Janosky. "Otitis Media in 2253 Pittsburgh-Area Infants: Prevalence and Risk Factors during the First Two Years of Life." Pediatrics 99, no. 3 (1997): 318–33.

Parascandola, M. "Objectivity and the Neutral Expert." Journal of Epidemiology and Community Health 57 (2003): 3–4.

Parascandola, M., and D. L. Weed. "Causation in Epidemiology." Journal of Epidemiology and Community Health 55 (2001): 905–12.

Parker, Rozsika. Mother Love / Mother Hate: The Power of Maternal Ambivalence. New York: Basic Books, 1995.

Parker, Ruth M., Michael S. Wolf, and Irwin Kirsch. "Preparing for an Epidemic of Limited Health Literacy: Weathering the Perfect Storm." Journal of General Internal Medicine 23, no. 8 (2008): 1273–76.

Paul, Pamela. Parenting, Inc.: How We Are Sold on $800 Strollers, Fetal Education, Baby Sign Language, Sleeping Coaches, Toddler Couture, and Diaper Wipe Warmers—and What It Means for Our Children. New York: Times Books, 2008.

Pawluch, Dorothy. The New Pediatrics: A Profession in Transition. New York: Aldine de Gruyter, 1996.

Pearce, Neil. "Epidemiology as a Population Science." International Journal of Epidemiology 28 (1999): S1015–18.

———. "Traditional Epidemiology, Modern Epidemiology, and Public Health." American Journal of Public Health 86 (1996): 678–83.

Pearce, Neil, and John B. McKinlay. "Back to the Future in Epidemiology and Public Health: Response to Dr. Gori." Journal of Clinical Epidemiology 51, no. 8 (1998): 643–46.

Pellechia, Marianne G. "Trends in Science Coverage: A Content Analysis of Three U.S. Papers." Public Understanding of Science 6, no. 1 (1997): 49–68.

Perdiguero, E., J. Bernabeau, R. Huertas, and E. Rodriguez-Ocaña. "History of Health, a Valuable Tool in Public Health." Journal of Epidemiology and Community Health 55 (2001): 667–73.

Persad, Malini D., and Janell L. Mensinger. "Maternal Breastfeeding Attitudes: Association with Breastfeeding Intent and Socio-Demographics among Urban Primiparas." Journal of Community Health 33 (2007): 53–60.

Petersen, Alan R. "Risk and the Regulated Self: The Discourse of Health Promotion as Politics of Uncertainty." Australian & New Zealand Journal of Sociology 32, no. 1 (1996): 44–57.

Petersen, Alan R., and Robin Bunton, eds. Foucault, Health and Medicine. New York: Routledge, 1997.

Petersen, Alan R., and Deborah Lupton. The New Public Health: Health and Self in the Age of Risk. London: Sage, 1996.

Peterson, Linda A. "A Value-Laden Issue." MCN, the American Journal of Maternal/Child Nursing 21 (1996): 105.

Peterson, Melody. "Breastfeeding Ads Delayed by a Dispute over Content." New York Times, December 4, 2003.

———. "Pediatric Book on Breast-Feeding Stirs Controversy with Its Cover." New York Times, September 18, 2002.

Petterson, Stephen M., and Alison Burke Albers. "Effects of Poverty and Maternal Depression on Early Child Development." Child Development 72, no. 6 (2001): 1794–1813.

Pettitt, David J., Michele R. Forman, Robert L. Hanson, William C. Knowler, and Peter H. Bennett. "Breastfeeding and Incidence of Non-Insulin-Dependent Diabetes Mellitus in Pima Indians." The Lancet 350 (1997): 166–68.

Phillips, Carl V. "The Economics of 'More Research Is Needed.'" International Journal of Epidemiology 30 (2001): 771–76.

Pickering, Andrew. Science as Practice and Culture. Chicago: University of Chicago Press, 1992.

Pinelli, Janet, Saroj Saigal, and Stephanie A. Atkinson. "Effect of Breastmilk Consumption on Neurodevelopmental Outcomes at 6 and 12

Months of Age in VLBW Infants." *Advances in Neonatal Care* 3, no. 2 (2003): 76–87.

Pitkin, Roy M., Mary Ann Branagan, and Leon F. Burmeister. "Accuracy of Data in Abstracts of Published Research Articles." *Journal of the American Medical Association* 281, no. 12 (1999): 1110–11.

Pollitt, Katha. "'Fetal Rights': A New Assault on Feminism." In *"Bad" Mothers: The Politics of Blame in Twentieth-Century America*, ed. Molly Ladd-Taylor and Lauri Umansky, 285–98. New York: New York University Press, 1998.

Poothullil, John M., Richie Poulton, Sheila Williams, Mary L. Hediger, W. June Ruan, Mary D. Overpeck, and Robert J. Kuczmarski. "Breastfeeding and Risk of Overweight." *Journal of the American Medical Association* 286, no. 12 (2001): 1448–50.

Porter, Donna V. "Breast-Feeding: Impact on Health, Employment and Society." Congressional Research Service Report RL32002, July 18, 2003.

Power, Michael. "The Nature of Risk: The Risk Management of Everything." *Balance Sheet* 12, no. 5 (2004): 19–28.

Presser, Harriet B. "Are the Interests of Women Inherently at Odds with the Interests of Children or the Family? A Viewpoint." In *Gender and Family Change in Industrialized Countries*, ed. Karen Oppenheim Mason and An-Magrit Jensen, 297–319. Oxford: Clarendon Press, 1995.

Proctor, Sandra B., and Carol Ann Holcomb. "Breastfeeding Duration and Childhood Overweight among Low-Income Children in Kansas, 1998–2002." *American Journal of Public Health* 98, no. 1 (2008): 106–10.

Public Health Leadership Society. "Principles of the Ethical Practice of Public Health" (2002). Available at www.apha.org/NR/rdonlyres/1CED3CEA-287E-4185-9CBD-BD405FC60856/0/ethicsbrochure.pdf.

Quigley, Maria A., Yvonne J. Kelly, and Amanda Sacker. "Breastfeeding and Hospitalization for Diarrheal and Respiratory Infection in the United Kingdom Millennium Cohort Study." *Pediatrics* 119, no. 4 (2007): 837–42.

Rabin, Roni Caryn. "Breast-Feed or Else." *New York Times*, June 13, 2006.

———. "Despite Worries over Toxins, Breast-Feeding Still Best for Infants." *New York Times*, December 20, 2008.

———. "It Seems the Fertility Clock Ticks for Men, Too." *New York Times*, February 27, 2007.

Ragoné, Heléna, and France Winddance Twine, eds. *Ideologies and Technologies of Motherhood: Race, Class, Sexuality, Nationalism.* New York: Routledge, 2000.

Raisler, Jeanne, Cheryl Alexander, and Patricia O'Campo. "Breast-Feeding and Infant Illness: A Dose-Response Relationship?" *American Journal of Public Health* 89 (1999): 25–30.

Raphael, Dennis. "The Question of Evidence in Health Promotion." *Health Promotion International* 15, no. 4 (2000): 355–67.

Rapp, Rayna. "The Power of 'Positive' Diagnosis: Medical and Maternal Discourses on Amniocentesis." In *Representations of Motherhood*, ed. Donna Bassin, Margaret Honey, and Meryle Mahrer Kaplan, 204–19. New Haven, CT: Yale University Press, 1994.

———. *Testing the Woman, Testing the Fetus: The Social Impact of Amniocentesis in America.* New York: Routledge, 1999.

Reaney, Patricia. "Breastfeeding Cuts Cardiovascular Risk—Study." Reuters, May 13, 2004.

Rees, Daniel I., and Joseph J. Sabia. "The Effect of Breast Feeding on Educational Attainment: Evidence from Sibling Data." *Journal of Human Capital* 3, no. 1 (2009): 43–72.

Reichenberg, Abraham, Raz Gross, Mark Weiser, Michealine Bresnahan, Jeremy Silverman, Susan Harlap, Jonathan Rabinowitz, Cory Shulman, Dolores Malaspina, Gad Lubin, Haim Y. Knobler, Michael Davidson, and Ezra Susser. "Advancing Paternal Age and Autism." *Archives of General Psychiatry* 63 (2006): 1026–32.

Richard, Patricia Bayer. "The Tailor-Made Child: Implications for Women and the State." In *Expecting Trouble: Surrogacy, Fetal Abuse, & New Reproductive Technologies*, ed. Patricia Boling, 9–24. Boulder, CO: Westview Press, 1995.

Riordan, Janice M. "The Cost of Not Breastfeeding: A Commentary." *Journal of Human Lactation* 13, no. 2 (1997): 93–97.

Rivers, Caryl. *Selling Anxiety: How the News Media Scare Women*. Hanover, NH: University Press of New England, 2007.

Roan, Shari. "Living for Two." *Los Angeles Times*, November 12, 2007.

Roberts, Dorothy E. *Killing the Black Body: Race, Reproduction, and the Meaning of Liberty*. New York: Vintage Books, 1997.

———. "Mothers Who Fail to Protect Their Children: Accounting for Private and Public Responsibility." In *Mother Troubles: Rethinking Contemporary Maternal Dilemmas*, ed. Julia E. Hanigsberg and Sara Ruddick, 31–49. Boston: Beacon Press, 1999.

Roberts, Marc J., and Michael R. Reich. "Ethical Analysis in Public Health." *The Lancet* 359 (2002): 1055–59.

Rochon, Paula A., Lisa A. Bero, Ari M. Bay, Jennifer L. Gold, Julie M. Dergal, Malcolm A. Binns, David L. Streiner, and Jerry H. Gurwitz. "Comparison of Review Articles Published in Peer-Reviewed and Throwaway Journals." *Journal of the American Medical Association* 287, no. 21 (2002): 2853–55.

Rodricks, Joseph V. "Some Attributes of Risk Influencing Decision-Making by Public Health and Regulatory Officials." *American Journal of Epidemiology* 154, no. 12 (2001): S7–S12.

Rogan, Walter J. "Pollutants in Breast Milk." *Archives of Pediatric and Adolescent Medicine* 150 (1996): 981–90.

Rogan, Walter J., Patricia J. Blanton, Christopher J. Portier, and Eric Stallard. "Should the Presence of Carcinogens in Breast Milk Discourage Breast Feeding?" *Regulatory Toxicology and Pharmacology* 13, no. 3 (1991): 228–40.

Rogan, Walter J., and Beth C. Gladen. "Breast-Feeding and Cognitive Development." *Early Human Development* 31 (1993): 181–93.

Rogers, Anne, and David Pilgrim. "The Risk of Resistance: Perspectives on the Mass Childhood Immunisation Programme." In *Medicine, Health and Risk: Sociological Approaches*, ed. Jonathan Gabe, 73–90. Oxford: Blackwell, 1995.

Roloff, Michael E., ed. *Communication Yearbook*. Vol. 23. Thousand Oaks, CA: Sage, 2000.

Romm, Aviva Jill. *The Natural Pregnancy Book: Herbs, Nutrition, and Other Holistic Choices*. Berkeley, CA: Celestial Arts, 2003.

Ropeik, David, and George Gray. *Risk: A Practical Guide for Deciding What's Really Safe and What's Really Dangerous in the World around You*. Boston: Houghton Mifflin, 2002.

Rose, Hilary. "Risk, Trust and Scepticism in the Age of the New Genetics." In *The Risk Society and Beyond: Critical Issues for Social Theory*, ed. Barbara Adam, Ulrich Beck, and Joost Van Loon, 63–77. London: Sage, 2000.

Rose, Nikolas. "The Politics of Life Itself." *Theory, Culture & Society* 18, no. 6 (2001): 1–30.

Rosenberg, Charles E. "Banishing Risk: Or the More Things Change the More They Remain the Same." *Perspectives in Biology and Medicine* 39, no. 1 (1995): 28–42.

———. *No Other Gods: On Science and American Social Thought*. Baltimore: Johns Hopkins University Press, 1997.

Ross, Brian. "Milk Money." *20/20*, ABC News, June 4, 2004.

Roth, Rachel. *Making Women Pay: The Hidden Costs of Fetal Rights*. Ithaca, NY: Cornell University Press, 2000.

Rothenberg, Karen H., and Elizabeth J. Thompson, eds. *Women and Prenatal Testing: Facing the Challenges of Genetic Technology*. Columbus: Ohio State University Press, 1994.

Rothman, Alexander J., and Peter Salovey. "Shaping Perceptions to Motivate Healthy Behavior: The Role of Message Framing." *Psychological Bulletin* 121, no. 1 (1997): 3–19.

Rothman, Barbara Katz. "Beyond Mothers and Fathers: Ideology in a Patriarchal Society." In *Mothering: Ideology, Experience, and Agency*, ed. Evelyn Nakano Glenn, Grace Chang, and Linda Rennie Forcey, 139–57. New York: Routledge, 1994.

———. *The Tentative Pregnancy: How Amniocentesis Changes the Experience of Motherhood*. New York: Norton, 1993.

Rothschild, Joan. *The Dream of the Perfect Child*. Bloomington: Indiana University Press, 2005.

Rothschild, Michael L. "Ethical Considerations in the Use of Marketing for the Management of Public Health and Social Issues." In *Ethics in Social Marketing*, ed. Alan R. Andreasen, 17–38. Washington, DC: Georgetown University Press, 2001.

Rothstein, William G. *Public Health and the Risk Factor: A History of an Uneven Medical Revolution*. Rochester, NY: University of Rochester Press, 2003.

Rothwell, Peter M., and Meena Bhatia. "Reporting of Observational Studies." *British Medical Journal* 335 (2007): 783–84.

Rousselot, Susan. *Avoiding Miscarriage: Everything You Need to Know to Feel More Confident in Pregnancy*. New York: Sea Change Press, 2006.

Ruhl, Lealle. "Dilemmas of the Will: Uncertainty, Reproduction, and the Rhetoric of Control." *Signs* 27, no. 3 (2002): 641–63.

Rumbelow, Helen. "Exposing the Myths of Breastfeeding" and "Benefits of Breastfeeding 'Being Oversold by NHS.'" *Times of London*, July 20, 2009.

Rust, G. S., C. J. Thompson, P. Minor, W. Davis-Mitchell, K. Holloway, and V. Murray. "Does Breastfeeding Protect Children from Asthma? Analysis of NHANES III Survey Data." *Journal of the National Medical Association* 93, no. 4 (2001): 139–48.

Ryan, Alan S. "Breastfeeding and the Risk of Childhood Obesity." *Collegium Antropologicum* 31 (2007): 19–28.

———. "The Resurgence of Breastfeeding in the United States." *Pediatrics* 99, no. 4 (1997): e12.

———. "The Truth about the Ross Mothers Survey." *Pediatrics* 113 (2004): 626–27.

Ryan, Alan S., Zhou Wenjun, and Andrew Acosta. "Breastfeeding Continues to Increase into the New Millennium." *Pediatrics* 110, no. 6 (2002): 1103–9.

Saarinen, Ulla M., and Merja Kajosaari. "Breastfeeding as Prophylaxis Against Atopic Disease: Prospective Follow-up Study until 17 Years Old." *The Lancet* 346, no. 8982 (1995): 1065–69.

Sachs, Lisbeth. "Causality, Responsibility and Blame—Core Issues in the Cultural Construction and Subtext of Prevention." *Sociology of Health and Illness* 18, no. 5 (1996): 632–52.

Saguy, Abigail C., and Kevin W. Riley. "Weighing Both Sides: Morality, Mortality, and Framing Contests over Obesity." *Journal of Health Politics, Policy and Law* 30, no. 5 (2005): 869–921.

Saha, Somnath, Sanjay Saint, and Dimitri A. Christakis. "Impact Factor: A Valid Measure of Journal Quality?" *Journal of the Medical Library Association* 91, no. 1 (2003): 42–46.

Saint, Sanjay, Dimitri A. Christakis, Somnath Saha, Joann G. Elmore, Deborah E. Welsh, Paul Baker, and Thomas D. Koepsell. "Journal Reading Habits of Internists." *Journal of General Internal Medicine* 15 (2000): 881–84.

Salsberry, Pamela J., and Patricia B. Reagan. "Dynamics of Early Childhood Overweight." *Pediatrics* 116, no. 6 (2005): 1329–38.

Samet, Jonathan M. "Epidemiology and Policy: The Pump Handle Meets the New Millennium." *Epidemiologic Reviews* 22, no. 1 (2000): 145–54.

Samet, Jonathan M., and Nora L. Lee. "Bridging the Gap: Perspectives on Translating Epidemiologic Evidence into Policy." *American Journal of Epidemiology* 154, no. 12 (2001): S1–S4.

Sandman, Peter M. "Emerging Communication Responsibilities of Epidemiologists." *Journal of Clinical Epidemiology* 4 (1991): 41–50.

Sanghavi, Darshak. "Why Do We Focus on the Least Important Causes of Cancer?" www.slate.com, April 25, 2008.

———. "Womb Raider: Do Future Health Problems Begin during Gestation?" Available at www.slate.com/id/2201788/ (accessed October 13, 2008).

Sanson, Gill. *The Osteoporosis 'Epidemic': Well Women and the Marketing of Fear*. New York: Penguin, 2001.

Sargent, James, Madeline Dalton, and Lisa Schwarz. "Health Benefits of Breastfeeding Promotion." *Journal of the American Medical Association* 285, no. 19 (2001): 2446.

Savitz, D. A., C. Poole, and W. C. Miller. "Reassessing the Role of Epidemiology in Public Health." *American Journal of Public Health* 89, no. 8 (1999): 1158–61.

Sayer, Liana C., Suzanne M. Bianchi, and John P. Robinson. "Are Parents Investing Less in Children? Trends in Mothers' and Fathers' Time with Children." *American Journal of Sociology* 110, no. 1 (2004): 1–43.

Scariati, Paula D., Laurence M. Grummer-Strawn, and Sara Beck Fein. "A Longitudinal Analysis of Infant Morbidity and the Extent of Breastfeeding in the United States." *Pediatrics* 99, no. 6 (1997): e5–e9.

Scarr, Sandra. "American Child Care Today." *American Psychologist* 53, no. 2 (1998): 95–108.

———. "Why Child Care Has Little Impact on Most Children's Development." *Current Directions in Psychological Science* 6, no. 5 (1997): 143–48.

Scarr, Sandra, Deborah Phillips, and Kathleen McCartney. "Facts, Fantasies and the Future of Child Care in the United States." *Psychological Science* 1, no. 1 (1990): 26–35.

Schack-Nielsen, Lene, Thorkild I. A. Sørensen, Erik Lykke Mortensen, and Kim Fleischer Michaelsen. "Late Introduction of Complementary Feeding, Rather Than Duration of Breastfeeding, May Protect against Adult Overweight." *American Journal of Clinical Nutrition*, electronic publication (2009): 109.

Schaefer-Graf, Ute M., Reinhard Hartmann, Julia Pawliczak, Doerte Passow, Michael Abou-Dakn, Klaus Vetter, and Olga Kordonouri. "Association of Breast-Feeding and Early Childhood Overweight in Children from Mothers with Gestational Diabetes Mellitus." *Diabetes Care* 29, no. 5 (2006): 1105–7.

Scher, Jonathan, and Carol Dyx. *Preventing Miscarriage: The Good News*. New York: HarperCollins, 2005.

Schmied, Virginia, and Deborah Lupton. "Blurring the Boundaries: Breastfeeding and Maternal Subjectivity." *Sociology of Health and Illness* 23, no. 2 (2001): 234–50.

Schmierbach, Mike. "Method Matters: The Influence of Methodology on Journalists' Assessment of Social Science Research." *Science Communication* 26, no. 3 (2005): 269–87.

Scholtens, Salome, Ulrike Gehring, Bert Brunekreef, Henriette A. Smit, Johan C. De Jongste, Marjan Kerkhof, Jorrit Gerritsen, and Alet H. Wijga. "Breastfeeding, Weight Gain in Infancy, and Overweight at Seven Years." *American Journal of Epidemiology* 165 (2007): 919–26.

Scholtens, S., A. H. Wijga, B. Brunekreef, M. Kerkhov, M. O. Hoekstra, J. Gerritsen, R. Aalberse, J. C. de Jongste, and H. A. Smit. "Breast Feeding, Parental Allergy and Asthma in Children Followed for 8 Years: The PIAMA Birth Cohort Study." *Thorax* 64, no. 7 (2009): 604–9.

Schwartz, Adria. "Taking the Nature out of Mother." In *Representations of Motherhood*, ed. Donna Bassin, Margaret Honey, and Meryle Mahrer Kaplan, 240–55. New Haven, CT: Yale University Press, 1994.

Schwartz, Barry. *The Paradox of Choice*. New York: Ecco, 2004.

Schwartz, Lisa M., and Steven Woloshin. "The Case for Letting Information Speak for Itself." *Effective Clinical Practice* 4 (2001): 76–79.

———. "Marketing Medicine to the Public: A Reader's Guide." *MSJAMA* 287, no. 6 (2002): 774–75.

Schwartz, Lisa M., Steven Woloshin, and Linda Baczek. "Media Coverage of Scientific Meetings: Too Much, Too Soon?" *Journal of the American Medical Association* 287, no. 21 (2002): 2859–63.

Schwartz, S., E. Susser, and M. Susser. "A Future for Epidemiology?" *Annual Review of Public Health* 20 (1999): 15–33.

Sclater, Shelley Day, Fatemah Ebtehaj, Emily Jackson, and Martin Richards, eds. *Regulating Autonomy: Sex, Reproduction, and Family*. Oxford: Hart Publishing, 2009.

Scott, Alan. "Risk Society or Angst Society: Two Views of Risk, Consciousness and Community." In *The Risk Society and Beyond: Critical Issues for Social Theory*, ed. Barbara Adam, Ulrich Beck, and Joost Van Loon, 33–46. London: Sage, 2000.

Scott, Joan W. "Deconstructing Equality-versus-Difference: Or, the Use of Poststructuralist Theory for Feminism." *Feminist Studies* 14, no. 1 (1988): 33–50.

———. "Gender: A Useful Category of Analysis." *American Historical Review* 91, no. 5 (1986): 1053–75.

Sears, Malcolm R., Justina M. Greene, Andrew R. Willan, Elizabeth M. Wiecek, D. Robin Taylor, Erin M. Flannery, Jan O. Cowan, G. Peter Herbison, Phil A. Silva, and Richie Poulton. "A Longitudinal, Population-Based, Cohort Study of Childhood Asthma Followed to Adulthood." *New England Journal of Medicine* 349, no. 15 (2003): 1414–22.

Sears, Martha, and William Sears. *The Breastfeeding Book: Everything You Need to Know about Nursing Your Child from Birth through Weaning.* Boston: Little, Brown, 2000.

Sears, Martha, William Sears, and Linda Hughey Holt. *The Pregnancy Book: Everything You Need to Know from America's Baby Experts.* Boston: Little, Brown, 1997.

Sears, William, and Martha Sears. *The Attachment Parenting Book: A Commonsense Guide to Understanding and Nurturing Your Baby.* Boston: Little, Brown, 2001.

———. *The Baby Book: Everything You Need to Know about Your Baby—From Birth to Age Two.* 1st ed. Boston: Little, Brown, 1992.

———. *The Birth Book: Everything You Need to Know to Have a Safe and Satisfying Birth.* Boston: Little, Brown, 1994.

———. *The Discipline Book: How to Have a Better-Behaved Child from Birth to Age Ten.* Boston: Little, Brown, 1995.

Sears, William, Martha Sears, Robert Sears, and James Sears. *The Baby Book: Everything You Need to Know about Your Baby from Birth to Age 2.* Updated and rev. ed. Boston: Little, Brown, 2003.

Semchyshyn, Stefan, and Carol Colman. *How to Prevent Miscarriage and Other Crises of Pregnancy: A Leading High-Risk Doctor's Prescription for Carrying Your Baby to Term.* Indianapolis: Wiley, 1990.

Sewell, William H. Jr. *Logics of History: Social Theory and Social Transformation.* Chicago: University of Chicago Press, 2005.

Shi, Leiyu, and Gregory D. Stevens. "Disparities in Access to Care and Satisfaction among U.S. Children: The Roles of Race/Ethnicity and Poverty Status." *Public Health Reports* 120 (2005): 431–41.

Shonkoff, Jack P. "Science, Policy, and Practice: Three Cultures in Search of a Shared Mission." *Child Development* 71, no. 1 (2000): 181–87.

Shu, Xiao Ou, Martha S. Linet, Michael Steinbuch, Wan Qing Wen, Jonathan D. Buckley, Joseph P. Neglia, John D. Potter, Gregory H. Reaman, and Leslie L. Robison. "Breastfeeding and Risk of Childhood Acute Leukemia." *Journal of the National Cancer Institute* 91, no. 20 (1999): 1765–72.

Shuchman, Miriam, and Michael S. Wilkes. "Medical Scientists and Health News Reporting: A Case of Miscommunication." *Annals of Internal Medicine* 126, no. 12 (1997): 976–82.

Siegel, Marc. *False Alarm: The Truth about the Epidemic of Fear.* Hoboken, NJ: Wiley, 2005.

Siegel, Michael. "Mass Media Antismoking Campaigns: A Powerful Tool for Health Promotion." *Annals of Internal Medicine* 129, no. 2 (1998): 128–32.

Silverman, Jay G., Michele R. Decker, Elizabeth Reed, and Anita Raj. "Intimate Partner Violence Victimization prior to and during Pregnancy among Women Residing in 26 U.S. States: Associations with Maternal and Neonatal Health." *American Journal of Obstetrics and Gynecology* 195 (2006): 140–48.

Silvers, Karen M., and Michael J. Epton. "Study Was Not Designed to Test the Hypothesis." *British Medical Journal* 335 (2007): 899.

Simmons, David. "NIDDM and Breastfeeding." *The Lancet* 350 (1997): 157–58.

Simoes, Eric A. F. "Environmental and Demographic Risk Factors for Respiratory Syncytial Virus Lower Respiratory Tract Disease." *Journal of Pediatrics* 143 (2003): S118–26.

Singer, Eleanor, and Phyllis M. Endreny. *Reporting on Risk: How the Mass Media Portray Accidents, Diseases, Disasters, and Other Hazards.* New York: Russell Sage Foundation, 1993.

Singh, Ilina. "Bad Boys, Good Mothers, and the 'Miracle' of Ritalin." *Science in Context* 15, no. 4 (2002): 577–603.

Singhal, Atul, Tim J. Cole, Mary Fewtrell, and Alan Lucas. "Breastmilk Feeding and Lipoprotein Profile in Adolescents Born Preterm: Follow-up of a Prospective Randomized Study." *The Lancet* 363 (2004): 1571–78.

Singhal, Atul, and Alan Lucas. "Early Origins of Cardiovascular Disease: Is There a Unifying Hypothesis?" *The Lancet* 363 (2004): 1642–45.

Sinha, Anushua, Jeanne Madden, Dennis Ross-Dengan, Stephen Soumerai, and Richard Platt. "Reduced Risk of Neonatal Respiratory Infections among Breastfed Girls but Not Boys." *Pediatrics* 112, no. 4 (2003): e303–7.

Sipos, Attila, Finn Rasmussen, Glynn Harrison, Per Tynelius, Glyn Lewis, David A. Leon, and David Gunnell. "Paternal Age and Schizophrenia: A Population Based Cohort Study." *British Medical Journal* 329 (2004): 1070–74.

Sirovich, Brenda E., and H. Gilbert Welch. "Cervical Cancer Screening among Women without a Cervix." *Journal of the American Medical Association* 291, no. 24 (2004): 2990–93.

Sjöberg, Lennart. "Worry and Risk Perception." *Risk Analysis* 18, no. 1 (1998): 85–93.

Skenazy, Lenore. *Free-Range Kids: Giving Our Children the Freedom We Had without Going Nuts with Worry.* San Francisco: Jossey-Bass, 2009.

Skrabanek, Petr. "The Epidemiology of Errors." *The Lancet* 342, nos. 8886/8887 (1993): 1502.

———."Risk-Factor Epidemiology: Science or Non-Science?" In Social Affairs Unit / Manhattan Institute, *Health, Lifestyle and Environment: Countering the Panic,* 46–56. London: SAU/MI, 1991.

Slovic, Paul. *The Perception of Risk.* London: Earthscan, 2000.

Slykerman, R. F., J. M. D. Thompson, D. M. O. Becroft, E. Robinson, J. E. Pryor, P. M. Clark, C. J. Wild, and E. A. Mitchell. "Breastfeeding and Intelligence of Preschool Children." *Acta Paediatrica* 94 (2005): 832–37.

Smith, Mick. "Sociology and Ethical Responsibility." *Sociology* 39, no. 3 (2005): 543–50.

Smith, Ted J., S. Robert Lichter, and Louis Harris and Associates. *What the People Want from the Press.* Washington, DC: Center for Media and Public Affairs, 1997.

Smith, William A. "Ethics and the Social Marketer: A Framework for Practitioners." In *Ethics in Social Marketing,* ed. Alan R. Andreasen, 1–16. Washington, DC: Georgetown University Press, 2001.

Snijders, Bianca E. P., Carel Thijs, Peter C. Dagnelie, Foekje F. Stelma, Monique Mommers, Ischa Kummeling, John Penders, Ronald van Ree, and Piet A. van den Brandt. "Breast-Feeding Duration and Infant Atopic Manifestations, by Maternal Allergic Status, in the First 2 Years of Life (KOALA Study)." *Journal of Pediatrics* 151 (2007): 347–51.

Snipes, Robin L., Michael S. LaTour, and Sara J. Bliss. "A Model of the Effects of Self-Efficacy on the Perceived Ethicality and Performance of Fear Appeals in Advertising." *Journal of Business Ethics* 19 (1999): 273–85.

Social Affairs Unit / Manhattan Institute. *Health, Lifestyle and Environment: Countering the Panic.* London: SAU/MI, 1991.

Sokal, Alan. *Beyond the Hoax: Science, Philosophy and Culture.* Oxford: Oxford University Press, 2008.

Solomon, Gina M., and Pilar M. Weiss. "Chemical Contaminants in Breast Milk: Time Trends and Regional Variability." *Environmental Health Perspectives* 110, no. 6 (2002): A339–47.

Sommer, Alfred. "How Public Health Policy Is Created: Scientific Processes and Political Reality." *American Journal of Epidemiology* 154, no. 12 (2001): S4–S6.

Sontag, Susan. *Illness as Metaphor and AIDS and Its Metaphors.* New York: Anchor Books, 1989.

Spencer, Nick. "Social, Economic, and Political Determinants of Child Health." *Pediatrics* 112, no. 3 (2003): 704–6.

Spock, Benjamin. *The Common Sense Book of Baby and Child Care.* New York: Duell, Sloan and Pearce, 1946.

Stabile, Carol A. "Shooting the Mother: Fetal Photography and the Politics of Disappearance." *Camera Obscura* 28 (1992): 178–205.

Standing Committee on Nutrition of the British Paediatric Association. "Is Breastfeeding Beneficial in the UK?" *Archives of Disease in Childhood* 71 (1994): 376–80.

Stanworth, Michelle, ed. *Reproductive Technologies: Gender, Motherhood and Medicine.* Minneapolis: University of Minnesota Press, 1987.

Stehr, Nico. *The Fragility of Modern Societies: Knowledge and Risk in the Information Age.* London: Sage, 2001.

Steinbrook, Robert. "Medical Journals and Medical Reporting." *New England Journal of Medicine* 342, no. 22 (2000): 1668–71.

Steinem, Gloria. "If Men Could Menstruate." *Ms.,* October 1978.

Stenvig, Thomas E. "Objectivity and Advocacy Are Not Contradictory Goals." *American Journal of Public Health* 90, no. 6 (2000): 987.

Sterene, George G., Alan Hinman, and Susan Schmid. "Potential Health Benefits of Child Day Care Attendance." *Reviews of Infectious Diseases* 8, no. 4 (1986): 660–62.

Stern, Paul C., and Harvey V. Fineberg, eds. *Understanding Risk: Informing Decisions in a Democratic Society.* Washington, DC: National Academy Press, 1996.

Stettler, Nicolas, Virginia A. Stallings, Andrea B. Troxel, Jing Zhao, Rita Schinnar, Steven E. Nelson, Ekhard

E. Ziegler, and Brian L. Strom. "Weight Gain in the First Week of Life and Overweight in Adulthood." *Circulation* 111 (2005): 1897–1903.

Stirling, Andy, and David Gee. "Science, Precaution, and Practice." *Public Health Reports* 117 (2002): 521–33.

Stobbe, Mike. "Breastfeeding Won't Deter Obesity." Associated Press, April 24, 2007.

Stone, Pamela. *Opting Out: Why Women Really Quit Careers and Head Home.* Berkeley: University of California Press, 2007.

Stossel, John. "Are We Scaring Ourselves to Death?" *ABC News* Special Report, September 9, 1996.

Strathearn, Lane, Abdullah A. Mamun, Jake M. Najman, and Michael J. O'Callaghan. "Does Breastfeeding Protect against Substantiated Child Abuse and Neglect? A 15-Year Cohort Study." *Pediatrics* 123, no. 2 (2009): 483–93.

Strauss, Richard. "Breast Milk and Childhood Obesity: The Czechs Weigh In." *Journal of Pediatric Gastroenterology and Nutrition* 37, no. 2 (2003): 210–11.

Štrbák, V., M. Škultétyová, M. Hromadová, A. Randuškova, and L. Macho. "Late Effects of Breast-Feeding and Early Weaning: Seven-Year Prospective Study in Children." *Endocrine Regulations* 25 (1991): 53–57.

Strong, Thomas H. *Expecting Trouble: The Myth of Prenatal Care in America.* New York: New York University Press, 2000.

Stuart-Macadam, Patricia, and Katherine A. Dettwyler, eds. *Breastfeeding: Biocultural Perspectives.* New York: Aldine de Gruyter, 1995.

Sullivan, Dana, and Maureen Connolly, eds. *Unbuttoned: Women Open up about the Pleasures, Pains, and Politics of Breastfeeding.* Boston: Harvard Common Press, 2009.

Sunstein, Cass R. *Laws of Fear: Beyond the Precautionary Principle.* Cambridge: Cambridge University Press, 2005.

Susser, Mervyn. "Does Risk Factor Epidemiology Put Epidemiology at Risk? Peering into the Future." *Journal of Epidemiology and Community Health* 52 (1998): 608–11.

———. "Should the Epidemiologist Be a Social Scientist or a Molecular Biologist?" *International Journal of Epidemiology* 28 (1999): S1019–22.

Szalavitz, Maia. "10 Ways We Get the Odds Wrong." *Psychology Today,* January/February 2008.

Szklo, Moyses. "The Evaluation of Epidemiologic Evidence for Policy-Making." *American Journal of Epidemiology* 154, no. 12 (2001): S13–S17.

———. "Issues in Publication and Interpretation in Research Findings." *Journal of Clinical Epidemiology* 4 (1991): 109–13.

Tanner, Andrea H. "Agenda Building, Source Selection, and Health News at Local Television Stations." *Science Communication* 25, no. 4 (2004): 350–63.

Taubes, Gary. "Epidemiology Faces Its Limits." *Science* 269 (July 14, 1995): 164–69.

Taveras, Elise M., Angela M. Capra, Paula A. Braveman, Nancy G. Jensvold, Gabriel J. Escobar, and Tracy A. Lieu. "Clinician Support and Psychosocial Risk Factors Associated with Breastfeeding Discontinuation." *Pediatrics* 112, no. 1 (2003): 108–15.

Taveras, Elise M., Sheryl L. Rifas-Shihman, Kelley S. Scanlon, Laurence M. Grummer-Strawn, Bettylou Sherry, and Matthew W. Gillman. "To What Extent Is the Protective Effect of Breastfeeding on Future Overweight Explained by Decreased Maternal Feeding Restriction?" *Pediatrics* 118, no. 6 (2006): 2341–48.

Taveras, Elise M., Kelley S. Scanlon, Leann Birch, Sheryl L. Rifas-Shiman, Janet W. Rich-Edwards, and Matthew W. Gillman. "Association of Breastfeeding with Maternal Control of Infant Feeding at Age 1 Year." *Pediatrics* 114, no. 5 (2004): 577–83.

Taylor, Daniel J., Kenneth L. Lichstein, H. Heith Durrence, Brant W. Reidel, and Andrew J. Bush. "Epidemiology of Insomnia, Depression, and Anxiety." *Sleep* 28, no. 11 (2005): 1457–64.

Taylor, Verta. *Rock-a-Bye Baby: Feminism, Self-Help, and Postpartum Depression.* New York: Routledge, 1996.

Tenepoir, Carol, Donald W. Kind, Michael T. Clarke, Kyoungsik Na, and Xiang Zhou. "Journal Reading Patterns and Preferences of

Pediatricians." *Journal of the American Medical Association* 95, no. 1 (2007): 56–63.

Tenner, Edward. *Our Own Devices: The Past and Future of Body Technology.* New York: Knopf, 2003.

Teret, Stephen. "Policy and Science: Should Epidemiologists Comment on the Policy Implications of Their Research?" *Epidemiology* 12, no. 4 (2001): 374–75.

Thaler, Richard H., and Cass R. Sunstein. *Nudge: Improving Decisions about Health, Wealth, and Happiness.* New Haven, CT: Yale University Press, 2008.

Thomas, James C., Michael Sage, Jack Dillenberg, and V. James Guillory. "A Code of Ethics for Public Health." *American Journal of Public Health* 92, no. 7 (2002): 1057–59.

Thorne, Barrie, and Marilyn Yalom, eds. *Rethinking the Family: Some Feminist Questions.* New York: Longman, 1982.

Thurer, Shari L. *The Myths of Motherhood.* New York: Penguin, 1994.

Tierney, Kathleen J. "Toward a Critical Sociology of Risk." *Sociological Forum* 14, no. 2 (1999): 215–42.

Tommasi, Mariano, and Kathryn Ierulli, eds. *The New Economics of Human Behavior.* Cambridge: Cambridge University Press, 1995.

Toschke, André, Jane Vignerova, Lida Lhotska, Katerina Osancova, Berthold Koletzko, and Rüdger von Kries. "Overweight and Obesity in 6- to 14-Year-Old Czech Children in 1991:

Protective Effect of Breastfeeding." *Journal of Pediatrics* 141 (2002): 764–69.

Traister, Rebecca. "Baby, We Were Born to Breast-Feed." Available at www.salon.com/mwt/broadsheet/2005/12/19/breastfed/index.html (accessed April 3, 2006).

Tsing, Anna Lowenhaupt. "Monster Stories: Women Charged with Perinatal Endangerment." In *Uncertain Terms: Negotiating Gender in American Culture,* ed. Faye Ginsburg and Anna Lowenhaupt Tsing, 282–99. Boston: Beacon Press, 1990.

Tulloch, John, and Deborah Lupton. "Consuming Risk, Consuming Science: The Case of GM Foods." *Journal of Consumer Culture* 2, no. 3 (2002): 363–83.

Turkheimer, Eric, Andreana Haley, Mary Waldron, Brian D'Onofrio, and Irving I. Gottesman. "Socioeconomic Status Modifies Heritability of IQ in Young Children." *Psychological Science* 14, no. 6 (2003): 623–28.

Uauy, Ricardo, and Patricio Peirano. "Breast Is Best: Human Milk Is the Optimal Food for the Brain." *American Journal of Clinical Nutrition* 70 (1999): 433–34.

Umansky, Lauri. "Breastfeeding in the 1990s: The Karen Carter Case and the Politics of Maternal Sexuality." In *"Bad" Mothers: The Politics of Blame in Twentieth-Century America,* ed. Molly Ladd-Taylor and Lauri Umansky, 299–309. New York: New York University Press, 1998.

Ungar, Sheldon. "Misplaced Metaphor: A Critical Analysis of the 'Knowledge Society.'" *Canadian Review of Sociology and Anthropology* 40, no. 3 (2003): 331–47.

Ungar, Sheldon, and Dennis Bray. "Silencing Science: Partisanship and the Career of a Publication Disputing the Dangers of Secondhand Smoke." *Public Understanding of Science* 14, no. 1 (2005): 5–23.

U.S. Department of Health and Human Services. *Blueprint for Action on Breastfeeding*. Washington, DC: U.S. Department of Health and Human Services, Office on Women's Health, 2000.

———. "Follow-up Report: The Surgeon General's Workshop on Breastfeeding and Human Lactation." 1985, DHHS Publication no. HRS-D-MC 85-2.

———. *Healthy People 2010: Understanding and Improving Health*. 2nd ed. Washington, DC: U.S. Government Printing Office, November 2000.

———. "Report of the Surgeon General's Workshop on Breastfeeding and Human Lactation." 1984. DHHS Publication no. HRS-D-MC 84-2.

U.S. Department of Health and Human Services, Centers for Disease Control and Prevention, National Center for Chronic Disease Prevention and Health Promotion, Office on Smoking and Health. *The Health Consequences of Smoking: A Report of the Surgeon General*. Washington, DC: U.S. Department of Health and Human Services, 2004.

U.S. Department of Health and Human Services, National Institutes of Health, National Institute of Diabetes and Digestive and Kidney Diseases, Weight-Control Information Network. "Statistics Related to Overweight and Obesity." October 2006, 1–9.

U.S. General Accounting Office. "Food Assistance: Potential to Serve More WIC Infants by Reducing Formula Costs." Report to the House and Senate Committees on Appropriations, Subcommittees on Agriculture, GAO-03-331, 2003.

Uttal, Lynet. *Making Care Work: Employed Mothers in the New Childcare Market*. New Brunswick, NJ: Rutgers University Press, 2002.

Vandell, Deborah Lowe. "Early Child Care: The Known and the Unknown." *Merrill-Palmer Quarterly* 50, no. 3 (2004): 387–414.

van Esterik, Penny. *Beyond the Breast-Bottle Controversy*. New Brunswick, NJ: Rutgers University Press, 1989.

Vaughan, Christopher. *How Life Begins: The Science of Life in the Womb*. New York: Times Books / Random House, 1996.

Victora, Cesar G., Fernando Barros, Rosângela C. Lima, Bernardo L. Horta, and Jonathan Wells. "Anthropometry and Body Composition of 18 Year Old Men according to Duration of Breastfeeding: Birth Cohort Study from Brazil." *British Medical Journal* 327 (2003): 901–5.

Victora, Cesar G., Jean-Pierre Habicht, and Jennifer Bryce. "Evidence-Based Public Health: Moving beyond Randomized Trials." *American Journal of Public Health* 94, no. 3 (2004): 400.

Virtanen, Suvi M., and Mikael Knip. "Nutritional Risk Predictors of ß Cell Autoimmunity and Type 1 Diabetes at a Young Age." *American Journal of Clinical Nutrition* 78 (2003): 1053–67.

von Bubnoff, Andreas. "Numbers Can Lie." *Los Angeles Times*, September 17, 2007.

Von Ehrenstein, Ondine S., Suzanne E. Fenton, Kayoko Kato, Zsuzsanna Kuklenyik, Antonia M. Calafat, and Erin P. Hines. "Polyfluoroalkyl Chemicals in the Serum and Milk of Breastfeeding Women." *Reproductive Toxicology* 27 (2009): 239–45.

Von Elm, Erik, Douglas G. Altman, Matthias Egger, Stuart J. Pocock, Peter C. Gøtzsche, and Jan P. Vandenbroucke. "Strengthening the Reporting of Observational Studies in Epidemiology (STROBE) Statement: Guidelines for Reporting Observational Studies." *The Lancet* 370 (2007): 1453–57.

von Kries, R., B. Koletzko, T. Sauerwald, and E. von Mutius. "Does Breastfeeding Protect against Childhood Obesity?" *Advances in Experimental and Biological Medicine* 478 (2000): 29–39.

von Kries, Rüdiger, Berthold Koletzko, Thorsten Sauerwald, Erika von Mutius, Dietmar Barnert, Veit Grunert, and Hubertus von Voss. "Breast Feeding and Obesity: Cross Sectional Study." *British Medical Journal* 319 (1999): 147–50.

Voss, Melinda. "Checking the Pulse: Midwestern Reporters' Opinions on Their Ability to Report Health Care News." *American Journal of Public Health* 92, no. 7 (2002): 1158–60.

Walker, Marsha. "When Women Decide Not to Breastfeed: Breastfeeding: Lifestyle, Not a Health Issue?" *MCN, the American Journal of Maternal/Child Nursing* 21 (1996): 64.

Wall, Glenda. "Moral Constructions of Motherhood in Breastfeeding Discourse." *Gender & Society* 15, no. 4 (2001): 592–610.

Wang, Youfa, May A. Beydoun, Lan Liang, Benjamin Caballero, and Shiriki K. Kumanyika. "Will All Americans Become Overweight or Obese? Estimating the Progression and Cost of the US Obesity Epidemic." *Obesity* 16, no. 10 (2008): 2323–30.

Ward, Julia DeJager. *La Leche League: At the Crossroads of Medicine, Feminism, and Religion.* Chapel Hill: University of North Carolina Press, 2000.

Weed, Douglas L. "Commentary: A Radical Future for Public Health." *International Journal of Epidemiology* 30 (2001): 440–41.

———. "Science, Ethics Guidelines, and Advocacy in Epidemiology." *Annals of Epidemiology* 4, no. 2 (1994): 166–71.

Weed, D. L., and R. E. McKeown. "Science, Ethics, and Professional Public Health Practice." *Journal of Epidemiology and Community Health* 57 (2003): 4–5.

Weigold, Michael F. "Communicating Science: A Review of the Literature." *Science Communication* 23, no. 2 (2001): 164–93.

Weimer, Jon. "The Economic Benefits of Breastfeeding: A Review and Analysis." Food and Rural Economics Division, Economic Research Service, U.S. Department of Agriculture. Food Assistance and Nutrition Research Report no. 13, 2001.

Weir, Lorna. *Pregnancy, Risk and Biopolitics: On the Threshold of the Living Subject.* London: Routledge, 2006.

Weisman, Carol S. *Women's Health Care: Activist Traditions and Institutional Change.* Baltimore: Johns Hopkins University Press, 1998.

Weiss, Barry D. "Outside the Clinician-Patient Relationship: A Call to Action for Health Literacy." In *Health Literacy: A Prescription to End Confusion,* ed. Lynn Nielsen-Bohlman,, Allison M. Panzer, and David A. Kindig, 285–99. Washington, DC: National Academies Press, 2004.

Weiss, Noel S. "Policy Emanating from Epidemiologic Data: What Is the Proper Forum." *Epidemiology* 124, no. 4 (2001): 373–74.

Weissman, Myrna M., Judith Weissman, Elizabeth Kagan Arleo, Erik Lykke Mortensen, Kim Fleischer Michaelsen, Stephanie A. Sanders, and June Machover Reinish. "Breastfeeding and Later Intelligence." *Journal of the American Medical Association* 288, no. 7 (2002): 828–30.

Welch, H. Gilbert, Lisa Schwartz, and Steven Woloshin. "What's Making Us Sick Is an Epidemic of Diagnoses." *New York Times,* January 2, 2007.

Wendler, David, Leah Belsky, Kimberly M. Thompson, and Ezekiel J. Emmanual. "Quantifying the Federal Minimum Risk Standard." *Journal of the American Medical Association* 294, no. 7 (2005): 826–32.

Wertz, Richard W., and Dorothy C. Wertz. *Lying-in: A History of Childbirth in America.* New Haven, CT: Yale University Press, 1977.

Weyermann, Maria, Herman Brenner, and Dietrich Rothenbacher. "Adipokines in Human Milk and Risk of Overweight in Early Childhood." *Epidemiology* 18, no. 6 (2007): 722–29.

Wicks, Robert H. "Message Framing and Constructing Meaning: An Emerging Paradigm in Mass Communication Research." *Communication Yearbook* 29 (2005): 333–61.

Wiemann, Constance M., Jacqueline C. Dubois, and Abbey B. Berenson. "Racial/Ethnic Differences in the Decision to Breastfeed among Adolescent Mothers." *Pediatrics* 101, no. 6 (1998): e11–18.

Wiessinger, Diane. "Watch Your Language!" *Journal of Human Lactation* 12, no. 1 (1996): 1–4.

Wilkes, Michael S. "The Public Dissemination of Medical Research: Problems and Solutions." *Journal of Health Communication* 2, no. 1 (1997): 3–15.

Wilkinson, Iain. *Anxiety in a Risk Society*. New York: Routledge, 2001.

Wilkoff, Will. *The Maternity Leave Breastfeeding Plan*. New York: Simon & Schuster, 2002.

Williams, Joan. *Unbending Gender: Why Family and Work Conflict and What to Do about It*. Oxford: Oxford University Press, 2000.

Williams, Patti, and Jennifer L. Aaker. "Can Mixed Emotions Peacefully Coexist?" *Journal of Consumer Research* 28 (2002): 636–49.

Williams, Simon J., Jonathan Gabe, and Michael Calnan, eds. *Health, Medicine and Society: Key Theories, Future Agendas*. London: Routledge, 2000.

Willis, Jim, with Albert Adelowo Okunade. *Reporting on Risks: The Practice and Ethics of Health and Safety Communication*. Westport, CT: Praeger, 1997.

Wilson, Nicole L., Leanne J. Robinson, Anne Donnet, Lionel Bovetto, Nicolle H. Packer, and Niclas G. Karlsson. "Glycoproteomics of Milk: Differences in Sugar Epitopes on Human and Bovine Milk Fat Globule Membranes." *Journal of Proteome Research* 7, no. 9 (2008): 3687–96.

Wilson, William Julius. *The Bridge over the Racial Divide: Rising Inequality and Coalition Politics*. Berkeley: University of California Press, 2001.

Wimmer, Jeffrey, and Thorsten Quandt. "Living in the Risk Society: An Interview with Ulrich Beck." *Journalism Studies* 7, no. 2 (2006): 336–47.

Windish, Donna M., Stephen J. Huot, and Michael L. Green. "Medicine Residents' Understanding of the Biostatistics and Results in the Medical Literature." *Journal of the American Medical Society* 298, no. 9 (2007): 1014–16.

Winker, Margaret A. "The Need for Concrete Improvement in Abstract Quality." *Journal of the American Medical Association* 281, no. 12 (1999): 1129–30.

Wirth, Frederick. *Prenatal Parenting: The Complete Psychological and Spiritual Guide to Loving Your Unborn Child*. New York: HarperCollins, 2001.

Witte, Kim. "The Manipulative Nature of Health Communication Research." *American Behavioral Scientist* 38, no. 2 (1994): 285–93.

Witte, Kim, and Mike Allen. "A Meta-Analysis of Fear Appeals: Implications for Effective Public Health Campaigns." *Health Education & Behavior* 27, no. 5 (2000): 591–615.

Witte, Kim, Judy M. Berkowitz, Kenzie A. Cameron, and Janet K. McKeon. "Preventing the Spread of Genital Warts: Using Fear Appeals to Promote Self-Protective Behaviors." *Health Education and Behavior* 25, no. 5 (1998): 571–85.

Wolf, Jacqueline H. *Don't Kill Your Baby: Public Health and the Decline of Breastfeeding in the Nineteenth and Twentieth Centuries*. Columbus: Ohio State University Press, 2001.

———. "Low Breastfeeding Rates and Public Health in the United States." *American Journal of Public Health* 93, no. 12 (2003): 2000–2010.

Wolf, Joan B. "Commentary—Rejoinder to Judy M. Hopkinson." *Journal of Health Politics, Policy and Law* 32, no. 4 (2007): 649–54.

———. "Is Breast Really Best? Risk and Total Motherhood in the National Breastfeeding Awareness Campaign." *Journal of Health Politics, Policy, and Law* 32, no. 4 (2007): 595–636.

Woloshin, Steven, and Lisa M. Schwartz. "Press Releases: Translating Research into News." *Journal of the American Medical Association* 287, no. 21 (2002): 2856–58.

Woloshin, Steven, Lisa M. Schwartz, and H. Gilbert Welch. "The Risk of Death by Age, Sex, and Smoking Status in the United States: Putting Health Risks in Context." *Journal of the National Cancer Institute* 100, no. 12 (2008): 845–53.

Woo, Jessica G., Lawrence M. Dolan, Ardythe L. Morrow, Sheela R. Geraghty, and Elizabeth Goodman. "Breastfeeding Helps Explain Racial and Socioeconomic Status Disparities in Adolescent Adiposity." *Pediatrics* 121, no. 3 (2008): e458–65.

Wood, David. "Effect of Child and Family Poverty on Child Health in the United States." *Pediatrics* 112, no. 3, suppl. (2003): 707–11.

Woodward, Kathleen. "Statistical Panic." *differences* 11, no. 2 (1999): 177–203.

Wright, Peter, and Ian J. Deary. "Breastfeeding and Intelligence." *The Lancet* 339 (1992): 612–14.

Wynne, Brian. "May the Sheep Safely Graze? A Reflexive View of the Expert-Lay Knowledge Divide." In *Risk, Environment and Modernity: Towards a New Ecology,* ed. Scott Lash, Bronislaw Szerszynski, and Brian Wynne, 44–83. London: Sage, 1996.

———. "Misunderstood Misunderstanding: Social Identities and Public Uptake of Science." *Public Understanding of Science* 1, no. 3 (1992): 281–304.

Xu, Xiaohui, Amy B. Dailey, Natalie C. Freeman, Barbara A. Curbow, and Evelyn O. Talbott. "The Effects of Birthweight and Breastfeeding on Asthma among Children Aged 1–5 Years." *Journal of Paediatrics and Child Health* 45 (2009): 646–51.

Yadlon, Susan. "Skinny Women and Good Mothers: The Rhetoric of Risk, Control, and Culpability in the Production of Knowledge about Breast Cancer." *Feminist Studies* 23, no. 3 (1997): 645–77.

Yalom, Marilyn. *A History of the Breast.* New York: Knopf, 1998.

Yang, Li, and Kathryn H. Jacobsen. "A Systematic Review of the Association between Breastfeeding and Breast Cancer." *Journal of Women's Health* 17, no. 10 (2008): 1635–45.

Yoder, Scot D. "Individual Responsibility for Health: Decision, Not Discovery." *Hastings Center Report* 32, no. 2 (2002): 22–31.

Young, T. Kue, Patricia J. Martens, Shayne P. Taback, Elizabeth A. C. Sellers, Heather J. Dean, Mary Cheang, and Bertha Flett. "Type 2 Diabetes Mellitis in Children: Prenatal and Early Infancy Risk Factors among Native Canadians." *Archives of Pediatric Adolescent Medicine* 156, no. 7 (2002): 651–55.

Zacharoulis, Stergios, Nudrat Nauman, Michael Marlowe, Rima Fawaz, and Allan S. Cunningham. "Questions about AAP Breastfeeding Statement." *Pediatrics* 102, no. 6 (1998): 1495–96.

Ziegler, Anette G., Sandra Schmidt, Doris Huber, Michael Hummel, and Ezio Bonifacio. "Early Infant Feeding and Risk of Developing Type 1 Diabetes-Associated Autoantibodies." *Journal of the American Medical Association* 290, no. 13 (2003): 1721–28.

Ziliak, Stephen T., and Deirdre McCloskey. *The Cult of Statistical Significance: How the Standard Error Costs Us Jobs, Justice, and Lives.* Ann Arbor: University of Michigan Press, 2008.

Index

About the Author

JOAN B. WOLF is Assistant Professor of Women's Studies at Texas A&M University and the author of *Harnessing the Holocaust: The Politics of Memory in France.*